Nutrition and Liver Disease

Special Issue Editors

Pietro Vajro
Claudia Mandato

MDPI • Basel • Beijing • Wuhan • Barcelona • Belgrade

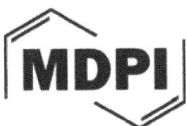

MDPI

Special Issue Editors

Pietro Vajro

Dept of Medicine, Surgery and Dentistry "Scuola Medica Salernitana"—Salerno
Italy

Claudia Mandato

Pediatric Liver and Nutrition consultant AORN Santobono-Pausilipon
Italy

Editorial Office

MDPI

St. Alban-Anlage 66

Basel, Switzerland

This edition is a reprint of the Special Issue published online in the open access journal *Nutrients* (ISSN 2072-6643) from 2017–2018 (available at: http://www.mdpi.com/journal/nutrients/special issues/nutrients liverdisease).

For citation purposes, cite each article independently as indicated on the article page online and as indicated below:

Lastname, F.M.; Lastname, F.M. Article title. *Journal Name* **Year**, *Article number*, page range.

First Editon 2018

ISBN 978-3-03842-923-4 (Pbk)
ISBN 978-3-03842-924-1 (PDF)

Table of Contents

About the Special Issue Editors

Pietro Vajro is Professor of Pediatrics at the Dept of Medicine, Surgery and Dentistry "Scuola Medica Salernitana" of the University of Salerno, Italy, Director of the Clinical Pediatrics Division of the University Hospital of Salerno and of the Pediatric Residency Program. Professor Vajro trained as "Assistant Etranger " at the Pediatric Hepatology Unit of Bicetre, France (under Prof. Daniel Alagille) and as Advanced NATO Fellow at the Liver Center of the University of California—San Francisco, California (under Professors R. Schmid, M.M. Thaler, and N. Blanckaert). His main clinical and research interests are focused on the reciprocal interaction between pediatric GI, nutrition, liver and biliary tract disorders. He is the author of over 200 full papers published in prestigious international, peer reviewed journals, and book chapters. He is/has been a member of the Editorial Board of high ranking pediatric and/or GI, nutrition and liver journals, and served as Secretary of the Liver Section of the Italian (SIGENP) and European (ESPGHAN) Societies for Pediatric Gastroenterology, Hepatology and Nutrition.

Claudia Mandato is a pediatrician working in the largest pediatric Hospital of South of Italy. She is an expert pediatric liver and nutrition consultant, and her research is mainly focused on nutrition in liver disease, particularly in the field of genetic and metabolic hepatopathies. She achieved her clinical and research experience at King's College Hospital, London and at the University of Naples Federico II and Salerno. She has authored over 30 articles, published in peer reviewed international journals, in the field of nutrition in children.

Preface to "Nutrition and Liver Disease"

Malnutrition in children and adults with end-stage liver disease is a challenging issue due to its multifactorial nature, which includes hypermetabolism, increased energy needs, malabsorption, and anorexia. Despite advances in both assessment and management of malnutrition, an adequate nutritional support is often limited in these patients. The complicated underlying metabolic scenario finally leads to catabolism and loss of skeletal muscular mass (SMM). The subsequent sarcopenia affects quality of life and clinical outcome: strict interdependence exists between the prevention of depletion of SMM, the early diagnosis of and curative therapy for hepatocellular carcinoma, the preservation of liver functional reserve, and improved liver disease outcomes. Moreover, sarcopenia impacts on growth and psycomotor development in children. As a consequence, a correct SMM assessment plays a central role and the pros and cons of different techniques, including bioelectric impedance analysis (BIA) or imaging, have to be considered. Hand-grip dynamometry, an easy-to-measure and sensitive technique, appears to be a promising marker for depletion of SMM in hepatopatic patients.

Strategies of nutritional intervention should consider the fine line between the need for a hypercaloric diet rich in proteins and the risk of hepatic encephalopathy and hyperammonemia in sarcopenic, chronically malnourished patients with end-stage liver disease. A global clinical and nutritional assessment represents the starting point of targeted nutritional intervention. Again, different approaches have been investigated in adults and children who are candidates for liver transplantation. In these patients, nutrient supplementation including synbiotics, micronutrients, branched-chain amino acids, and immunonutrients have been considered for both adult and pediatric patients.

Nutritional management is mandatory in certain inherited metabolic/genetic defects. In these patients, specific dietary restrictions/supplementations represent a challenge for pediatricians and for adult hepatologists at the time of transition of care, to guarantee liver health along with optimal growth and brain development. A dietician familiar with metabolic disorders is often needed on the team that is caring for these patients. Dietary intervention is an evolving and increasingly used therapy also for the novel group of Congenital Disorders of Glycosylation (CDG). Monosaccharide supplements are increasingly being evaluated in trials for a number of subtypes of CDG. Monosaccharides, in fact, have relatively high safety, especially compared to experimental drugs, and are easy to administer. Very recent data are presented regarding nutritional therapy, by evaluating many of the different options that have somehow been associated with a positive effect on liver function in CDG.

A number of liver diseases driven by primary nutritional/intestinal tract diseases (e.g., inflammatory bowel disease, celiac disease, cystic fibrosis, alcoholic steatohepatitis, non-alcoholic steatohepatitis, parenteral nutrition-associated liver disease), are now included under the umbrella term "gut–liver axis dysfunction". One of the prominent factors of pathogenesis appears to be increased permeability of the intestinal barrier, which facilitates translocation of bacterial toxins and microorganisms into the portal circulation, mesenteric lymph nodes, and liver, and the overall proinflammatory status of the compromised intestine. Nutritional strategies that focus on improving the composition of the microbiota are attractive areas of investigation. A nutraceutical approach, which investigated hepatoprotective effects of specific nutrients has also been proposed, mainly in obesity-related liver disease and alcoholic liver disease.

In conclusion, to improve quality of life and prevent nutrition-related medical complications, patients diagnosed with advanced liver disease should have their nutritional status promptly assessed and be supported by appropriate dietary interventions. Furthermore, a dietary approach that uses specific food supplements and/or restriction diets is often necessary for patients with hepatic conditions associated with an underlying metabolic, nutritional or intestinal disease, due to the hepatoprotective, and/or anti-oxidant, and/or anti-inflammatory effects of these measures.

Pietro Vajro, Claudia Mandato

Special Issue Editors

nutrients

MDPI

Review
Nutrition and Liver Disease

Claudia Mandato [1], Antonella Di Nuzzi [2] and Pietro Vajro [2,*]

[1]   Pediatrics, Santobono - Pausilipon Pediatric Hospital, 80100 Naples, Italy; cla.mandato@gmail.com
[2]   Department of Medicine, Surgery and Dentistry "Scuola Medica Salernitana", Pediatrics Section,
      University of Salerno, 84081 Baronissi (Salerno), Italy; antonelladinuzzi@gmail.com
*   Correspondence: pvajro@unisa.it; Tel.: +39-339-2361-008

Received: 20 December 2017; Accepted: 20 December 2017; Published: 23 December 2017

Abstract: Malnutrition in children and adults with advanced liver disease represents a tremendous challenge as the nutritional problems are multifactorial. This Editorial comments the articles appearing in this special issue of *Nutrients*, "Nutrition and Liver disease" dealing with multiple diagnostic and therapeutic features that relate the outcomes of liver disease to nutrition. To improve quality of life and prevent nutrition-related medical complications, patients diagnosed with advanced liver disease should have their nutritional status promptly assessed and be supported by appropriate dietary interventions. Furthermore specific food supplements and/or restriction diets are often necessary for those with hepatic conditions associated with an underlying metabolic or nutritional or intestinal disease.

Keywords: nutrition; liver disease; cholestasis; liver transplantation; assessment; support

Despite advances in both the assessment and management of patients with liver disease, the provision of appropriate nutritional support for these patients is frequently lacking, an omission that has a large impact on clinical outcomes and quality of life. Except for elimination diets indicated for some hereditary or metabolic diseases that affect the liver, the general nutritional recommendations for most cases of compensated liver disease are analogous to the customary recommendations for a balanced diet. Malnutrition in children and adults with advanced liver disease, however, remains a tremendous challenge. The nutritional problems of these patients are multifactorial, and commonly include decreased intake due to anorexia, hypermetabolism, increased energy loss, and increased energy needs (Figure 1). The complicated underlying metabolic scenario is characterized by reduced glycogen stores, reduced protein synthesis, decreased branched-chain amino acid (BCAA)/aromatic amino acid (AAA) or BCCA/tyrosine (BT) ratios (3.5:1→1:1), and disturbances in fat metabolism during fasting.

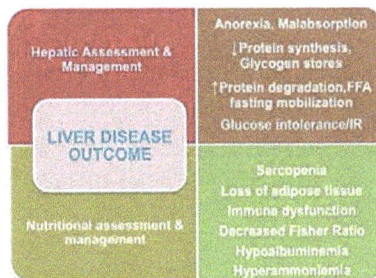

Figure 1. Diagnostic and therapeutic issues that link outcomes of liver diseases to nutrition.

In this special issue of *Nutrients*, which focuses on "Nutrition and Liver Disease," a number of contributors have presented novel information and additional perspectives on multiple diagnostic and therapeutic features that relate the outcomes of patients with liver disease to nutrition.

1. Skeletal Muscle Mass

Skeletal muscle mass (SMM) is determined by the balance between protein synthesis and breakdown. Skeletal muscle loss (SML) is a major complication of liver cirrhosis (LC). In clinical settings, the assessment of skeletal muscle mass (SMM) to identifysevere SML (or sarcopenia) has long represented a very simple and objective bedside clinical measure of liver disease severity, because SML is associated with liver disease prognosis. It has now recently enhanced thanks to the support of various new imaging methods for assessing core SMM.

In this issue of *Nutrients*, the prognostic value of SMM was reported by studies in various categories of hepatic conditions, and the information has furthered our knowledge on the following issues:

- Strict interdependence exists between (1) the prevention of depletion of SMM,(2) the early diagnosis of and curative therapy for hepatocellular carcinoma (HCC),(3) the preservation of liver functional reserve, and (4) improved liver disease outcomes [1]. Age of male patients, female gender, a Child–Pugh score, and increased tumor size were significantly related to the SMM index, as measured at the third lumbar vertebra by transverse computed tomography (CT) imaging, which is a commonly used tool for HCC in the clinical setting. The results of the study by Imai et al. overall confirmed that sarcopenia negatively impacts the survival of patients with HCC, and is a valuable prognostic factor that might be impacted by liver functional reserve and the clinical stage of HCC.
- Therelationship between the loss of SMM, as assessed by bioelectric impedance analysis (BIA), and liver fibrosis, as measured by virtual-touch-quantification (VTQ) and acoustic-radiation-force-impulse elastography in patients with chronic liver disease (CLD), was reported by Nishikawa et al. [2]. Interestingly, BCAAs-to-tyrosine ratio (BTR) showed the second strongest correlation with the VTQ level, and was an independent predictor for decreased SMM index.
- BothBTR and SMM, as evaluated by BIA, were also confirmed to be reliable predictors of outcome in patients with liver diseases in another study, which found that increased values of BTR and SMM were associated with the resolution of chronic hepatitis C in patients treated with interferon-free direct-acting-antiviral therapy [3].
- However, all that glitters is not gold, and these studies have both strengths and limitations. The study by Imai et al. [1] was based on imaging techniques, and, although these assessments are objective and not affected by defects in hepatic synthesis or retention of NaCl and water, they are either expensive or involve radiation and cannot easily be repeated to monitor progress. The other twostudies [2,3] that used BIA, which is based on a two-component model of body composition (fat and fat-free mass), may have drawbacks. As recently emphasized by Amodio et al. [4] the validity of this technique is in fact critically dependent on assumptions relating to tissue density and hydration.

In future clinical and research settings, hand-grip dynamometry, which can provide measures for risk stratification for all-cause death, cardiovascular death, and cardiovascular disease in the general population [5], should be also implemented for the assessment of muscle strength. Indeed, for patients with cirrhosis, muscle strength, as assessed by hand-grip dynamometry, appears to be an easy-to-measure, sensitive, and specific marker for depletion of SMM [6] and ispositively correlated with total body protein [5,7].

2. Nutritional Assessment and Support

Another major issue concerns the fine line between the need for a hypercaloric diet rich in proteins and the risk of hepatic encephalopathy and hyperammonemia in sarcopenic, chronically malnourished patients with end-stage liver disease. The appropriate nutritional support of adult cirrhosis before and after liver transplantation was the focus of three articles in this issue.

- The first article [8] recommends the performance of an accurate multidisciplinary assessment of malnutrition in order to optimize nutritional support, especially for those patients with elevated risk for malnutrition because of the severity of their native liver disease. The recommended daily requirements for nutrients and energy intake should be achieved through oral intake, oral supplementation, and enteral nutrition. Parenteral nutrition (PN) should be used for moderately or severely malnourished patients with cirrhosis who cannot be fed orally or enterally, or if they have fasted longer than 72 h [9].
- The important and difficult issues concerned with the careful assessment of nutritional status of patients who are candidates for liver transplantation were also emphasized in the articles by Ahmed Hammad et al. [10] and Yang et al. [11]. The perioperative nutritional interventions, including the use of synbiotics, micronutrients, branched-chain amino acid (BCAA) supplements, and immunonutrients; fluid and electrolyte balance, the partial substitution of conventional fats with medium-chain triglycerides, and carefully monitored supplementation using fat soluble vitamins for cholestasis were reviewed for both adult and pediatric patients. Children with chronic liver disease are particularly vulnerable to malnutrition, which can compromise growth and brain development. They should benefit from early intervention provided by a multidisciplinary team. Yang et al. in particular have focused on the nutritional needs and support of children with chronic liver disease [11]; they revised the issues by providing conclusions that are consistent with the most recent guidelines of the European Society of Paediatric Gastroenterology Hepatology and Nutrition (ESPGHAN) [12].

3. Hepatopathies due to Inherited Metabolic/Genetic Defects

A number of inherited metabolic/genetic defects, including those that require (a) specific well established dietary restrictions (galactosemia, hereditary fructose intolerance, inborn errors of the urea cycle such as citrin deficiency and related metabolic pathways),(b) the addition of specific drugs (e.g., tyrosinemia; Wilson disease), or (c) special food supplements such as uncooked starch (e.g., glycogen storage diseases), represent a further challenge not only for pediatricians but also for adult hepatologists at the time of transition of care [13]. A dietician familiar with metabolic disorders is often needed on the team caring for these patients [14].

Dietary intervention is an evolving and increasingly used therapy also for the novel group of Congenital Disorders of Glycosylation (CDG). Glycosylation consists in the covalent binding ofan oligosaccharide chain to the polypeptide side chains of a glycoprotein. The carbohydrate consists of a simple sugar (e.g., glucose, galactose, mannose, and xylose), an amino sugar (e.g., *N*-acetylglucosamine or *N*-acetylgalactosamine), or an acidic sugar (e.g., sialic acid or *N*-acetylneuraminic acid). Monosaccharide supplements are being evaluated in trials for more and more subtypes of CDG, because monosaccharides have relatively high safety, especially compared to experimental drugs, and are easy to administer. The mechanism is still poorly understood, although in CDG-Ib, alimentary addition of mannose appear to bypass the defective step (conversion of fructose-6-phosphate to mannose-6-phosphate) by allowing for the formation of mannose-6-phosphate via the action of hexokinase [15]. In their article, Morava and her group presented an accurate overview of very recent data on the contributions of nutritional therapy by evaluating many of the different options for nutritional therapy that have somehow been associated with a positive effect on liver function in CDG [16]. The questions these authors, however, pose include whether or not these dietary interventions are sufficient and whether these dietary interventions are the most efficient therapies for CDG. They remind the reader that mannose therapy for patients with mannose phosphate isomerase (MPI)-CDG has not only been found to be possibly hazardous at higher doses, but unfortunately also cannot prevent progressive fibrotic liver disease in about one third of affected patients. In addition, recent experience with galactose therapy has been found beneficial for several CDGs [17–19] without, however, completely alleviating all clinical symptoms. While recognizing the progress this approach represents, they also suggest that future therapy for CDG therapy will most likely include administration of activated monosaccharides instead of single dietary sugars. The efficacy and toxicity of these novel drugs, however, remain to be investigated in human trials as well after careful preliminary evaluations in animal models are made.

4. Hepatopathies Driven by Primary Nutritional/Intestinal Tract Diseases

A number of liver diseases that are driven by primary nutritional/intestinal tract diseases (e.g., inflammatory bowel disease (IBD), celiac disease, cystic fibrosis (CF), alcoholic steatohepatitis (ASH), and non-alcoholic steatohepatitis (NASH) parenteral nutrition-associated liver disease(PNALD)), which are included under the umbrella term *gut-liver axisdysfunction* [20,21], also represent specific challenges. Investigations of the associations between the liver and diseased intestine are still preliminary, and further studies are essential for the clinical management of these complicated conditions (Figure 2).

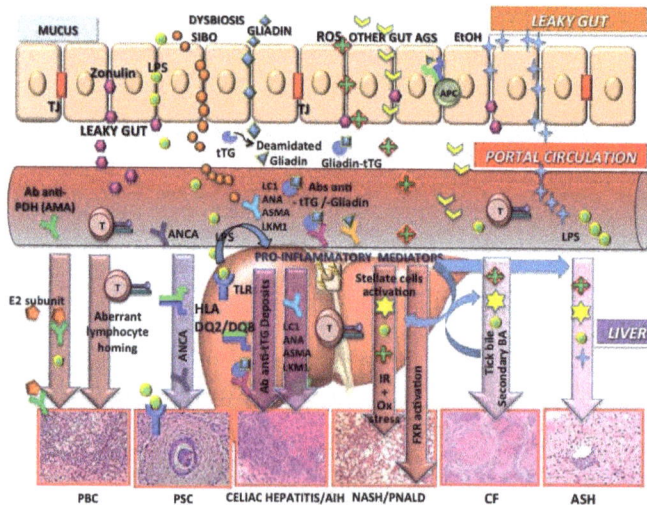

Figure 2. Gut-liver axis and liver diseases. Increased intestinal permeability and dysbiosis are common features linking the liver to a number of nutritional/gastrointestinal (GI) diseases depicted in the figure. The toll-like receptor (TLR)–bacterial lipopolysaccharide (LPS) interaction is one of the mechanisms involved in the release of proinflammatory mediators (cytokines), leading to liver inflammation and stellate-cell-activation-dependent fibrosis. Emerging therapeutic approaches that target the gut-liver axis therefore represent promising therapies to prevent or halt liver disease progression.

Genetic predisposition and environmental stimulation determine the loss of tolerance in primary biliary cholangitis (PBC) where antimitochondrial antibodies (AMAs) cross-react with proteins from intestinal bacteria (E2 subunit), possibly because of molecular mimicry. Aberrant homing of intestinal lymphocytes also occurs. The association between celiac disease and PBC is also well established.

Closely associated with inflammatory bowel disease, primary sclerosing cholangitis (PSC) is also a heterogeneous disease that involves marked interactions between altered immune status (human leucocyte antigen (HLA)), altered bile composition, and host microbiome. Some subgroups of antineutrophil cytoplasmic antibodies (ANCAs) in the blood and bile are associated with increased liver enzyme levels and are biomarkers of liver disease with a possible role in the pathogenesis of the disease as well.

In celiac disease, immunoactive molecules generated from cross-linking between tissue transglutaminase and food/bacterial antigens reach the liver through the portal circulation and are responsible for transglutaminase antigen (tTG)–antibody complex hepatic deposits. The liver may respond to gluten either as a reactive "celiac hepatitis" or a true autoimmune hepatitis (with anti-liver cytosol (LC1), anti-nuclear antibodies (ANA), anti-smoot muscle antibodies (ASMA), anti-liver kidney microsomes (LKM1)) based on the DQ2 strong linkage disequilibrium with the DR3 and DR4, the latter being the major HLA risk factor for autoimmune liver disease.

Increased levels of bacterial endotoxin in the portal circulation suggest a role for gut-derived toxins also in the alcoholic liver diseasesteatohepatitis (ASH), non-alcoholic fatty liver disease (NAFLD/NASH), and parenteral nutrition liver disease (PNALD). Alcohol (EtOH) consumption and endogenous alcohol production by gut bacteria in obese individuals can disrupt the tight junctions (TJ) of the intestinal epithelial barrier, resulting in increased gut permeability. The bacterial endotoxin (lypopolisaccharides, LPS) contributes to inflammation through activation of toll-like receptor 4 (TLR4). Oxidative stress with reactive oxygen species (ROS), insulin resistance (IR), secondary bile acids (BAs), and farnesoid X receptor activation (FXR) represent major mechanisms of pathogenesis.

Animals with cystic fibrosis transmembrane conductance regulator defects and patients with cystic fibrosis have microbiomes that are different from individuals without CF, which might be accounted for by altered bile properties, prolonged small bowel transit, frequent antibiotic exposure, and small intestinal bacterial overgrowth (SIBO) (adapted and modified from [20]).

For celiac disease [22] and NASH [23,24], nutritional correction of the underlying gastrointestinal/nutritional disease may be effective in preventing the progression of liver disease. Readers are also referredto the 2017 *Nutrients* issue (ISSN 2072-6643) edited by Nobili and Alisi, where specific measures for the treatment of obesity-related NAFLD are specifically discussed.

Unfortunately, for some nutritional/intestinal conditions such as IBD and CF, the liver disease does not seem to be affected by decreases in the inflammatory activity in the intestinal tract [25] or improved function of the pancreas/respiratory tract [26].

Impaired intestinal function, directly or indirectly associated with gut dysbiosis, may also be one of the main pathogenic mechanisms of PNALD [27] (Figure 2).

- In this issue of *Nutrients*, Cahova et al. [28] reviewed studies of animal models and humans that suggested that chronic parenteral nutrition-related liver damage depends on intestinal failure and associated complications rather than PN administration per se. The prominent factors appear to be increased permeability of the intestinal barrier, which facilitates translocation of bacterial toxins and microorganisms into the portal circulation, mesenteric lymph nodes, and liver, and the overall proinflammatory status of the compromised intestine. The gut microbiota play a weighty role in the maintenance of the functional intestinal barrier and the establishment of either an immunotolerant or inflammatory intestinal setting [23,27]. Therapeutic strategies that focus on improving the composition of the microbiota through the targeted delivery of beneficial microbiota or by supplementation with immunomodulators are attractive areas of investigation.
- Alcoholic liver disease (ALD) is a strong predictor of malnutrition because of the numerous risk factors for malnutrition that are associated with both acute and chronic alcohol abuse. Due to complicated pathogenetic mechanisms, therapies for ALD and especially for severe alcoholic hepatitis (AH) are thorny problems in clinical practice. For severe acute AH, specific drug treatments, including glucocorticoids and pentoxifylline, have been identified and currently are recommended by international guidelines. However, further elucidation of the mechanisms of pathogenesis is still needed [29]. In this context, the article by Xuchong Tang et al. [30] in this issue of *Nutrients* is particularly welcome. The study revealed that an artichoke extract exhibited

significant preventive hepatoprotective effects not only for the carbon-tetrachloride-induced hepatoxicity [31,32] and NAFLD/NASH [33] as previously demonstrated but also against acute alcohol-induced liver injury (ASH). The effects probably depend on the ability of components of the extract not only to attenuate oxidative stress but also to suppress the toll-like receptor 4/nuclear factor kappa-light-chain-enhancer of activated Bcells (TLR4/NFkB) inflammatory pathway, a signaling pathway suggested to be one of the mechanisms of pathogenesis also of NAFLD through the overexpression of hepcidin [34].

5. Conclusions

In conclusion, to improve quality of life and prevent nutrition-related medical complications, patients diagnosed with advanced liver disease should have their nutritional status promptly assessed and be supported by appropriate dietary interventions. Furthermore, a dietary approach that uses specific food supplements and/or restriction diets is often necessary for patients with hepatic conditions associated with an underlying metabolic or nutritional or intestinal disease, due to the hepatoprotective and/or anti-oxidant and/or anti-inflammatory effects of these measures.

Author Contributions: The authors contributed equally.

Conflicts of Interest: The authors declare no conflict of interest.

References

1. Imai, K.; Takai, K.; Watanabe, S.; Hanai, T.; Suetsugu, A.; Shiraki, M.; Shimizu, M. Sarcopenia Impairs Prognosis of Patients with Hepatocellular Carcinoma: The Role of Liver Functional Reserve and Tumor-Related Factors in Loss of Skeletal Muscle. *Nutrients* **2017**, *9*, 1054. [CrossRef] [PubMed]
2. Nishikawa, H.; Nishimura, T.; Enomoto, H.; Iwata, Y.; Ishii, A.; Miyamoto, Y.; Ishii, N.; Yuri, Y.; Takata, R.; Hasegawa, K.; et al. Impact of Virtual Touch Quantification in Acoustic Radiation Force Impulse for Skeletal Muscle Mass Loss in Chronic Liver Diseases. *Nutrients* **2017**, *9*, 620. [CrossRef] [PubMed]
3. Yoh, K.; Nishikawa, H.; Enomoto, H.; Ishii, A.; Iwata, Y.; Miyamoto, Y.; Ishii, N.; Yuri, Y.; Hasegawa, K.; Nakano, C.; et al. Predictors Associated with Increase in Skeletal Muscle Mass after Sustained Virological Response in Chronic Hepatitis C Treated with Direct Acting Antivirals. *Nutrients* **2017**, *9*, 1135. [CrossRef] [PubMed]
4. Amodio, P.; Bemeur, C.; Butterworth, R.; Cordoba, J.; Kato, A.; Montagnese, S.; Uribe, M.; Vilstrup, H.; Morgan, M.Y. The nutritional management of hepatic encephalopathy in patients with cirrhosis: International Society for Hepatic Encephalopathy and Nitrogen Metabolism Consensus. *Hepatology* **2013**, *58*, 325–336. [CrossRef] [PubMed]
5. Leong, D.P.; Teo, K.K.; Rangarajan, S.; Lopez-Jaramillo, P.; Avezum, A., Jr.; Orlandini, A.; Seron, P.; Ahmed, S.H.; Rosengren, A.; Kelishadi, R.; et al. Prognostic value of grip strength: Findings from the Prospective Urban Rural Epidemiology (PURE) study. *Lancet* **2015**, *386*, 266–273. [CrossRef]
6. Huisman, E.J.; Trip, E.J.; Siersema, P.D.; van Hoek, B.; van Erpecum, K.J. Protein energy malnutrition predicts complications in liver cirrhosis. *Eur. J. Gastroenterol. Hepatol.* **2011**, *23*, 982–989. [CrossRef] [PubMed]
7. Dasarathy, S. Consilience in sarcopenia of cirrhosis. *J. Cachexia Sarcopenia Muscle* **2012**, *3*, 225–237. [CrossRef] [PubMed]
8. Perumpail, B.J.; Li, A.A.; Cholankeril, G.; Kumari, R.; Ahmed, A. Optimizing the Nutritional Support of Adult Patients in the Setting of Cirrhosis. *Nutrients* **2017**, *9*, 1114. [CrossRef] [PubMed]
9. Plauth, M.; Cabré, E.; Campillo, B.; Kondrup, J.; Marchesini, G.; Schütz, T.; Shenkin, A.; Wendon, J.; ESPEN. ESPEN Guidelines on Parenteral Nutrition: Hepatology. *Clin. Nutr.* **2009**, *28*, 436–444. [CrossRef] [PubMed]
10. Hammad, A.; Kaido, T.; Aliyev, V.; Mandato, C.; Uemoto, S. Nutritional Therapy in Liver Transplantation. *Nutrients* **2017**, *9*, 1126. [CrossRef] [PubMed]
11. Yang, C.H.; Perumpail, B.J.; Yoo, E.R.; Ahmed, A.; Kerner, J.A., Jr. Nutritional Needs and Support for Children with Chronic Liver Disease. *Nutrients* **2017**, *9*, 1127. [CrossRef] [PubMed]

12. McLin, V.A.; Allen, U.; Boyer, O.; Bucuvalas, J.; Colledan, M.; Cuturi, M.C.; d'Antiga, L.; Debray, D.; Dezsofi, A.; Goyet, J.V.; et al. Early and Late Factors Impacting Patient and Graft Outcome in Pediatric Liver Transplantation: Summary of an ESPGHAN Monothematic Conference. *J. Pediatr. Gastroenterol. Nutr.* **2017**, *65*, 53–59. [CrossRef] [PubMed]

13. Guercio Nuzio, S.; Ann Tizzard, S.; Vajro, P. Tips and hints for the transition: What adult hepatologists should know when accept teens with a pediatric hepatobiliary disease. *Clin. Res. Hepatol. Gastroenterol.* **2014**, *38*, 277–283. [CrossRef] [PubMed]

14. Thompson, R.J.; Azevedo, R.A.; Galoppo, C.; Lewindon, P.; McKiernan, P. Cholestatic and metabolic liver diseases: Working Group report of the second World Congress of Pediatric Gastroenterology, Hepatology, and Nutrition. *J. Pediatr. Gastroenterol. Nutr.* **2004**, *39*, 611–615. [CrossRef]

15. Péanne, R.; de Lonlay, P.; Foulquier, F.; Kornak, U.; Lefeber, D.J.; Morava, E.; Pérez, B.; Seta, N.; Thiel, C.; Van Schaftingen, E.; et al. Congenital disorders of glycosylation (CDG): Quo vadis? *Eur. J. Med. Genet.* **2017**. [CrossRef]

16. Witters, P.; Cassiman, D.; Morava, E. Nutritional Therapies in Congenital Disorders of Glycosylation (CDG). *Nutrients* **2017**, *9*, 1222. [CrossRef] [PubMed]

17. Morelle, W.; Potelle, S.; Witters, P.; Wong, S.; Climer, L.; Lupashin, V.; Matthijs, G.; Gadomski, T.; Jaeken, J.; Cassiman, D.; et al. Galactose supplementation in patients with tmem165-CDG rescues the glycosylation defects. *J. Clin. Endocrinol. Metab.* **2017**, *102*, 1375–1386. [CrossRef] [PubMed]

18. Morava, E. Galactose supplementation in phosphoglucomutase-1 deficiency; review and outlook for a novel treatable CDG. *Mol. Genet. Metab.* **2014**, *112*, 275–279. [CrossRef] [PubMed]

19. Wong, S.Y.; Gadomski, T.; van Scherpenzeel, M.; Honzik, T.; Hansikova, H.; Holmefjord, K.S.B.; Mork, M.; Bowling, F.; Sykut-Cegielska, J.; Koch, D.; et al. Oral D-galactose supplementation in PGM1-CDG. *Genet. Med.* **2017**, *19*, 1226–1235. [CrossRef] [PubMed]

20. Poeta, M.; Pierri, L.; Vajro, P. Gut-Liver Axis Derangement in Non-Alcoholic Fatty Liver Disease. *Children* **2017**, *4*, 66. [CrossRef] [PubMed]

21. Troisi, J.; Pierri, L.; Landolfi, A.; Marciano, F.; Bisogno, A.; Belmonte, F.; Palladino, C.; Guercio Nuzio, S.; Campiglia, P.; Vajro, P. Urinary Metabolomics in Pediatric Obesity and NAFLD Identifies Metabolic Pathways/Metabolites Related to Dietary Habits and Gut-Liver Axis Perturbations. *Nutrients* **2017**, *9*, 485. [CrossRef] [PubMed]

22. Marciano, F.; Savoia, M.; Vajro, P. Celiac disease-related hepatic injury: Insights into associated conditions and underlying pathomechanisms. *Dig. Liver Dis.* **2016**, *48*, 112–119. [CrossRef] [PubMed]

23. Vajro, P.; Paolella, G.; Fasano, A. Microbiota and gut-liver axis: Their influences on obesity and obesity-related liver disease. *J. Pediatr. Gastroenterol. Nutr.* **2013**, *56*, 461–468. [CrossRef] [PubMed]

24. Ma, J.; Zhou, Q.; Li, H. Gut Microbiota and Nonalcoholic Fatty Liver Disease: Insights on Mechanisms and Therapy. *Nutrients* **2017**, *9*, 1124. [CrossRef] [PubMed]

25. Vavricka, S.R.; Schoepfer, A.; Scharl, M.; Lakatos, P.L.; Navarini, A.; Rogler, G. Extraintestinal Manifestations of Inflammatory Bowel Disease. *Inflamm. Bowel Dis.* **2015**, *21*, 1982–1992. [CrossRef] [PubMed]

26. Debray, D.; Narkewicz, M.R.; Bodewes, F.A.J.A.; Colombo, C.; Housset, C.; de Jonge, H.R.; Jonker, J.W.; Kelly, D.A.; Ling, S.C.; Poynard, T.; et al. Cystic Fibrosis–related Liver Disease: Research Challenges and Future Perspectives. *J. Pediatr. Gastroenterol. Nutr.* **2017**, *65*, 443–448. [CrossRef] [PubMed]

27. Orso, G.; Mandato, C.; Veropalumbo, C.; Cecchi, N.; Garzi, A.; Vajro, P. Pediatric parenteral nutrition-associated liver disease and cholestasis: Novel advances in pathomechanisms-based prevention and treatment. *Dig. Liver Dis.* **2016**, *48*, 215–222. [CrossRef] [PubMed]

28. Cahova, M.; Bratova, M.; Wohl, P. Parenteral Nutrition-Associated Liver Disease: The Role of the Gut Microbiota. *Nutrients* **2017**, *9*, 987. [CrossRef] [PubMed]

29. Abenavoli, L.; Masarone, M.; Federico, A.; Rosato, V.; Dallio, M.; Loguercio, C.; Persico, M. Alcoholic Hepatitis: Pathogenesis, Diagnosis and Treatment. *Rev. Recent. Clin. Trials.* **2016**, *11*, 159–166. [CrossRef] [PubMed]

30. Tang, X.; Wei, R.; Deng, A.; Lei, T. Protective Effects of Ethanolic Extracts from Artichoke, an Edible Herbal Medicine, against Acute Alcohol-Induced Liver Injury in Mice. *Nutrients* **2017**, *9*, 1000. [CrossRef] [PubMed]

31. Colak, E.; Ustuner, M.C.; Tekin, N.; Colak, E.; Burukoglu, D.; Degirmenci, I.; Gunes, H.V. The hepatocurative effects of *Cynara scolymus* L. leaf extract on carbon tetrachloride-induced oxidative stress and hepatic injury in rats. *Springerplus* **2016**, *5*, 216. [CrossRef] [PubMed]

32. Mehmetçik, G.; Ozdemirler, G.; Koçak-Toker, N.; Cevikbaş, U.; Uysal, M. Effect of pretreatment with artichoke extract on carbon tetrachloride-induced liver injury and oxidative stress. *Exp. Toxicol. Pathol.* **2008**, *60*, 475–480. [CrossRef] [PubMed]

33. Rangboo, V.; Noroozi, M.; Zavoshy, R.; Rezadoost, S.A.; Mohammadpoorasl, A. The Effect of Artichoke Leaf Extract on Alanine Aminotransferase and Aspartate Aminotransferase in the Patients with Nonalcoholic Steatohepatitis. *Int. J. Hepatol.* **2016**. [CrossRef] [PubMed]

34. Chen, W.; Wang, X.; Huang, L.; Liu, B. Hepcidin in non-alcoholic fatty liver disease regulated by the TLR4/NF-κB signaling pathway. *Exp. Ther. Med.* **2016**, *11*, 73–76. [CrossRef] [PubMed]

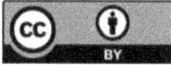

nutrients

MDPI

Review

Optimizing the Nutritional Support of Adult Patients in the Setting of Cirrhosis

Brandon J. Perumpail [1], Andrew A. Li [2], George Cholankeril [2], Radhika Kumari [2] and Aijaz Ahmed [2,*]

1   Department of Medicine, Drexel University College of Medicine, Philadelphia, PA 19129, USA; bjp63@drexel.edu
2   Division of Gastroenterology and Hepatology, Stanford University School of Medicine, Stanford, CA 94305, USA; andrewli@stanford.edu (A.A.L.); georgetc@stanford.edu (G.C.); rkumari@stanford.edu (R.K.)
*   Correspondence: aijazahmed@stanford.edu; Tel.: +1-650-498-6091; Fax: +650-498-5692

Received: 28 August 2017; Accepted: 9 October 2017; Published: 13 October 2017

Abstract: Aim: The aim of this work is to develop a pragmatic approach in the assessment and management strategies of patients with cirrhosis in order to optimize the outcomes in this patient population. Method: A systematic review of literature was conducted through 8 July 2017 on the PubMed Database looking for key terms, such as malnutrition, nutrition, assessment, treatment, and cirrhosis. Articles and studies looking at associations between nutrition and cirrhosis were reviewed. Results: An assessment of malnutrition should be conducted in two stages: the first, to identify patients at risk for malnutrition based on the severity of liver disease, and the second, to perform a complete multidisciplinary nutritional evaluation of these patients. Optimal management of malnutrition should focus on meeting recommended daily goals for caloric intake and inclusion of various nutrients in the diet. The nutritional goals should be pursued by encouraging and increasing oral intake or using other measures, such as oral supplementation, enteral nutrition, or parenteral nutrition. Conclusions: Although these strategies to improve nutritional support have been well established, current literature on the topic is limited in scope. Further research should be implemented to test if this enhanced approach is effective.

Keywords: nutrition; cirrhosis; end-stage liver disease; Child-Turcotte-Pugh; malnutrition; dietary intervention; improved oral intake

1. Introduction

Malnutrition has become increasingly common in end-stage liver disease [1]. The prevalence of malnutrition has been reported in a significant proportion of patients with cirrhosis and ranges from 10% to 100%, contingent on severity of hepatic decompensation in the setting of cirrhosis [2,3]. However, even with this high occurrence, malnutrition is still under-diagnosed and ineffectively treated [4]. More specifically, many patients who are awaiting liver transplantation develop various nutritional deficiencies [1]. Malnutrition is a predictor of morbidity and mortality in patients with cirrhosis [3]. Malnutrition related to liver disease has been linked to a risk of infections, complications associated with surgery, poor candidacy for liver transplantation, and a prolonged length of stay in the hospital or intensive care unit [2,5]. Routine screening of patients with end-stage liver disease for malnutrition can facilitate prompt diagnosis leading to timely initiation of treatment and improved outcomes [6,7].

2. Malnutrition in End-Stage Liver Disease

In the presence of cirrhosis, malnutrition is diagnosed and defined as a deficiency in nutrients [8]. Under normal post-prandial conditions, ingested carbohydrates are metabolized by the liver and stored as glycogen. Subsequently, during the normal fasting period glycogen can be broken down (glycogenolysis) to glucose (gluconeogenesis) to maintain stable blood glucose levels (glucose homeostasis). Patients with cirrhosis have a compromised ability to store glycogen and blunted gluconeogenesis. Therefore, cirrhotic patients may enter a starvation state between dinner and breakfast, stimulating lipid oxidation, thus shifting from carbohydrate to fat as the main source of energy metabolism. A complex interaction of many factors are involved in increasing the risk of malnutrition in cirrhosis [9]. Poor calorie intake is a common contributor in these patients, which often stems from a lack of appetite or anorexia. The molecular mechanisms involved in malnutrition in the cirrhotic state are not fully understood and include zinc deficiency, early satiety resulting from an increased amount of leptin and tumor necrosis factor-alpha in the blood, etc. [8,9]. In addition, many patients may develop a poor appetite due to ascites or hepatic encephalopathy [10]. The resulting dietary restriction of salt may make food unpalatable, further escalating poor nutritional status [11]. Another cause of malnutrition is impaired absorption and digestion resulting from a host of factors, such as decreased bile-salt, bacterial overgrowth, and portal hypertension [8]. Finally, hypermetabolism leads to malnutrition through increased energy expenditure and is an independent predictor of both transplant-free and post-transplant survival [8,10,12]. This is mainly caused by changes in nutrient utilization due to the lack of available carbohydrates for energy, which places the body in a state of starvation, especially overnight [12]. Infection and ascites also contribute to the hypermetabolic state [10]. In the setting of cirrhosis, protein-energy malnutrition (PEM) is noted in up to two-thirds of affected individuals and correlates with Child-Turcotte-Pugh classification. PEM is associated with poor survival in this patient population. The contributing factors to PEM include hypermetabolism, poor caloric intake, malabsorption, increased intestinal permeability leading to protein loss, and decreased hepatic protein synthesis. In addition, PEM leads to muscle wasting manifested by a reduction in skeletal muscle volume and strength (secondary sarcopenia related to cirrhosis). Secondary sarcopenia associated with cirrhosis is an independent predictor of poor survival. Furthermore, certain disease-specific issues impacting the management of malnutrition must be individualized. For example, alcohol abuse associated with low socio-economic status and poor psycho-social support may pose a complex challenge in the management of malnutrition.

In order to fully address the issue of malnutrition in end-stage liver disease, improvement must be made in promptly diagnosing patients in need for nutritional support.

3. Improved Assessment of Malnutrition

A systematic approach to screen for malnutrition in cirrhotic patients must be established to more directly address the growing problem of malnutrition. During the initial evaluation (stage 1 assessment), cirrhotic patients with immediate need for nutritional support must be identified. Subsequently, these selected patients must undergo a standardized evaluation (stage 2 assessment) leading to individualized patient care with a focus to optimize the nutritional status. This two-stage approach is summarized in Figure 1.

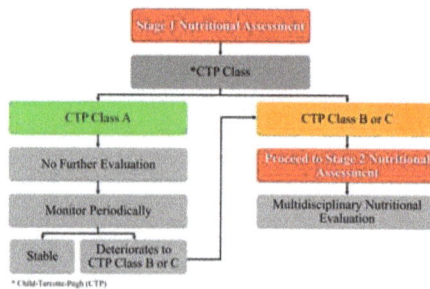

Figure 1. Two-stage approach to nutritional assessment in cirrhosis.

3.1. Stage 1 Assessment for Malnutrition: Define Immediate-Need Populations

The goal of a two-stage approach is to maximize the allocation of time and resources to those who need it the most to improve overall outcomes. Not every patient needs an immediate full evaluation (stage 2 assessment) for malnutrition; patients who are the most at risk should be targeted first and assessed. Malnutrition severity is strongly associated with the severity of hepatic decompensation (liver failure) in the setting of cirrhosis [3,13]. A Chinese study evaluating malnutrition in patients with chronic liver disease found that patients with the highest rate of nutritional risk were also those with the greatest degree of liver failure (patients in Child-Turcotte-Pugh (CTP) classes B and C) [13]. The two-stage approach uses the association between malnutrition and severity of liver failure to identify the patient population in immediate need of nutritional assessment using the CTP scoring system. This classification, created by Child and Turcotte in 1964 and later adjusted in 1973 by Pugh, is a commonly-used tool for measuring the severity of liver failure in cirrhotic patients and to estimate the risk of surgical procedures [14–16]. The CTP system scores 1–3 points, with one being the most normal and three being the most abnormal, in five different categories (albumin, bilirubin, prothrombin prolongation time, and hepatic encephalopathy) to grade patients into three classes: A (5–6 points), B (7–9 points), and C (10–15 points), with classes B and C being the most severe [17]. This constitutes the 'stage 1 assessment' and identifies patients with cirrhosis at the highest risk of malnutrition, namely CTP classes B and C [13]. Another study evaluated of cirrhotic patients for malnutrition categorized by the three CTP classes and noted malnourishment in more than half the patients in the CTP class B and C groups, 77.3% and 94.4% respectively, while less than half of the patients in CTP class A developed malnutrition [3]. In a study that compared the Subjective Global Assessment (SGA) of patients' nutrition with their CPT class, only patients in class B and C were indicated to have levels of malnutrition ranging from moderate to severe [11]. Thus, cirrhotic patients with CTP class B and C have been shown to be the most likely to develop malnutrition and require comprehensive 'stage 2 assessment' for poor nutritional status.

3.2. Stage 2 Assessment for Malnutrition: Multidisciplinary Nutritional Assessment

A more thorough and comprehensive evaluation of the nutritional status can be achieved and a focused individualized approach can be pursued. This not only allows for proper apportionment of resources and time, but also provides a more targeted approach in which patients can be prioritized based on the severity of malnutrition. A study evaluating protein depletion in patients with cirrhosis concluded that the utilization of multiple nutritional assessment tools were crucial in making an accurate assessment of severity of malnutrition [18]. End-stage liver disease is a confounding factor that affects the results of multiple nutritional assessment tools and, thus, there has to be confirmation across many techniques to diagnose malnutrition [5]. For example, weight and albumin concentrations could be unreliable measurements alone due to other complications from cirrhosis, such as ascites or low protein synthesis, respectively [10,18,19]. Other cross-sectional studies looking at nutritional assessment techniques found that the use of a variety of techniques, such as the SGA, biochemical tests, and anthropometry, lead to a better understanding of nutritional status [2,20–22]. A variety of tests should be used to evaluate different aspects and severity of nutrition rather than any single nutritional screening tool, thus creating a multidisciplinary approach shown in Figure 2 [1,19].

A standard nutritional evaluation often used in hospitals is the SGA [23]. It is an attractive test due to its accuracy while also being cheap, non-invasive, and simple to execute [23]. Multiple studies compare the SGA results with other nutritional measurement tools and have found it to provide consistent results, validating the SGA's precision and specificity [2,22,24]. It was also studied in the context of liver transplantation and was shown to predict complications during transplantation, as well as post-operative outcomes [5]. The SGA is a questionnaire with two main components, history and physical examination [25]. The history portion asks questions regarding previous weight changes over time, recent alterations of food intake, recent functionality, and symptoms affecting intake [25]. The physical examination measures fat loss, muscle wasting, and the presence of edema and ascites [25].

A score is calculated based on the evaluation and the patient is assigned to one of three stages—Stage A, well nourished; Stage B, moderately malnourished; or Stage C, severely malnourished, with each stage having a list of features characterizing the multiple categories assessed [25].

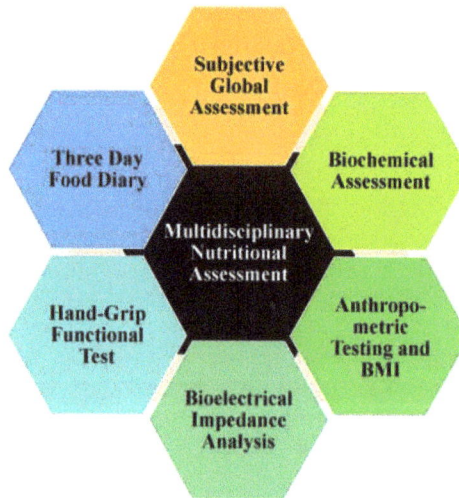

Figure 2. Multidisciplinary nutritional assessment.

A biochemical assessment for markers of malnutrition is commonly used for monitoring nutrition [1]. The test should include many factors, such as hemoglobin, albumin, white blood cell count, retinol-binding protein, transferrin, liver function exams, glucose, cholesterol, urea nitrogen, C-reactive protein, pre-albumin, nitrogen balance, creatinine, sodium, magnesium, zinc, potassium, and others [19,20]. Serum albumin is a common tool used to measure nutritional status and can help categorize the level of malnutrition [20]. However, one issue is that albumin also declines due to hepatic damage, making it an unreliable marker [19,26]. Pre-albumin and transferrin are impacted by malnutrition and hepatic damage similarly, but respond faster and, therefore, could also be used as early indications of malnutrition [26]. Retinol binding protein (RBP) relies on the presence of other nutrients, such as vitamin A and zinc, in order to carry out its function. Thus, micronutrient deficiency due to malnutrition would affect the blood levels of RBP as well [27]. Nitrogen balance is a good measure of dietary protein intake and protein metabolism [28]. Deficiency occurs when protein metabolism is greater than protein intake, as indicated by a negative nitrogen balance [28].

Furthermore, anthropometric testing and body mass index (BMI) are necessary tools when assessing nutritional body composition [29]. Anthropometric testing measures height, weight, mid-arm circumference, mid-arm muscle circumference, triceps skin fold thickness, and biceps skin fold thickness [20,21]. BMI and anthropometric measures can be used to assess skeletal muscle mass and adipose deposit levels [30–32]. A recent study found that thigh muscle thickness when used with BMI can be an important tool in identifying sarcopenia and malnutrition [31]. A potential problem with BMI is that edema and ascites could increase the measured weight and make BMI inaccurate; however, dry BMI can be measured by using corrective factors for dry weight that account for the level of edema. Five, ten, or fifteen percent are subtracted from the measured weight for mild, moderate, or severe ascites, and an extra 5% would be subtracted if edema is present [30,31]. Another way to account for ascites is to use the established BMI standards for ascites where BMI below or equal to 22 with no ascites, a BMI of 23 kg/m [2] with mild ascites, or a BMI of 25 kg/m [2] with tension ascites is considered a state of malnutrition [33]. Another useful tool to measure body composition is bioelectrical impedance analysis (BIA) [33–35]. BIA is swift, simple, and non-invasive, which makes it an attractive new technique that is gaining interest [35–37]. It conducts an electric current through the body and calculates its electric impedance, which is made up of two components—resistance, which measures body water, and reactance, which measures body cell mass (BCM). Based on this information, measurements about body composition can be estimated, such as BCM, BCM%, extracellular mass, mass that is not from body fat, body fat mass, phase angle, and total body water [34,37,38]. This information can be utilized to understand various aspects of body composition and determine how they change over time with intervention [33]. For example, BIA can calculate body water, which could be indicative of edema or ascites [33]. Furthermore, recent research has found that phase angle is a better predictor of nutritional status in cirrhosis than anthropomethric evaluation tools and can even be used for early diagnosis of malnutrition [35].

Functional testing is another important evaluation when assessing nutrition; this allows for a means of testing the strength and ability of the skeletal muscle [2]. A longitudinal study found that although muscle strength and muscle mass both deteriorate with malnutrition, the former declines at a much quicker rate [39]. Additionally, muscle strength can decrease without a loss in muscle mass [39]. Hand-grip strength is a tool used to assess muscle strength and has been validated as an independent method of identifying malnutrition and muscle capability [40]. Moreover, a comparative study found that when tested against other nutritional assessment tools, such as SGA, BMI, and anthropometric measurements, the hand-grip strength test had the highest accuracy for detecting the presence of nutritional compromise in the context of liver disease [41]. Another study found that not only does hand-grip strength correlate with nutritional level, it also predicts hospital outcomes, such as post-operative complications, length of hospitalization, risk of re-hospitalization, and physical ability.

The final portion of the assessment is an evaluation of dietary intake [2]. The best method to record this is through a three-day food diary with specific instructions given to the patient on how to complete the diary so that accurate information on food consumption can be documented [2]. Many studies have validated the three-day food diary as an effective measure of dietary intake and it has been shown to be more accurate than other methods such as the food frequency questionnaire and 24-h recall [42,43]. The food diary helps physicians and dieticians understand the different food habits, dietary choices, and overall consumption levels (calories and protein content) of the patient over time so that they can assess nutrition in an individualized manner [44]. The use of multiple tools and tests to evaluate the patient's nutritional status creates a well-rounded image of the patient's health so that an assessment of malnutrition are both thorough and specific. An initial assessment stage that filters patients based on severity of hepatic decompensation in the setting of cirrhosis allows only the malnourished or most at-risk for malnutrition to proceed to the next stage. Furthermore, this individualized approach results in pragmatic utilization and allocation of restricted resources.

4. Treatment Options for Malnourished Patients

Malnutrition in the setting of cirrhosis has been noted as a reliable indicator of quality of life and key predictor of inpatient outcomes (morbidity and mortality) [3]. Studies have indicated that these outcomes can be improved by optimizing the nutritional status of a patient with cirrhosis [7]. Unfortunately, malnutrition remains an alarmingly prevalent problem, especially in patients with cirrhosis [3,45]. Therefore, it is very important to develop an objective and standardized initial and follow-up evaluation pathway/management protocol to assess the nutritional status of patients with cirrhosis. In particular, patients with hepatic decompensation/liver failure awaiting liver transplantation require an ongoing evaluation of their nutritional status in the era of donor organ shortage and longer waiting times on transplant waitlists.

4.1. Proper Dietary Recommendations and Education

In patients with cirrhosis, the recommendation for different macromolecules has changed over time and health care practitioners need to be aware of these changes so that patients are properly managed [12]. Gastroenterology and hepatology fellowships do not always offer a comprehensive training in nutritional assessment and treatment; therefore, physicians may not always know the best methods available for diagnosing or treating patients who face malnourishment [9]. The most important aspect of malnourishment management is ensuring that the patient's rehabilitative diet has the correct amount of each essential nutrient or macromolecule according to the current regulations [12]. Furthermore, diet plays a substantial role in cirrhosis and the related severity of hepatic decompensation/liver failure. Inadequate diets have been associated with further progression of liver disease and increased risk of cirrhosis. However, proper diet alterations have been noted to not only prevent disease progression, but also to reduce the severity of liver failure [46,47]. The recommendation for malnourished patients with cirrhosis is 35–40 kcal/kg/day to promote anabolism [33,48]. Protein deficiency is a significant problem in malnutrition which can be addressed through an intake of 1.2–1.5 g/kg/day [48,49]. Furthermore, hepatic damage causes an increase in aromatic amino acids (AAA) and decreases branched-chain amino acids (BCAA) which can lead to hepatic encephalopathy and other neurological complications [29]. Studies have found that increasing the BCAA to AAA ratio through improved dietary BCAA intake has led to normalization and increased survival [12,50]. The guideline for carbohydrates is 50–70% of daily calories [51]. However, simple sugars, especially fructose, should be avoided as much as possible [6]. The recommendation for lipids is 10–20% of calories with the majority being monounsaturated and polyunsaturated fatty acids [6,11]. Special considerations have to be taken for hepatic encephalopathy and ascites [33]. In hepatic encephalopathy, there should be an increased emphasis on BCAAs and fiber with decreased ammonia [33]. Previous recommendations for hepatic encephalopathy included decreased protein intake, but more recent data have shown that this practice is outdated and incorrect [6,9,10]. Patients with ascites should be on a low-sodium diet (less than or equal to 2 g/day) and should also have water restriction when edema is present or if hyponatremia occurs [33]. Ensuring patients meet these requirements, organized in Table 1, is the first step in optimizing nutritional support in patients with end-stage liver disease. In patients with cirrhosis associated with nonalcoholic steatohepatitis caloric restriction, but not protein restriction, can be recommended. Furthermore, patients with fluid retention must be educated to restrict their sodium intake to less than 2 g per day and fluid intake of 2 L per day.

Table 1. Nutritional recommendations for malnutrition in cirrhosis.

Nutritional Recommendations for Malnutrition in Cirrhosis	
Daily Calories	35–40 kcal/kg/day
Proteins	1.2–1.5 g/kg/day with increased BCAAs
Carbohydrates	50–70% of daily calories with decreased simple sugars—especially fructose
Lipids	10–20% of daily calories with increased MUFAs and PUFAs
Special Considerations	
Hepatic Encephalopathy	Maintain protein intake, increase BCAAs and decreased ammonia intake
Ascites	Low-sodium diet ($\leq$2 g/day) and water restriction when necessary

4.2. Techniques to Promote Oral Intake

In general, adequate oral intake has been a difficult task for many patients facing malnutrition related to cirrhosis and other chronic ailments [52]. Patients with malnutrition are unable to maintain their daily caloric targets and requirements for nutrients despite institution of reinforced diet plans [52]. Many studies have reported that patients with malnutrition have significant amounts of calories wasted with each partially-ingested meal [53,54]. One study questioned patients after meals at the hospital in an attempt to understand the reasoning behind incomplete meal intake and suspected that meal sensory perception affected eating capability despite hunger [55]. Patients responded regarding various aspects of their meal experience (appearance, aroma, taste, texture, temperature, and food variety) and requested that more attention be paid to provide a more individualized eating experience [55]. These factors should be continuously re-evaluated to reflect the preferences of the patients as their appetite changes based on the severity of hepatic decompensation [55]. In addition to this study, others have shown that meal presentation and appearance impacts the desire to eat; patients ate more from a neatly-arranged plate rather than a disorganized one [54,55]. Additionally, overwhelming odors from food discouraged eating [55]. For example, when feeling nauseous, patients desired meals that had neutral tastes [55]. Often softer foods that were easier to ingest were associated with increased intake [55,56]. A hot meal versus a cold meal was more likely to be ingested [55]. Another study assessing issues with oral intake showed that interruptions during meal times by nurses, physicians, or tests led to missed meals that were never served later; patients were also unaware of the options available for extra snacks between meals [53]. This suggests that patients should have scheduled meal times that are protected and nursing staff should ensure that the patients eat during the dedicated meal period without interruption, plus improving patient awareness regarding additional accessible snacks can increase caloric intake [53]. Studies to improve intake noted that smaller meals, increased meal frequency, and fortified nutrition within these meals were effective in instituting increased nutritional support [57]. Furthermore, studies in the setting of cirrhosis found that 4–6 meals high in carbohydrates with an evening snack fortified with BCAAs prevented hypoglycemia and led to increased nutrition due to reduced catabolism overnight [8]. Another important factor found in studies was the level of nursing education [58]. Poulsen and colleagues [58] noticed increased nutrition and oral intake in patients when nurses were given a short class on nutritional care to provide individualized nutritional support. Figure 3 summarizes the various interventions that can be used to promote oral intake and improve nutritional status of patients with cirrhosis.

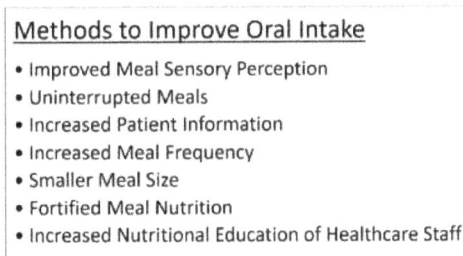

Methods to Improve Oral Intake

- Improved Meal Sensory Perception
- Uninterrupted Meals
- Increased Patient Information
- Increased Meal Frequency
- Smaller Meal Size
- Fortified Meal Nutrition
- Increased Nutritional Education of Healthcare Staff

Figure 3. Methods to improve oral intake.

4.3. Alternative Feeding Methods

Although oral intake of food is the preferred route of nutrition, factors, such as patient weakness or inability to eat, may necessitate pursuit of alternative methods for nutrient delivery [10,59]. Oral supplements should be used in an individualized approach to fulfill any specific nutrient deficiencies a patient may have [10,59]. A clinical trial noted that patients given oral supplements between meals met the recommended nutritional intakes [59]. Other options for patients unable to handle oral intake are enteral nutrition through a nasogastric tube and, if necessary, parenteral nutrition [10]. Both of these have been shown to be effective in various studies assessing malnutrition [10,60]. Complications of cirrhosis and end-stage liver disease associated with gut microbiota dysfunction, such as hepatic encephalopathy, are effectively managed with prebiotics, probiotics and synbiotics. Optimal management of hepatic encephalopathy and favorable gut microbiota may lead to improved nutritional status in patients with cirrhosis. Herbal remedies and supplements should be avoided with cirrhosis due to increased risk of hepatotoxicity with marginal hepatic reserve.

5. Conclusions

Malnutrition is a growing problem, especially in cirrhotic patients with end-stage liver disease. The enhancement of methods to assess and treat malnutrition is the key to optimizing patient outcomes. Assessment of malnutrition should be done in two stages, the first to identify patients at risk for malnutrition based on cirrhosis and the second to run a complete multidisciplinary nutritional evaluation on these patients. Treatments for malnutrition should make sure patients reach the recommended daily caloric and nutrient goals by increasing oral intake or by using other measures, such as oral supplementation, enteral nutrition, or parenteral nutrition. Further prospective data are needed from dedicated studies to optimize the nutritional status and outcomes in patients with cirrhosis improved through proper nutritional support of patients with advanced liver disease [7]. Therefore, standardized protocols to screen for malnutrition associated with cirrhosis and timely intervention with nutritional support is a pivotal step in reducing the risk of morbidity and mortality.

Author Contributions: All authors designed the project. First prepared the manuscript. Manuscript was reviewed and edited by all authors. The last author (senior author) supervised the project.

Conflicts of Interest: The authors declare no conflict of interest.

References

1. Lim, H.S.; Kim, H.C.; Park, Y.H.; Kim, S.K. Evaluation of Malnutrition Risk after Liver Transplantation Using the Nutritional Screening Tools. *Clin. Nutr. Res.* **2015**, *4*, 242–249. [CrossRef] [PubMed]
2. Marr, K.J.; Shaheen, A.A.; Lam, L.; Stapleton, M.; Burak, K.; Raman, M. Nutritional status and the performance of multiple bedside tools for nutrition assessment among patients waiting for liver transplantation: A Canadian experience. *Clin. Nutr. ESPEN* **2017**, *17*, 68–74. [CrossRef] [PubMed]
3. Maharshi, S.; Sharma, B.C.; Srivastava, S. Malnutrition in cirrhosis increases morbidity and mortality. *J. Gastroenterol. Hepatol.* **2015**, *30*, 1507–1513. [CrossRef] [PubMed]
4. Cheung, K.; Lee, S.S.; Raman, M. Prevalence and mechanisms of malnutrition in patients with advanced liver disease, and nutrition management strategies. *Clin. Gastroenterol. Hepatol.* **2012**, *10*, 117–125. [CrossRef] [PubMed]
5. Stephenson, G.R.; Moretti, E.W.; El-Moalem, H.; Clavien, P.A.; Tuttle-Newhall, J.E. Malnutrition in liver transplant patients: Preoperative subjective global assessment is predictive of outcome after liver transplantation. *Transplantation* **2001**, *72*, 666–670. [CrossRef] [PubMed]
6. McClain, C.J. Nutrition in patients with cirrhosis. *Gastroenterol. Hepatol.* **2016**, *12*, 507–510.
7. Alberda, C.; Gramlich, L.; Jones, N.; Jeejeebhoy, K.; Day, A.G.; Dhaliwal, R.; Heyland, D.K. The relationship between nutritional intake and clinical outcomes in critically ill patients: Results of an international multicenter observational study. *Intensive Care Med.* **2009**, *35*, 1728–1737. [CrossRef] [PubMed]
8. Ye, Q.; Yin, W.; Zhang, L.; Xiao, H.; Qi, Y.; Liu, S.; Qian, B.; Wang, F.; Han, T. The value of grip test, lysophosphatidlycholines, glycerophosphocholine, ornithine, glucuronic acid decrement in assessment of nutritional and metabolic characteristics in hepatitis B cirrhosis. *PLoS ONE* **2017**, *12*, e0175165. [CrossRef] [PubMed]
9. Patton, H.M. Nutritional assessment of patients with chronic liver disease. *Gastroenterol. Hepatol.* **2012**, *8*, 687–690.
10. Patel, J.J.; McClain, C.J.; Sarav, M.; Hamilton-Reeves, J.; Hurt, R.T. Protein requirements for critically Ill patients with renal and liver failure. *Nutr. Clin. Pract.* **2017**, *32* (Suppl. 1), 101S–111S. [CrossRef] [PubMed]
11. Teiusanu, A.; Andrei, M.; Arbanas, T.; Nicolaie, T.; Diculescu, M. Nutritional status in cirrhotic patients. *Maedica* **2012**, *7*, 284–289. [PubMed]
12. Eghtesad, S. Malnutrition in liver cirrhosis: The influence of protein and sodium. *Middle East J. Dig. Dis.* **2013**, *5*, 65–75. [PubMed]
13. Shi, S.; Han, J.; Yan, M.; Wang, K.; Yu, H.; Meng, Q. Nutritional risk assessment in patients with chronic liver disease. *Zhonghua Gan Zang Bing Za Zhi* **2014**, *22*, 536–539. [PubMed]
14. Child, C.G.; Turcotte, J.G. Surgery and portal hypertension. *Major Probl. Clin. Surg.* **1964**, *1*, 1–85. [PubMed]

15. Pugh, R.N.; Murray-Lyon, I.M.; Dawson, J.L.; Pietroni, M.C.; Williams, R. Transection of the oesophagus for bleeding oesophageal varices. *Br. J. Surg.* **1973**, *60*, 646–649. [CrossRef] [PubMed]

16. Zhou, C.; Hou, C.; Cheng, D.; Tang, W.; Lv, W. Predictive accuracy comparison of MELD and Child-Turcotte-Pugh scores for survival in patients underwent TIPS placement: A systematic meta-analytic review. *Int. J. Clin. Exp. Med.* **2015**, *8*, 13464–13472. [PubMed]

17. Raszeja-Wyszomirska, J.; Wasilewicz, M.P.; Wunsch, E.; Szymanik, B.; Jarosz, K.; Wójcicki, M.; Milkiewicz, P. Assessment of a modified Child-Pugh-Turcotte score to predict early mortality after liver transplantation. *Transplant. Proc.* **2009**, *41*, 3114–3116. [CrossRef] [PubMed]

18. Prijatmoko, D.; Strauss, B.J.; Lambert, J.R.; Sievert, W.; Stroud, D.B.; Wahlqvist, M.L.; Katz, B.; Colman, J.; Jones, P.; Korman, M.G. Early detection of protein depletion in alcoholic cirrhosis: Role of body composition analysis. *Gastroenterology* **1993**, *105*, 1839–1845. [CrossRef]

19. Bharadwaj, S.; Ginoya, S.; Tandon, P.; Gohel, T.D.; Guirguis, J.; Vallabh, H.; Jevenn, A.; Hanouneh, I. Malnutrition: Laboratory markers vs nutritional assessment. *Gastroenterol. Rep.* **2016**, *4*, 272–280. [CrossRef] [PubMed]

20. Tai, M.L.; Goh, K.L.; Mohd-Taib, S.H.; Rampal, S.; Mahadeva, S. Anthropometric, biochemical and clinical assessment of malnutrition in Malaysian patients with advanced cirrhosis. *Nutr. J.* **2010**, *9*, 27. [CrossRef] [PubMed]

21. Nunes, F.F.; Bassani, L.; Fernandes, S.A.; Deutrich, M.E.; Pivatto, B.C.; Marroni, C.A. Food consumption of cirrhotic patients, comparison with the nutritional status and disease staging. *Arq. Gastroenterol.* **2016**, *53*, 250–256. [CrossRef] [PubMed]

22. Filipovic, B.F.; Gajic, M.; Milinic, N.; Milovanović, B.; Filipović, B.R.; Cvetković, M.; Sibalić, N. Comparison of two nutritional assessment methods in gastroenterology patients. *World J. Gastroenterol.* **2010**, *16*, 1999–2004. [CrossRef] [PubMed]

23. Da Silva Fink, J.; Daniel de Mello, P.; Daniel de Mello, E. Subjective global assessment of nutritional status—A systematic review of the literature. *Clin. Nutr.* **2015**, *34*, 785–792. [CrossRef] [PubMed]

24. Mourao, F.; Amado, D.; Ravasco, P.; Vidal, P.M.; Camilo, M.E. Nutritional risk and status assessment in surgical patients: A challenge amidst plenty. *Nutr. Hosp.* **2004**, *19*, 83–88. [PubMed]

25. Detsky, A.S.; McLaughlin, J.R.; Baker, J.P.; Johnston, N.; Whittaker, S.; Mendelson, R.A.; Jeejeebhoy, K.N. What is subjective global assessment of nutritional status? *JPEN J. Parenter. Enteral Nutr.* **1987**, *11*, 8–13. [CrossRef] [PubMed]

26. Fuhrman, M.P.; Charney, P.; Mueller, C.M. Hepatic proteins and nutrition assessment. *J. Am. Diet. Assoc.* **2004**, *104*, 1258–1264. [CrossRef] [PubMed]

27. Chaves, G.V.; Peres, W.A.; Goncalves, J.C.; Ramalho, A. Vitamin A and retinol-binding protein deficiency among chronic liver disease patients. *Nutrition* **2015**, *31*, 664–668. [CrossRef] [PubMed]

28. Rand, W.M.; Pellett, P.L.; Young, V.R. Meta-analysis of nitrogen balance studies for estimating protein requirements in healthy adults. *Am. J. Clin. Nutr.* **2003**, *77*, 109–127. [PubMed]

29. Johnson, T.M.; Overgard, E.B.; Cohen, A.E.; DiBaise, J.K. Nutrition assessment and management in advanced liver disease. *Nutr. Clin. Pract.* **2013**, *28*, 15–29. [CrossRef] [PubMed]

30. Tandon, P.; Ney, M.; Irwin, I.; Ma, M.M.; Gramlich, L.; Bain, V.G.; Esfandiari, N.; Baracos, V.; Montano-Loza, A.J.; Myers, R.P. Severe muscle depletion in patients on the liver transplant wait list: Its prevalence and independent prognostic value. *Liver Transpl.* **2012**, *18*, 1209–1216. [CrossRef] [PubMed]

31. Tandon, P.; Low, G.; Mourtzakis, M.; Zenith, L.; Myers, R.P.; Abraldes, J.G.; Shaheen, A.A.; Qamar, H.; Mansoor, N.; Carbonneau, M.; et al. A model to identify sarcopenia in patients with cirrhosis. *Clin. Gastroenterol. Hepatol.* **2016**, *14*, 1473–1480. [CrossRef] [PubMed]

32. Ponziani, F.R.; Gasbarrini, A. Sarcopenia in patients with advanced liver disease. *Curr. Protein Pept. Sci.* **2017**. [CrossRef] [PubMed]

33. Moctezuma-Velazquez, C.; Garcia-Juarez, I.; Soto-Solis, R.; Hernandez-Cortes, J.; Torre, A. Nutritional assessment and treatment of patients with liver cirrhosis. *Nutrition* **2013**, *29*, 1279–1285. [CrossRef] [PubMed]

34. Verney, J.; Metz, L.; Chaplais, E.; Cardenoux, C.; Pereira, B.; Thivel, D. Bioelectrical impedance is an accurate method to assess body composition in obese but not severely obese adolescents. *Nutr. Res.* **2016**, *36*, 663–670. [CrossRef] [PubMed]

35. Fernandes, S.A.; de Mattos, A.A.; Tovo, C.V.; Marroni, C.A. Nutritional evaluation in cirrhosis: Emphasis on the phase angle. *World J. Hepatol.* **2016**, *8*, 1205–1211. [CrossRef] [PubMed]

36. Dehghan, M.; Merchant, A.T. Is bioelectrical impedance accurate for use in large epidemiological studies? *Nutr. J.* **2008**, *7*, 26. [CrossRef] [PubMed]

37. Walter-Kroker, A.; Kroker, A.; Mattiucci-Guehlke, M.; Glaab, T. A practical guide to bioelectrical impedance analysis using the example of chronic obstructive pulmonary disease. *Nutr. J.* **2011**, *10*, 35. [CrossRef] [PubMed]

38. Lee, Y.; Kwon, O.; Shin, C.S.; Lee, S.M. Use of bioelectrical impedance analysis for the assessment of nutritional status in critically ill patients. *Clin. Nutr. Res.* **2015**, *4*, 32–40. [CrossRef] [PubMed]

39. Goodpaster, B.H.; Park, S.W.; Harris, T.B.; Kritchevsky, S.B.; Nevitt, M.; Schwartz, A.V.; Simonsick, E.M.; Tylavsky, F.A.; Visser, M.; Newman, A.B. The loss of skeletal muscle strength, mass, and quality in older adults: The health, aging and body composition study. *J. Gerontol. A Biol. Sci. Med. Sci.* **2006**, *61*, 1059–1064. [CrossRef] [PubMed]

40. Flood, A.; Chung, A.; Parker, H.; Kearns, V.; O'Sullivan, T.A. The use of hand grip strength as a predictor of nutrition status in hospital patients. *Clin. Nutr.* **2014**, *33*, 106–114. [CrossRef] [PubMed]

41. Sharma, P.; Rauf, A.; Matin, A.; Agarwal, R.; Tyagi, P.; Arora, A. Handgrip strength as an important bed side tool to assess malnutrition in patient with liver disease. *J. Clin. Exp. Hepatol.* **2017**, *7*, 16–22. [CrossRef] [PubMed]

42. Crawford, P.B.; Obarzanek, E.; Morrison, J.; Sabry, Z.I. Comparative advantage of 3-day food records over 24-h recall and 5-day food frequency validated by observation of 9- and 10-year-old girls. *J. Am. Diet. Assoc.* **1994**, *94*, 626–630. [CrossRef]

43. Yang, Y.J.; Kim, M.K.; Hwang, S.H.; Ahn, Y.; Shim, J.E.; Kim, D.H. Relative validities of 3-day food records and the food frequency questionnaire. *Nutr. Res. Pract.* **2010**, *4*, 142–148. [CrossRef] [PubMed]

44. Ortega, R.M.; Perez-Rodrigo, C.; Lopez-Sobaler, A.M. Dietary assessment methods: Dietary records. *Nutr. Hosp.* **2015**, *31* (Suppl. 3), 38–45. [PubMed]

45. Rojas-Loureiro, G.; Servin-Caamano, A.; Perez-Reyes, E.; Servin-Abad, L.; Higuera-de la Tijera, F. Malnutrition negatively impacts the quality of life of patients with cirrhosis: An observational study. *World J. Hepatol.* **2017**, *9*, 263–269. [CrossRef] [PubMed]

46. Pimentel, C.F.; Lai, M. Nutrition interventions for chronic liver diseases and nonalcoholic fatty liver disease. *Med. Clin. N. Am.* **2016**, *100*, 1303–1327. [CrossRef] [PubMed]

47. Kim, W. Treatment options in non-alcoholic fatty liver disease. *Korean J. Gastroenterol.* **2017**, *69*, 353–358. [CrossRef] [PubMed]

48. Chao, A.; Waitzberg, D.; de Jesus, R.P.; Bueno, A.A.; Kha, V.; Allen, K.; Kappus, M.; Medici, V. Malnutrition and nutritional support in alcoholic liver Disease: A review. *Curr. Gastroenterol. Rep.* **2016**, *18*, 65. [CrossRef] [PubMed]

49. Putadechakum, S.; Klangjareonchai, T.; Soponsaritsuk, A.; Roongpisuthipong, C. Nutritional status assessment in cirrhotic patients after protein supplementation. *ISRN Gastroenterol.* **2012**, *2012*, 690402. [CrossRef] [PubMed]

50. Hanai, T.; Shiraki, M.; Nishimura, K.; Ohnishi, S.; Imai, K.; Suetsugu, A.; Takai, K.; Shimizu, M.; Moriwaki, H. Sarcopenia impairs prognosis of patients with liver cirrhosis. *Nutrition* **2015**, *31*, 193–199. [CrossRef] [PubMed]

51. Anastácio, L.R.; Davisson Correia, M.I.T. Nutrition therapy: Integral part of liver transplant care. *World J. Gastroenterol.* **2016**, *22*, 1513–1522. [CrossRef] [PubMed]

52. Thibault, R.; Chikhi, M.; Clerc, A.; Darmon, P.; Chopard, P.; Genton, L.; Kossovsky, M.P.; Pichard, C. Assessment of food intake in hospitalised patients: A 10-year comparative study of a prospective hospital survey. *Clin. Nutr.* **2011**, *30*, 289–296. [CrossRef] [PubMed]

53. Van Bokhorst-de van der Schueren, M.A.; Roosemalen, M.M.; Weijs, P.J.; Langius, J.A. High waste contributes to low food intake in hospitalized patients. *Nutr. Clin. Pract.* **2012**, *27*, 274–280. [CrossRef] [PubMed]

54. Navarro, D.A.; Boaz, M.; Krause, I.; Elis, A.; Chernov, K.; Giabra, M.; Levy, M.; Giboreau, A.; Kosak, S.; Mouhieddine, M.; et al. Improved meal presentation increases food intake and decreases readmission rate in hospitalized patients. *Clin. Nutr.* **2016**, *35*, 1153–1158. [CrossRef] [PubMed]

55. Sorensen, J.; Holm, L.; Frost, M.B.; Kondrup, J. Food for patients at nutritional risk: A model of food sensory quality to promote intake. *Clin. Nutr.* **2012**, *31*, 637–646. [CrossRef] [PubMed]

56. Forde, C.G.; van Kuijk, N.; Thaler, T.; de Graaf, C.; Martin, N. Texture and savoury taste influences on food intake in a realistic hot lunch time meal. *Appetite* **2013**, *60*, 180–186. [CrossRef] [PubMed]

57. Lorefalt, B.; Wissing, U.; Unosson, M. Smaller but energy and protein-enriched meals improve energy and nutrient intakes in elderly patients. *J. Nutr. Health Aging* **2005**, *9*, 243–247. [PubMed]

58. Poulsen, I.; Vendel Petersen, H.; Rahm Hallberg, I.; Schroll, M. Lack of nutritional and functional effects of nutritional supervision by nurses: A quasi-experimental study in geriatric patients. *Scand. J. Food Nutr.* **2007**, *51*, 6–12. [CrossRef]

59. Campbell, K.L.; Webb, L.; Vivanti, A.; Varghese, P.; Ferguson, M. Comparison of three interventions in the treatment of malnutrition in hospitalised older adults: A clinical trial. *Nutr. Diet.* **2013**, *70*, 325–331. [CrossRef]

60. Kozeniecki, M.; Fritzshall, R. Enteral nutrition for adults in the hospital setting. *Nutr. Clin. Pract.* **2015**, *30*, 634–651. [CrossRef] [PubMed]

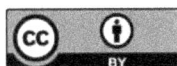

nutrients

MDPI

Review

Nutritional Needs and Support for Children with Chronic Liver Disease

Christine H. Yang [1], Brandon J. Perumpail [2], Eric R. Yoo [3], Aijaz Ahmed [4,*]and John A. Kerner Jr. [1]

[1]   Division of Pediatric Gastroenterology, Hepatology and Nutrition, Lucile Packard Children's Hospital, Palo Alto, Stanford, CA 94304, USA; christine.yang@stanford.edu (C.H.Y.); JKerner@stanfordhealthcare.org (J.A.K.J.)
[2]   Department of Medicine, Drexel University College of Medicine, Philadelphia, PA 19129, USA; bjp63@drexel.edu
[3]   Department of Medicine, Santa Clara Valley Medical Center, San Jose, CA 95128, USA; eric.r.yoo@gmail.com
[4]   Division of Gastroenterology and Hepatology, Stanford University School of Medicine, Stanford, CA 94305, USA
*   Correspondence: aijazahmed@stanford.edu; Tel.: +1-650-498-5691; Fax: +1-650-498-5692

Received: 22 August 2017; Accepted: 11 October 2017; Published: 16 October 2017

Abstract: Malnutrition has become a dangerously common problem in children with chronic liver disease, negatively impacting neurocognitive development and growth. Furthermore, many children with chronic liver disease will eventually require liver transplantation. Thus, this association between malnourishment and chronic liver disease in children becomes increasingly alarming as malnutrition is a predictor of poorer outcomes in liver transplantation and is often associated with increased morbidity and mortality. Malnutrition requires aggressive and appropriate management to correct nutritional deficiencies. A comprehensive review of the literature has found that infants with chronic liver disease (CLD) are particularly susceptible to malnutrition given their low reserves. Children with CLD would benefit from early intervention by a multi-disciplinary team, to try to achieve nutritional rehabilitation as well as to optimize outcomes for liver transplant. This review explains the multifactorial nature of malnutrition in children with chronic liver disease, defines the nutritional needs of these children, and discusses ways to optimize their nutritional.

Keywords: nutrition; chronic liver disease; children

1. Introduction

The liver plays a crucial role in many of the body's metabolic processes, including regulating protein, fat, and carbohydrate metabolism; vitamin storage and activation; and detoxification and excretion of waste products [1]. In children with chronic liver disease (CLD), disruption of these processes results in improper nutrient digestion, absorption, and usage, and ultimately malnutrition. CLD is defined as progressive destruction and regeneration of liver parenchyma leading to fibrosis and cirrhosis, which has been present for at least six months [2]. It results from hepatic injury leading to irreversible impairment of liver function, with changes in architecture and blood supply [3]. This results in impaired synthesis of serum proteins and clotting factors, compromised glycemic control and ammonia metabolism, and impaired bile secretion and cholestasis [4]. The prevalence and etiologies for CLD in children can vary by country and age of onset. In the United States, the prevalence of liver disease in children is unclear; however, it is estimated that 15,000 children are hospitalized for liver disease annually [5]. The overall incidence of liver disease in neonates in the United States is approximately 1 in every 2500 live births [6] with extrahepatic biliary atresia, metabolic disorders, and neonatal hepatitis being the most common causes of CLD in neonates [7]. In older children in the

United States, common causes of CLD include metabolic disorders, chronic intrahepatic cholestasis, obesity-related steatohepatitis, drug- and toxin-induced disorders, and viral hepatitis [5]. In Australia, the most common cause of CLD starting in the neonatal age in children is biliary atresia, occurring in approximately 1 in 8000 live births, with other common causes being alpha-1-antitrypsin deficiency and Alagille's syndrome [8,9]. Similarly, in Brazil, biliary atresia is the most common cause of CLD in children [10]. In contrast, a study in Pakistan found viral hepatitis to be the most common cause of neonatal onset CLD, followed by metabolic disorders and biliary atresia [11] while a study in India found metabolic disorders to be the most common cause of CLD in children [12].

Children are particularly susceptible to malnutrition due to their high energy needs for growth [13]. Approximately 25% of children diagnosed with CLD worldwide are undernourished, with the incidence being higher in developing countries [14]. Furthermore, many children with chronic liver disease will eventually require liver transplantation, and studies have noted that malnourishment during liver transplantation is associated with poorer outcomes, including increased risks for morbidity and mortality [15–17] as well as compromised neurocognitive development [18,19] and growth [20]. Otherwise unexplained clinical or laboratory nutritional deficiencies (such as iron deficiency, vitamin D deficiency/rickets, vitamin K deficiency/coagulopathy) should raise suspicion for CLD potentially complicating another diagnosis, such as celiac disease, inflammatory bowel disease, or chronic cholestasis [21]. This review discusses the multi-factorial mechanisms behind malnutrition in children with CLD, as well as strategies to optimize nutritional support in children with CLD.

2. Mechanisms of Malnutrition in Children with Cld

2.1. Decreased Energy Intake

Children with CLD are often unable to consume adequate calories for their energy needs (Figure 1) [22]. Contributing factors include anorexia, changes in taste perception, early satiety, and nausea and vomiting [13]. Anorexia is attributed to changes in amino acid metabolism, which results in increased tryptophan levels and subsequent increases in brain serotonergic activity. Tryptophan is the amino acid precursor to serotonin, which regulates eating behavior. Increased cerebrospinal concentrations of tryptophan have been associated with anorexia in patients with CLD [23]. Deficiency in zinc or magnesium contributes to changes in taste perception, which may be aggravated by supplementation with unpalatable formulas and also discourages intake [13]. Furthermore, pediatric CLD patients have decreased stomach volume and discomfort from ascites and organomegaly that result in early satiety [24]. Increased pro-inflammatory cytokines, common in children with CLD, results in nausea and vomiting [25]. Together, these factors lead to decreased consumption and reduced energy intake.

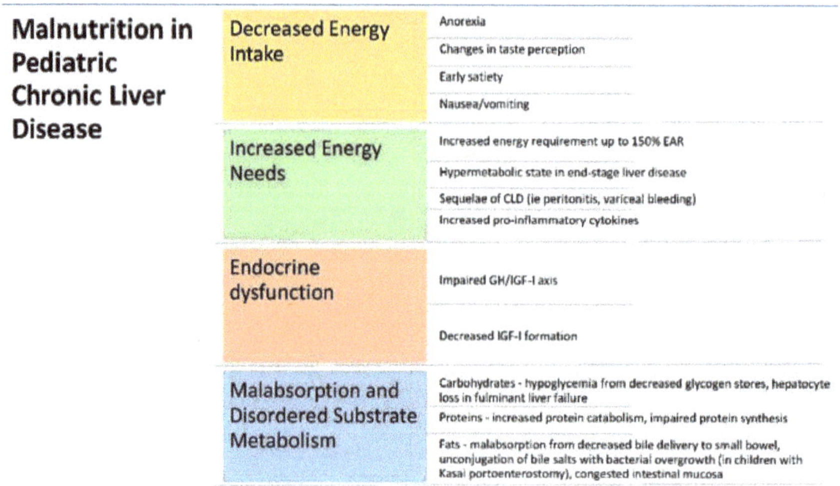

Figure 1. Mechanisms of malnutrition in children with CLD.

EAR: estimated average requirements; GH: growth hormone; IGF: insulin-like growth factor.

2.2. Increased Energy Needs

Children with CLD can have an increase in energy requirements of up to 140% compared to children without CLD [26–28]. Children with end-stage liver disease in particular are in a hypermetabolic state, in which there is increased metabolic activity and excess lipid oxidation [29]. Moreover, this is further aggravated by the sequelae of CLD, including episodes of sepsis from peritonitis or cholangitis, as well as variceal bleeding [13,30]. Children with CLD can also have higher levels of pro-inflammatory cytokines, which have been correlated with malnutrition due to increased energy consumption [31].

2.3. Endocrine Dysfunction

In addition to decreased energy intake and increased metabolism, growth failure in children with CLD is further aggravated by an impaired growth hormone (GH)/insulin-like growth factor (IGF-I) axis. IGF-I and its major circulating binding protein, IGF Binding Protein 3 (IGF-BP3), are synthesized in the liver, and protein malnutrition decreases IGF-I formation, as well as increases its serum clearance and degradation [32]. IGF-I levels are decreased further due to GH resistance in children with CLD caused by downregulation of the GH receptor [30].

2.4. Malabsorption and Disordered Substrate Metabolism

2.4.1. Carbohydrates

The liver receives glucose-rich blood via the portal vein, from which it creates glycogen to be stored in the liver. Glucose is also circulated from the liver to the muscles where lactate, pyruvate, and alanine are generated via glycolysis [33,34]. However, in children with CLD, glycogen stores are depleted from their longstanding condition, resulting in hypoglycemia. Significant hepatocyte loss, such as that in fulminant liver failure, can also cause hypoglycemia [35]. Infants and small children are particularly susceptible due to their lower reserve [13]. In contrast, adults with cirrhosis have increased insulin levels and can develop diabetes mellitus due to increased insulin secretion by the pancreas, decreased insulin degradation by the liver [36] and decreased glucose uptake by tissues [37].

These processes may also occur in children, but unlike adults, few children with CLD (aside from those with cystic fibrosis) develop diabetes mellitus [38].

2.4.2. Proteins

With reduced glycogen stores in CLD, proteins are increasingly utilized for gluconeogenesis [39]. However, the liver's capacity for protein synthesis in CLD is limited due to reduced substrate availability, decreased hepatocyte function, and increased catabolism. Consequently, hypoalbuminemia can develop, leading to peripheral edema, ascites, and decreased enteral intake due to discomfort [13]. Additionally, the liver is the site of synthesis for all coagulation factors with the exception of factor VIII, thus coagulopathy is also a consequence of CLD [30]. Increased protein catabolism also results in increased nitrogenous waste products such as ammonia, which is normally converted to urea by the liver for excretion. This conversion is compromised in CLD, resulting in increased ammonia levels. Abnormal protein use by the liver in CLD results in increased aromatic amino acids (AAAs) and decreased branched-chain amino acids (BCAAs) [40]. An abnormal ratio of BCAAs to AAAs correlates with both histologic damage and encephalopathy [40]. Increased cerebral uptake of AAAs results in formation of false neurotransmitters and causes neurologic dysfunction, along with increased ammonia levels [41]. That said, children with CLD usually do not require protein restriction due to their increased growth needs [42].

2.4.3. Fats

Cholestasis in CLD results in compromised absorption of fats due to decreased delivery of bile salts to the small bowel [43]. This can further be aggravated by small bowel bacterial overgrowth, such as in children who have undergone a Kasai portoenterostomy for biliary atresia, as the bacteria unconjugate bile salts [44]. Congested gastric and intestinal mucosa from portal hypertension further worsen fat malabsorption, and medications, such as cholestyramine to treat pruritus, bind bile salts, decreasing micellar solubilization and thus absorption of di- and monoglycerides from long-chain triglycerides (LCTs) [30]. Children with Alagille syndrome can also have pancreatic insufficiency and decreased lipase, which compromises the hydrolysis of triglycerides [45]. Due to these mechanisms, up to 50% of LCTs, fat-soluble vitamins, and essential polyunsaturated fatty acids (PUFAs) may not be absorbed well in children with CLD [46–48] and deficiencies in long-chain polyunsaturated fatty acids (LCPs) critical to neurologic growth and development, such as arachidonic acid and docosahexaenoic acid (DHA), can develop within 8–12 weeks [30]. Furthermore, children with CLD have increased fat oxidation, likely due to decreased carbohydrate stores. This increased oxidation further decreases fat stores, which then are difficult to replete given the presence of fat malabsorption [13,29]. Lastly, impaired bile flow from cholestasis can result in increased plasma concentration of triglycerides and cholesterol, which may then deposit in the hands, elbows, knees, ankles, and corneas as xanthomas [49].

2.5. Fat-Soluble Vitamins

CLD affects absorption, metabolism, and storage of fat-soluble vitamins. Decreased delivery of bile salts to the small bowel results in malabsorption of fat, as well as the fat-soluble vitamins A, D, E, and K. Without supplementation, fat-soluble vitamin deficiency can develop within 6–12 weeks of birth [30] and even after supplementation up to 30% of severely cholestatic children will remain deficient in all fat-soluble vitamins [50,51].

2.5.1. Vitamin A

Vitamin A has the activity of all-*trans* retinol. Retinol is required for rhodopsin formation (a pigment required for retina rod cell function and dark adaptation), as well as normal cell differentiation. In the diet, vitamin A is available as retinyl palmitate from animal sources (dairy, eggs, fish oils) and as carotenoids from plants (leafy green vegetables, orange-colored fruits, vegetables). Decreased bile salts in the intestine results in decreased hydrolysis of retinyl esters to retinol, as well as decreased formation of micelles, which are required for absorption. Retinol-binding protein (RBP), which is synthesized by the liver and transports vitamin A to peripheral tissues, is also decreased in CLD, thus impairing utilization. Vitamin A deficiency can result in night blindness, xerophthalmia, and keratomalacia [13].

2.5.2. Vitamin D

Vitamin D consists of a group of fat-soluble prohormones and their metabolites, the chief of which are vitamin D_2 (ergocalciferol) and vitamin D_3 (cholecalciferol). These must first undergo hydroxylation in the liver and kidney before they can be utilized by the body. Vitamin D helps regulate calcium and phosphorus, and is critical in bone homeostasis. It can be synthesized in the skin when exposed to sunlight, and can be consumed in the diet from fish oils and fortified dairy products. In CLD, vitamin D deficiency develops from malabsorption, decreased dietary intake and sunlight exposure, and compromised liver hydroxylation. Deficiency results in defective bone mineralization, and if untreated, rickets and fractures [13]. Infants are particularly susceptible, as their bone mineral content can decrease rapidly over the first two years of life [52]. Breastfed infants with CLD are at even higher risk, as breastmilk contains low amounts of vitamin D [53].

2.5.3. Vitamin E

Vitamin E, which consists of tocopherols and tocotrienols, has important anti-oxidant properties. Vitamin E is found in leafy green vegetables, vegetable oils, and nuts. Deficiency in vitamin E in CLD results from malabsorption, and consequences thereof include problems with nerve conduction, including peripheral neuropathy, myopathy, and spinocerebellar dysfunction. Vitamin E deficiency can also result in hemolytic anemia due to oxidative damage to the membranes of red blood cells [54].

2.5.4. Vitamin K

Vitamin K is necessary for carboxylation of glutamic residues on coagulation factors II, VII, IX, and X, as well as proteins C and S, within the liver. Vitamin K_1 [phylloquinone] is found in leafy green vegetables and dairy products, and vitamin K_2 [menaquinone] is synthesized by intestinal bacterial flora. Deficiency in vitamin K in CLD results from malabsorption and manifests as coagulopathy, with easy bleeding and bruising [13]. Due to limited ability of the body to store vitamin K, vitamin K deficiency is one of the earliest fat-soluble vitamin deficiencies to develop in children with CLD [55].

2.6. Trace Elements and Metals

Derangements in trace elements and metals can occur with CLD. Calcium and magnesium are often depleted in CLD, as vitamin D stimulates their absorption from the intestines. They also bind to unabsorbed fatty acids, which further decreases their absorption in children with CLD. Iron deficiency can occur from recurrent gastrointestinal bleeds [13]. Iron deficiency can result in compromised neurologic development in children [56] and multiple studies have found that children with CLD demonstrate delays in mental (-1 standard deviation) and motor (-2 standard deviations) function [6]. Zinc deficiency can develop due to malabsorption as well as increased urinary losses, as zinc is retained in the body by being bound to albumin [57]. Deficiency in zinc results in acrodermatitis, immunodeficiency, and altered protein metabolism; in addition, zinc deficiency, as well as selenium deficiency, can exacerbate growth failure and poor protein synthesis [22,58]. In contrast, copper and manganese levels may be increased in children with cholestasis and CLD, as they are excreted in the bile [59,60]. Thus, in children with CLD who are receiving total parenteral nutrition (TPN), the amount of manganese they receive should be closely monitored, as manganese toxicity in the form of deposition in the basal ganglia can develop [61,62].

3. Strategies to Manage Malnutrition in Cld

3.1. Nutritional Assessment

Accurate nutritional assessment is critical to the management of children with CLD. Standard weight and height measurements may be inaccurate in children with CLD, as they can be confounded by fluid overload, ascites, and organomegaly [30]. Body weight alone may underestimate the incidence of malnutrition in adults and children with CLD by up to 50% [63]. Linear growth is a more sensitive parameter, but stunting and growth deceleration do not occur until late in growth failure. Thus, other measurements, such as triceps or subscapular skinfolds, midarm circumference, and arm muscle measurements (midarm muscle area), should be used. Triceps, skinfolds, and midarm circumference are indicators of body fat and protein, and can reveal early loss in fat stores before height and weight are affected. In children with CLD, triceps skinfold thickness has been shown to be more sensitive for malnutrition compared to weight-for-height z scores [14,16]. Furthermore, these upper limb measurements are less affected by edema compared to truncal or lower limb measurements [13]. When growth data are documented, they should be charted as standard deviation scores related to the median value for the child's age and sex, where a z-score of 0 is equivalent to the 50th percentile. This will assist in evaluating whether nutritional interventions are effective. Children who are particularly at risk for developing malnutrition include those younger than two years in age with severe cholestasis (bilirubin > 4 mg/dL), progressive liver diseases (biliary atresia and severe familial intrahepatic cholestasis), end-stage liver disease awaiting liver transplantation, and recurrent complications of liver disease (ascites, bleeding varices) [30].

Protein markers, such as albumin and prealbumin, are of limited utility in children with CLD. Albumin may be depressed due to hepatic synthetic dysfunction, inflammation, or acute physiologic stress [64]. Prealbumin is a more sensitive marker of malnutrition compared to albumin, as it has a shorter half-life (2 days compared to 18–20 days); that said, prealbumin levels can be normal in chronic malnutrition [65]. On the other hand, essential fatty acid deficiency can be diagnosed with an increased serum triene to tetraene ratio (greater than 0.4). Essential fatty acid deficiency may exist in up to a third of children with end-stage liver disease awaiting liver transplant [22]. Although there are drawbacks to each of the individual assessment tools, a combination of the tools described can be used to more clearly evaluate malnutrition.

3.2. Supplementation of Specific Macronutrients and Micronutrients

Because of the increased energy needs of children with CLD, energy intake should be increased to 140–200% of estimated average requirements (EARs). In infants, this can be achieved by concentrating medium-chain triglyceride (MCT)-containing formulas (an example being Pregestimil by Mead Johnson Nutrition), so as to increase the number of kilocalories per ounce. Older children can be supplemented with high-calorie, nutrient-dense drinks (examples including Pediasure Peptide by Abbott Nutrition, Peptamen by Nestle Healthcare Nutrition). If a sufficient amount cannot be consumed orally, nasogastric (NG) feedings may be needed [30]. Despite disruption to the GH/IGF-I axis, GH therapy has not been found to have benefits in children with end-stage liver disease [66,67].

3.2.1. Carbohydrates

Carbohydrates are a major source of energy, and can be particularly useful for increasing caloric intake. They can be given as monomers, polymers, and starch. Complex carbohydrates such as maltodextrin and glucose polymers can be particularly useful, as their use restricts the osmolality of feeds, while maintaining a high-energy density greater than 1 kcal/mL. In infants, glucose polymers can be added to feeds, while in older children, a supplemental drink can be given, or mixed with fluids and foods [30].

3.2.2. Proteins

Protein restriction is rarely needed in children or adults with CLD [68]. Children with CLD require 2–3 g/kg/day of protein, but can tolerate up to 4 g/kg/day without developing encephalopathy [42]. Severe protein restriction (<2 g/kg/day) may be temporarily required in the context of acute encephalopathy, but should not be continued long-term, as this can lead to endogenous muscle protein consumption [27].

Given the abnormal AAA to BCAA ratio in children with CLD, there has been interest in whether BCAA-enriched formulas can have nutritional benefit. Specific hypercaloric formulas with low salt and lactose, high MCT and BCAA are available [27]. Thus far there is insufficient evidence to recommend routine use of BCAA-enriched formulas, though there have been studies showing potential benefit. One study which compared children receiving 32% BCAA formula compared to standard formula showed improved lean body mass, though no improvement in amino acid levels [69]. Another study evaluated infants receiving 50% BCAA formula compared to 22% BCAA formula, and demonstrated that infants receiving the 50% BCAA formula had improved protein retention due to suppressed endogenous protein catabolism and normalization of the plasma amino acid profile [28]. Animal models of biliary obstruction have increased weight gain, protein and muscle mass, body composition, and bone mineral density if given BCAAs [70]. That said, numerous studies in adults have not demonstrated a clear benefit to BCAA supplementation [71].

3.2.3. Fats

MCTs, unlike LCTs, do not require micellar solubilization to be transported into the enterocyte, and are transferred directly into the enterocyte and to the portal circulation without reesterification [72]. 95% of MCTs are absorbed even in very cholestatic children, thus MCTs are critical in managing nutrition in children with CLD, where absorption of LCTs is highly compromised [73]. Although 30–50% of total fat should be provided as MCTs [13], care should be taken to ensure LCTs are not eliminated from the diet, as they provide essential fatty acids. Thus, it is necessary to increase overall total fat intake, in both LCTs and MCTs. For older children, MCT oil and emulsions can be added to meals, and should be balanced by fats high in LCP content [30]. For infants, formulas containing up to 75% fat as MCT can be given, but formulas with >80% MCTs can lead to essential fatty acid deficiency. Increased MCT content can also worsen steatorrhea [74]. The minimal linoleic acid intake recommended for infants is 1–2% of total energy intake, with a ratio of linoleic to linolenic acid of 5:15.1 [75]. They can be supplemented in the form of walnut or fish oils, as well as dietary products rich in PUFAs, such as egg yolks [30].

3.3. Fat-Soluble Vitamins

In the presence of direct-reacting serum bilirubin levels greater than 2 mg/dL, the diet should be adequately supplemented with fat-soluble vitamins [76]. The role of serum bile acid as a surrogate marker to guide the monitoring of fat-soluble vitamin deficiency is still undefined. In infants with biliary atresia, total serum bilirubin appears to be a better predictor of fat-soluble vitamin deficiency compared to serum bile acids, though neither are perfect [77]. Serum vitamin and prothrombin levels should be monitored to allow proper adjustment of dosages to the specific needs of the patient [78].

3.3.1. Vitamin A

Serum retinol level is the most convenient and practical means of measuring vitamin A status, though retinol dose response (RDR) is believed to be more reliable but is not widely available (Figure 2). It is important to monitor levels in children receiving supplementation, as hypervitaminosis A can lead to potentially fatal hepatotoxicity [13]. Supplementation with 5000–10,000 IU/day may be needed in children with CLD [30].

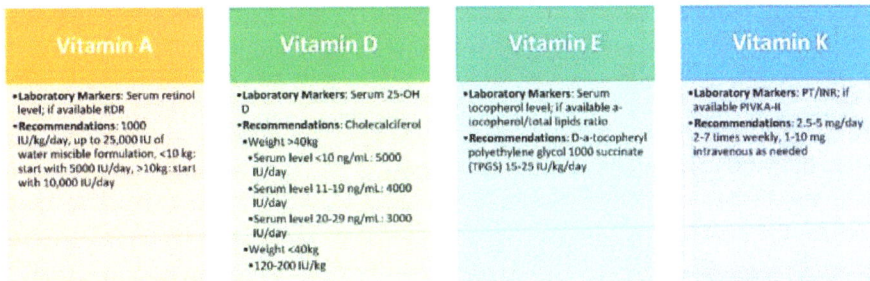

Figure 2. Management of fat-soluble vitamin deficiency in CLD. INR: international normalized ratio; IU: international unit; PIVKA-II: protein induced in vitamin K absence; PT: prothrombin time; RDR: retinol dose response.

3.3.2. Vitamin D

Serum 25-OH D is the most abundant vitamin D metabolite in the body, and can be used to monitor vitamin D status. Low levels of 25-OH D are associated with reduced bone mineral density in children with CLD [52]. It is important to optimize vitamin D levels before liver transplantation due to the use of corticosteroids post-transplant, which can compromise bone density [79]. Co-supplementation with a micellar vitamin E formulation can improve vitamin D absorption in children with cholestatic liver disease [80] and 25-OH D_3 is more water-soluble and thus better absorbed compared to vitamin D_2 [81]. 25-OH D levels, along with calcium and phosphorus, should be monitored to prevent vitamin D overdose. Up to 400 IU/day can be given as supplementation; however, children who are deficient may need substantially higher doses [13].

3.3.3. Vitamin E

The serum tocopherol level is commonly used to measure vitamin E status, though the alpha tocopherol/total lipids ratio is more specific [82]. D-alpha-tocopheryl polyethylene glycol 1000 succinate (TPGS) is the most readily absorbed form of vitamin E in cholestatic patients, as it can form micelles without the need for bile salts [13]. Unfortunately, correction of vitamin E deficiency may not reverse severe spinocerebellar degeneration [83], but it can reverse most other neurologic complications [84]. Supplementation with 50–400 IU/day of TPGS may be needed in children with CLD [30].

3.3.4. Vitamin K

The PIVKA-II [protein induced in vitamin K absence] assay is the most sensitive for measuring vitamin K deficiency, but it is not widely available [50,85]. Therefore, vitamin K status is usually evaluated by checking coagulation values, including prothrombin time (PT) and international normalized ratio (INR). Deficiency can be diagnosed if these values improve after a dose of parenteral vitamin K [13]. Supplementation with 2.5–5 mg/day of vitamin K may be needed [30], though oral vitamin K, even in micellar form, is poorly absorbed in children with CLD [86]. This is further exacerbated by medications commonly used to treat encephalopathy, such as lactulose, which reduces intestinal bacterial production of vitamin K. Thus, intermittent parenteral repletion may be required [13].

3.4. Water-Soluble Vitamins and Minerals

Water-soluble vitamins should also be supplemented in children with CLD in the form of a multivitamin. For minerals, including selenium, zinc, calcium, and magnesium, supplementation should be based from plasma levels. Iron may need to be supplemented in children with chronic blood loss from gastrointestinal bleeds [30]. Repletion of zinc and magnesium in particular may be helpful, as zinc plays a role in immune function and tissue repair [13], while magnesium may help improve bone status [87].

3.5. Mode of Delivery

Nutritional supplementation should be given enterally whenever possible. Enteral nutrition has numerous advantages over parenteral nutrition: it is cheaper, more physiologic, does not come with the risk of catheter-associated bloodstream infections, maintains gastrointestinal tract immunity as well as gut barrier integrity, and reduces bacterial overgrowth. However, as discussed in a previous section, many children with CLD are unable to orally consume sufficient calories to treat or prevent malnutrition. Therefore, NG tube feedings are often required. Gastrostomy tubes are generally avoided in children with CLD due to portal hypertension and the potential for stomal varices to develop, placement difficulty due to organomegaly, and risk of peritoneal infection with ascites [8,68]; they may be helpful in children with stable compensated liver disease such as cystic fibrosis [30]. With modern soft Silastic™ (Dow Corning Corporation, Midland, MI, USA) NG tubes, NG feeds are safe even in patients with esophageal varices [42,88–90]. Using a NG tube for nocturnal feeds is usually the first choice, as it allows for normal oral feeding during the day while supplementing overnight. Nocturnal feeding is also helpful in infants with severe CLD, as it prevents fasting hypoglycemia and reduces protein catabolism. Children with severe malabsorption or feeding intolerance may require continuous feeds [30]. Intensive enteral NG feeding can successfully reverse malnutrition in children with CLD, as well as decrease parental anxiety [42,73,91]. However, feeding aversion can also develop, especially in infants who have received long-term NG feeds. This is further aggravated by the need for often unpalatable medication and formulas. Thus, involvement of a multidisciplinary care team including dieticians, psychologists, and speech and occupational therapists is critical. Strategies to prevent feeding aversion include promoting daytime oral intake, as well as encouraging children to experiment with various age-appropriate flavors and textures [73].

Some children with CLD will require parenteral nutrition. These include children who cannot tolerate enteral nutrition due to feeding intolerance, or those with recurrent variceal bleeding. In the short-term, parenteral nutrition is not associated with hepatobiliary dysfunction or worsened cholestasis, though these certainly do occur with long-term use [92]. Standard amino acid and lipid formulations are well tolerated in patients with stable CLD, though triglyceride levels should be closely monitored in children with severe liver disease, hepatic encephalopathy, and sepsis. Amino acid levels should also be monitored. If encephalopathy does develop, the amino acid content can be decreased to 1–2 g/kg/day [30]. Manganese levels also need to be monitored given the potential for manganese toxicity to exacerbate CLD [93,94]. Parenteral nutrition is particularly helpful in children with acute fulminant liver failure, as these children are in a hypercatabolic state. In these children, standard formulations can be used, but the total volume should be restricted to 75% of maintenance, and concentration may need to be further increased to prevent hypoglycemia. Protein restriction should not be needed, especially if the patient is being electively ventilated [30].

4. Effect of Liver Transplantation on Nutritional Status [Figure 3]

Malnutrition is a significant risk factor for both morbidity and mortality related to liver transplantation, thus nutritional support is of utmost importance in children with CLD prior to undergoing transplant (Figure 3) [15,95,96]. Children who were malnourished prior to transplant may require support with parenteral nutrition peri-operatively, while children with normal nutritional status prior to transplant can start enteral feedings with rapid buildup of calories within 3–5 days postoperatively. Children after liver transplant require at least 120% of EAR post-operatively, which can be administered in the form of high-energy pediatric and infant formulas, either orally or via nasogastric tube [30]. Children with oral aversion pre-operatively will likely require nasogastric supplementation post-operatively for up to two months; regular diet for age is usually achieved by six months [97]. Energy intake should include 6–8 g/kg/day of carbohydrates, 2.5–3 g/kg/day of protein, and 5–6 g/kg/day of fat [30].

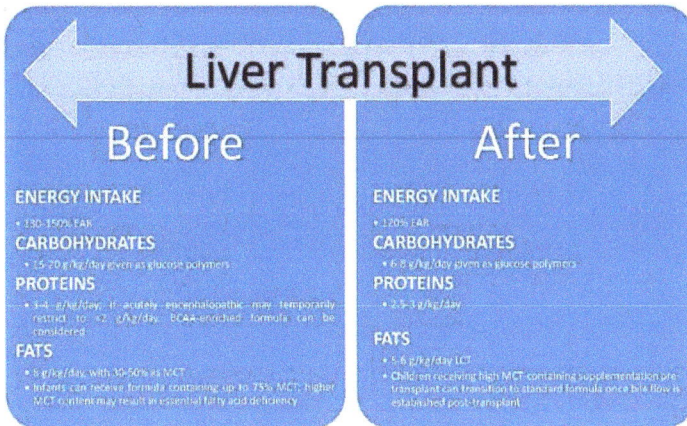

Figure 3. Nutritional needs of children with CLD before and after liver transplant. EAR: estimated average requirements; LCT: long-chain triglycerides; MCT: medium-chain triglycerides.

Preoperative nutritional status also affects postoperative growth. Children who are more stunted, with a height standard deviation score (SDS) >−2, grow more rapidly after a transplant, but may not achieve normal height. This is in contrast to children who are less stunted: while their initial growth velocity post-operatively is slower, they ultimately achieve normal growth velocity [98]. There is no difference in catch-up growth between genders or pre-transplantation liver disease; the exception being Alagille syndrome, which is associated with growth failure, both before and after a transplant, in up to 50% of patients [99,100]. Recombinant GH has been trialed in eight growth-retarded children after a transplant, and while there were increases in both median growth rate and height SDS, growth velocity was not maintained beyond the first year [101].

Ultimately, nutritional rehabilitation can be achieved with liver transplantation [73,102,103]. After transplantation, there is a rapid return to normal midarm muscle area and midarm fat within 3–6 months [103,104] and catch-up growth is usually achieved within 18 months [15]. However, it can take months to years for bone density to return to normal. Osteoporosis and fractures have been described within 3–6 months after a transplant, and can be exacerbated by glucocorticoid therapy required after a transplant [67]. Long-chain PUFA and BCAA metabolism also take time to normalize after a transplant [71,105] and abnormalities in IGF-binding proteins BP1, BP2, and BP3 persist for several months [106].

5. Conclusions

Malnutrition is common in children with CLD, and requires aggressive and appropriate management to correct nutritional deficiencies. Infants with CLD are particularly susceptible to malnutrition given their low reserves. Children with CLD would benefit from early intervention by a multi-disciplinary team, to try to achieve nutritional rehabilitation, as well as to optimize outcomes for liver transplantation.

Acknowledgments: No sources of funding were used for this work.

Conflicts of Interest: The authors declare no conflict of interest.

References

1. Pratt, C.A.; Garcia, M.G.; Kerner, J.A., Jr. Nutritional management of neonatal and infant liver disease. *NeoReviews* **2001**, *2*, e215–e222. [CrossRef]
2. Widodo, A.D.; Soelaeman, E.J.; Dwinanda, N.; Narendraswari, P.P.; Purnomo, B. Chronic liver disease is a risk factor for malnutrition and growth retardation in children. *Asia Pac. J. Clin. Nutr.* **2017**, *26* (Suppl. 1), S57–S60. [PubMed]
3. Young, S.; Kwarta, E.; Azzam, R.; Sentongo, T. Nutrition assessment and support in children with end-stage liver disease. *Nutr. Clin. Pract.* **2013**, *28*, 317–329. [CrossRef] [PubMed]
4. Sokal, E.M.; Goldstein, D.; Ciocca, M.; Lewindon, P.; Ni, Y.H.; Silveira, T.; Sibal, A.; Dhawan, A.; Mack, C.; Bucuvalas, J.; et al. End-stage liver disease and liver transplant: Current situation and key issues. *J. Pediatr. Gastroenterol. Nutr.* **2008**, *47*, 239–246. [CrossRef] [PubMed]
5. Arya, G.; Balistreri, W.F. Pediatric liver disease in the United States: Epidemiology and impact. *J. Gastroenterol. Hepatol.* **2002**, *17*, 521–525. [CrossRef] [PubMed]
6. Rodriguez-Baez, N.; Wayman, K.I.; Cox, K.L. Growth and development in chronic liver disease. *NeoReviews* **2001**, *2*, e211–e214. [CrossRef]
7. Danks, D.M.; Campbell, P.E.; Jack, I.; Rogers, J.; Smith, A.L. Studies of the aetiology of neonatal hepatitis and biliary atresia. *Arch. Dis. Child.* **1977**, *52*, 360–367. [CrossRef] [PubMed]
8. Baker, A.; Stevenson, R.; Dhawan, A.; Goncalves, I.; Socha, P.; Sokal, E. Guidelines for nutritional care for infants with cholestatic liver disease before liver transplantation. *Pediatr. Transplant.* **2007**, *11*, 825–834. [CrossRef] [PubMed]
9. Smart, K.M.; Alex, G.; Hardikar, W. Feeding the child with liver disease: A review and practical clinical guide. *J. Gastroenterol. Hepatol.* **2011**, *26*, 810–815. [CrossRef] [PubMed]
10. Pinto, R.B.; Schneider, A.C.; da Silveira, T.R. Cirrhosis in children and adolescents: An overview. *World J. Hepatol.* **2015**, *7*, 392–405. [CrossRef] [PubMed]
11. Tahir, A.; Malik, F.R.; Ahmad, I.; Akhtar, P. Aetiological factors of chronic liver disease in children. *J. Ayub Med. Coll. Abbottabad* **2011**, *23*, 12–14. [PubMed]
12. Dhole, S.D.; Kher, A.S.; Ghildiyal, R.G.; Tambse, M.P. Chronic Liver Diseases in Children: Clinical Profile and Histology. *J. Clin. Diagn. Res.* **2015**, *9*, SC04–SC07. [CrossRef] [PubMed]
13. Nightingale, S.; Ng, V.L. Optimizing nutritional management in children with chronic liver disease. *Pediatr. Clin. N. Am.* **2009**, *56*, 1161–1183. [CrossRef] [PubMed]
14. Sokol, R.J.; Stall, C. Anthropometric evaluation of children with chronic liver disease. *Am. J. Clin. Nutr.* **1990**, *52*, 203–208. [PubMed]
15. Chin, S.; Shepherd, R.; Cleghorn, G.; Patrick, M.; Javorsky, G.; Frangoulis, E.; Ong, T.H.; Balderson, G.; Koido, Y.; Matsunami, H.; et al. Survival, growth and quality of life in children after orthotopic liver transplantation: A 5 year experience. *J. Paediatr. Child Health* **1991**, *27*, 380–385. [CrossRef] [PubMed]
16. Shepherd, R.; Chin, S.; Cleghorn, G.; Patrick, M.; Ong, T.; Lynch, S.; Balderson, G.; Strong, R. Malnutrition in children with chronic liver disease accepted for liver transplanation: Clinical profile and effect on outcome. *J. Paediatr. Child Health* **1991**, *27*, 295–299. [CrossRef] [PubMed]
17. DeRusso, P.; Ye, W.; Shepherd, R.; Haber, B.; Shneider, B.; Whitington, P.; Schwarz, K.B.; Bezerra, J.A.; Rosenthal, P.; Karpen, S.; et al. Growth failure and outcomes in infants with biliary atresia: A report from the Biliary Atresia Research Consortium. *Hepatology* **2007**, *46*, 1632–1638. [CrossRef] [PubMed]
18. Wayman, K.; Cox, K.; Esquivel, C. Neurodevelopmental outcome of young children with extrahepatic biliary atresia 1 year after liver transplantation. *J. Pediatr.* **1997**, *131*, 894–898. [CrossRef]
19. Stewart, S.; Uauy, R.; Waller, D.; Kennard, B.; Benser, M.; Andrews, W. Mental and motor development, social competence, and growth one year after successful pediatric liver transplantation. *J. Pediatr.* **1989**, *114* (4 Pt 1), 574–581. [CrossRef]
20. Moukarzel, A.; Najm, I.; Vargas, J.; McDiarmid, S.; Busuttil, R.; Ament, M. Effect of nutritional status on outcome of orthotopic liver transplantation in pediatric patients. *Transplant. Proc.* **1990**, *22*, 1560–1563. [PubMed]
21. Vajro, P.; Maddaluno, S.; Veropalumbo, C. Persistent hypertransaminasemia in asymptomatic children: A stepwise approach. *World J. Gastroenterol.* **2013**, *19*, 2740–2751. [CrossRef] [PubMed]

22. Chin, S.; Shepherd, R.; Thomas, B.; Cleghorn, G.; Patrick, M.; Wilcox, J.; Ong, T.H.; Lynch, S.V.; Strong, R. The nature of malnutrition in children with end-stage liver disease awaiting orthotopic liver transplantation. *Am. J. Clin. Nutr.* **1992**, *56*, 164–168. [PubMed]

23. Laviano, A.; Cangiano, C.; Preziosa, I. Plasma tryptophan levels and anorexia in liver cirrhosis. *Int. J. Eat. Disord.* **1997**, *21*, 181–186. [CrossRef]

24. Aqel, B.; Scolapio, J.; Dickson, R.; Burton, D.; Bouras, E. Contribution of ascites to impaired gastric function and nutritonal intake in patients with cirrhosis and ascites. *Clin. Gastroenterol. Hepatol.* **2005**, *3*, 1095–1100. [CrossRef]

25. Aranda-Michel, J. Nutrition in hepatic failure and liver transplantation. *Curr. Gastroenterol. Rep.* **2001**, *3*, 362–370. [CrossRef] [PubMed]

26. Cortez, A.; de Morais, M.; Speridiao, P.G.; da Motta, M.R.; Calanca, F.; Neto, U. Food intake, growth and body composition of children and adolescents with autoimmune hepatitis. *J. Clin. Gastroenterol.* **2010**, *44*, 200–207. [CrossRef] [PubMed]

27. Pierro, A.K.; Carnielli, V.; Superina, R.; Roberts, E.; Filler, R.; Smith, J.; Heim, T. Resting energy expenditure is increased in infants and children with extrahepatic biliary atresia. *J. Pediatr. Surg.* **1989**, *24*, 534–538. [CrossRef]

28. Protheroe, S.; McKieran, P.; Kelly, D. Can measurement of dietary-induced thermogenesis (DIT) predict response to nutritional intervention in infants with liver disease? *Clin. Nutr.* **1996**, *15*, 39. [CrossRef]

29. Greer, R.; Lehnert, M.; Lewindon, P.; Cleghorn, G.; Shepherd, R. Body composition and components of energy expenditure in children with end-stage liver disease. *J. Pediatr. Gastroenterol. Nutr.* **2003**, *36*, 358–363. [CrossRef] [PubMed]

30. Kelly, D.A.; Proteroe, S.; Clarke, S. Acute and chronic liver disease. In *Nutrition in Pediatrics*, 5th ed.; Duggan, C., Watkins, J.B., Koletzko, B., Walker, W.A., Eds.; People's Medical Publishing House-USA: Shelton, CT, USA, 2016; pp. 851–863.

31. Santetti, D.; Wilasco, M.I.d.A.; Dornelles, C.T.L.; Werlang, I.C.R.; Fontella, F.U.; Kieling, C.O.; Luiz dos Santos, J.; Gonçalves Vieira, S.M.; Sueno Goldani, H.A. Serum proinflammatory cytokines and nutritional status in pediatric chronic liver disease. *World J. Gastroenterol.* **2015**, *21*, 8927–8934. [CrossRef] [PubMed]

32. Zamboni, G.; Dufillot, D.; Antoniazzi, F.; Valentini, R.; Gendrel, D.; Tato, L. Growth hormone-binding proteins and insulin-like grwoth factor-binding proteins in protein-energy malnutrition, before and after nutritonal rehabilitation. *Pediatr. Res.* **1996**, *39*, 410–414. [CrossRef] [PubMed]

33. Romjin, J.; Endert, E.; Suerwein, H. Glucose and fat metablism during short-term starvation in cirrhosis. *Gastroenterology* **1991**, *100*, 731–737. [CrossRef]

34. Hellerstein, M.; Munro, H. Interaction of liver, muscle and adipose tissue in the regulation of metabolism in response to nutritional and other factors. In *The Liver: Biology and Pathobiology*, 3rd ed.; Arias, I., Boyer, J., Fausto, N., Eds.; Raven Press: New York, NY, USA, 1994; pp. 1169–1191.

35. Changani, K.; Jalan, R.; Cox, I.; Ala-Korpela, M.; Bhakoo, K.; Taylor-Robinson, S.; Bell, J.D. Evidence for altered hepatic gluconeogenesis in patients with cirrhosis using in vivo 31-phosphorus magnetic resonance spectroscopy. *Gut* **2001**, *49*, 557–564. [CrossRef] [PubMed]

36. Petrides, A.; DeFronzo, R. Glucose and insulin metabolism in cirrhosis. *J. Hepatol.* **1989**, *8*, 107–114. [CrossRef]

37. Nielsen, M.; Caumo, A.; Aagaard, N.; Chandramouli, V.; Schumann, W.; Landau, B.; Schmitz, O.; Vilstrup, H. Contribution of defects in glucose uptake to carbohydrate intolerance in liver cirrhosis: Assessment during physiological glucose and insulin concentrations. *Am. J. Physiol. Gastrointest. Liver Physiol.* **2005**, *288*, G1135–G1143. [CrossRef] [PubMed]

38. Cleghorn, G. The role of basic nutritional research in pediatric liver disease: A historical perspective. *Gastroenterol. Hepatol.* **2009**, *24*, S93–S96. [CrossRef] [PubMed]

39. Swart, G.R.; van den Berg, J.W.; Wattimena, J.L.; Rietveld, T.; van Vuure, J.K.; Frenkel, M. Elevated protein requirements in cirrhosis of the liver investigated by whole body protein turnover studies. *Clin. Sci.* **1988**, *75*, 101–107. [CrossRef] [PubMed]

40. Protheroe, S.; Jones, R.; Kelly, D. Evaluation of the role of branched chain amino acids in the treatment of protein malnutrition in infants with liver disease. *Gut* **1995**, *37*, A350.

41. Munro, H.N.; Fernstrom, J.D.; Wurtman, R.J. Insulin, plasma amino acid imbalance, and hepatic coma. *Lancet* **1975**, *1*, 722–724. [CrossRef]

42. Charlton, C.P.; Buchanan, E.; Holden, C.E.; Preece, M.A.; Green, A.; Booth, I.W.; Tarlow, M.J. Intensive enteral feeding in advanced cirrhosis: Reversal of malnutrition without precipitation of hepatic encephalopathy. *Arch. Dis. Child.* **1992**, *67*, 603–607. [CrossRef] [PubMed]
43. Dietschy, J. The biology of bile acids. *Arch. Intern. Med.* **1972**, *130*, 473–474. [CrossRef] [PubMed]
44. Yamamoto, T.; Hamanak, Y.; Suzuki, T. Intestinal microflora and bile acids following biliary tract reconstruction. *Nippon Geka Gakkai Zasshi* **1991**, *92*, 1288–1291. [PubMed]
45. Emerick, K.; Rand, E.; Goldmuntz, E.; Krantz, I.; Spinner, N.; Piccoli, D. Features of Alagille syndrome in 92 patients: Frequency and relation to prognosis. *Hepatology* **1999**, *29*, 822–829. [CrossRef] [PubMed]
46. Greenberger, N.; Skillman, T. Medium-chain triglycerides. *N. Engl. J. Med.* **1969**, *280*, 1045–1058. [CrossRef] [PubMed]
47. Glasgow, J.; Hamilton, J.; Sass-Kortsak, A. Fat absorption in congenital obstructive liver disease. *Arch. Dis. Child.* **1973**, *48*, 601–607. [CrossRef] [PubMed]
48. Phan, C.; Tso, P. Intestinal lipid absorption and transport. *Front. Biosci.* **2001**, *6*, D299–D319. [CrossRef] [PubMed]
49. Sabesin, S.M. Cholestatic lipoproteins—Their pathogenesis and significance. *Gastroenterology* **1982**, *83*, 704–709. [PubMed]
50. Mager, D.R.; McGee, P.L.; Furuya, K.N.; Roberts, E.A. Prevalence of vitamin K deficiency in children with mild to moderate chronic liver disease. *J. Pediatr. Gastroenterol. Nutr.* **2006**, *42*, 71–76. [CrossRef] [PubMed]
51. Shneider, B.L.; Magee, J.C.; Bezerra, J.A.; Haber, B.; Karpen, S.J.; Raghunathan, T.; Rosenthal, P.; Schwarz, K.; Suchy, F.J.; Kerkar, N. Efficacy of fat-soluble vitamin supplementation in infants with biliary atresia. *Pediatrics* **2012**, *130*, e607–e614. [CrossRef] [PubMed]
52. Argao, E.A.; Specker, B.L.; Heubi, J.E. Bone mineral content in infants and children with chronic cholestatic liver disease. *Pediatrics* **1993**, *91*, 1151–1154. [PubMed]
53. Leerbeck, E.; Sondergaard, H. The total content of vitamin D in human milk and cow's milk. *Br. J. Nutr.* **1980**, *44*, 7–12. [CrossRef] [PubMed]
54. Sokol, R.J.; Heubi, J.E.; Iannaccone, S.; Bove, K.E.; Balistreri, W.F. Mechanism causing vitamin E deficiency during chronic childhood cholestasis. *Gastroenterology* **1983**, *85*, 1172–1182. [PubMed]
55. Usui, Y.; Tanimura, H.; Nishimura, N.; Kobayashi, N.; Okanoue, T.; Ozawa, K. Vitamin K concentrations in the plasma and liver of surgical patients. *Am. J. Clin. Nutr.* **1990**, *51*, 846–852. [PubMed]
56. Grantham-McGregor, S.; Ani, C. A review of studies on the effect of iron deficiency on cognitive development in children. *J. Nutr.* **2001**, *131*, 649S–666S. [PubMed]
57. Stamoulis, I.; Kouraklis, G.; Theocharis, S. Zinc and the liver: An active interaction. *Dig. Dis. Sci.* **2007**, *52*, 1595–1612. [CrossRef] [PubMed]
58. Umusig-Quitain, P.; Gregorio, G.V. High incidence of zinc deficiency among Filipino children with compensated and decompensated liver disease. *J. Gastroenterol. Hepatol.* **2010**, *25*, 387–390. [CrossRef] [PubMed]
59. Goksu, N.; Ozsoylu, S. Hepatic and serum levels of zinc, copper, and magnesium in childhood cirrhosis. *J. Pediatr. Gastroenterol. Nutr.* **1986**, *5*, 459–462. [CrossRef] [PubMed]
60. Bayliss, E.A.; Hambidge, K.M.; Sokol, R.J.; Stewart, B.; Lilly, J.R. Hepatic concentrations of zinc, copper and manganese in infants with extrahepatic biliary atresia. *J. Trace Elem. Med. Biol.* **1995**, *9*, 40–43. [CrossRef]
61. Fitzgerald, K.; Mikalunas, V.; Rubin, H.; McCarthey, R.; Vanagunas, A.; Craig, R.M. Hypermanganesemia in patients receiving total parenteral nutrition. *JPEN J. Parenter. Enter. Nutr.* **1999**, *23*, 333–336. [CrossRef] [PubMed]
62. Ikeda, S.; Yamaguchi, Y.; Sera, Y.; Ohshiro, H.; Uchino, S.; Yamashita, Y.; Ogawa, M. Manganese deposition in the globus pallidus in patients with biliary atresia. *Transplantation* **2000**, *69*, 2339–2343. [CrossRef] [PubMed]
63. Trocki, O.; Wotton, M.J.; Cleghorn, G.J.; Shepherd, R.W. Value of total body potassium in assessing the nutritional status of children with end-stage liver disease. *Ann. N. Y. Acad. Sci.* **2000**, *904*, 400–405. [CrossRef] [PubMed]
64. Klein, S. The myth of serum albumin as a measure of nutritional status. *Gastroenterology* **1990**, *99*, 1845–1846. [CrossRef]
65. Myron Johnson, A.; Merlini, G.; Sheldon, J.; Ichihara, K. Scientific Division Committee on Plasma Proteins IFoCC, Laboratory M. Clinical indications for plasma protein assays: Transthyretin (prealbumin) in inflammation and malnutrition. *Clin. Chem. Lab. Med.* **2007**, *45*, 419–426. [CrossRef] [PubMed]

66. Bucuvalas, J.C.; Horn, J.A.; Chernausek, S.D. Resistance to growth hormone in children with chronic liver disease. *Pediatr. Transplant.* **1997**, *1*, 73–79. [PubMed]

67. Hogler, W.; Baumann, U.; Kelly, D. Endocrine and bone metabolic complications in chronic liver disease and after liver transplantation in children. *J. Pediatr. Gastroenterol. Nutr.* **2012**, *54*, 313–321. [CrossRef] [PubMed]

68. Protheroe, S.M. Feeding the child with chronic liver disease. *Nutrition* **1998**, *14*, 796–800. [CrossRef]

69. Chin, S.E.; Shepherd, R.W.; Thomas, B.J.; Cleghorn, G.J.; Patrick, M.K.; Wilcox, J.A.; Ong, T.H.; Lynch, S.V.; Strong, R. Nutritional support in children with end-stage liver disease: A randomized crossover trial of a branched-chain amino acid supplement. *Am. J. Clin. Nutr.* **1992**, *56*, 158–163. [PubMed]

70. Sokal, E.M.; Baudoux, M.C.; Collette, E.; Hausleithner, V.; Lambotte, L.; Buts, J.P. Branched chain amino acids improve body composition and nitrogen balance in a rat model of extra hepatic biliary atresia. *Pediatr. Res.* **1996**, *40*, 66–71. [CrossRef] [PubMed]

71. Platell, C.; Kong, S.E.; McCauley, R.; Hall, J.C. Branched-chain amino acids. *J. Gastroenterol. Hepatol.* **2000**, *15*, 706–717. [CrossRef] [PubMed]

72. Carey, M.C.; Small, D.M.; Bliss, C.M. Lipid digestion and absorption. *Annu. Rev. Physiol.* **1983**, *45*, 651–677. [CrossRef] [PubMed]

73. Beath, S.V.; Booth, I.W.; Kelly, D.A. Nutritional support in liver disease. *Arch. Dis. Child.* **1993**, *69*, 545–547. [CrossRef] [PubMed]

74. Kaufman, S.S.; Scrivner, D.J.; Murray, N.D.; Vanderhoof, J.A.; Hart, M.H.; Antonson, D.L. Influence of portagen and pregestimil on essential fatty acid status in infantile liver disease. *Pediatrics* **1992**, *89*, 151–154. [PubMed]

75. Koletzko, B.; Agostoni, C.; Carlson, S.E.; Clandinin, T.; Hornstra, G.; Neuringer, M.; Uauy, R.; Yamashiro, Y.; Willatts, P. Long chain polyunsaturated fatty acids (LC-PUFA) and perinatal development. *Acta Paediatr.* **2001**, *90*, 460–464. [CrossRef] [PubMed]

76. Shneider, B.L.; Magee, J.C.; Karpen, S.J.; Rand, E.B.; Narkewicz, M.R.; Bass, L.M.; Schwarz, K.; Whitington, P.F.; Bezerra, J.A.; Kerkar, N.; et al. Total Serum Bilirubin within 3 Months of Hepatoportoenterostomy Predicts Short-Term Outcomes in Biliary Atresia. *J. Pediatr.* **2016**, *170*. [CrossRef] [PubMed]

77. Venkat, V.L.; Shneider, B.L.; Magee, J.C.; Turmelle, Y.; Arnon, R.; Bezerra, J.A.; Hertel, P.M.; Karpen, S.J.; Kerkar, N.; Loomes, K.M. Total serum bilirubin predicts fat-soluble vitamin deficiency better than serum bile acids in infants with biliary atresia. *J. Pediatr. Gastroenterol. Nutr.* **2014**, *59*, 702–707. [CrossRef] [PubMed]

78. Catzola, A.; Vajro, P. Management options for cholestatic liver disease in children. *Expert Rev. Gastroenterol. Hepatol.* **2017**, *11*, 1019–1030. [CrossRef] [PubMed]

79. Guichelaar, M.M.; Kendall, R.; Malinchoc, M.; Hay, J.E. Bone mineral density before and after OLT: Long-term follow-up and predictive factors. *Liver Transpl.* **2006**, *12*, 1390–1402. [CrossRef] [PubMed]

80. Argao, E.A.; Heubi, J.E.; Hollis, B.W.; Tsang, R.C. D-Alpha-tocopheryl polyethylene glycol-1000 succinate enhances the absorption of vitamin D in chronic cholestatic liver disease of infancy and childhood. *Pediatr. Res.* **1992**, *31*, 146–150. [CrossRef] [PubMed]

81. Heubi, J.E.; Hollis, B.W.; Specker, B.; Tsang, R.C. Bone disease in chronic childhood cholestasis. I. Vitamin D absorption and metabolism. *Hepatology* **1989**, *9*, 258–264. [CrossRef] [PubMed]

82. Sokol, R.J.; Heubi, J.E.; Iannaccone, S.T.; Bove, K.E.; Balistreri, W.F. Vitamin E deficiency with normal serum vitamin E concentrations in children with chronic cholestasis. *N. Engl. J. Med.* **1984**, *310*, 1209–1212. [CrossRef] [PubMed]

83. Perlmutter, D.H.; Gross, P.; Jones, H.R.; Fulton, A.; Grand, R.J. Intramuscular vitamin E repletion in children with chronic cholestasis. *Am. J. Dis. Child.* **1987**, *141*, 170–174. [CrossRef] [PubMed]

84. Sokol, R.J.; Butler-Simon, N.; Conner, C.; Heubi, J.E.; Sinatra, F.R.; Suchy, F.J.; Heyman, M.B.; Perrault, J.; Rothbaum, R.J.; Levy, J. Multicenter trial of D-alpha-tocopheryl polyethylene glycol 1000 succinate for treatment of vitamin E deficiency in children with chronic cholestasis. *Gastroenterology* **1993**, *104*, 1727–1735. [CrossRef]

85. Ferland, G.; Sadowski, J.A.; O'Brien, M.E. Dietary induced subclinical vitamin K deficiency in normal human subjects. *J. Clin. Invest.* **1993**, *91*, 1761–1768. [CrossRef] [PubMed]

86. Pereira, S.P.; Shearer, M.J.; Williams, R.; Mieli-Vergani, G. Intestinal absorption of mixed micellar phylloquinone [vitamin K1] is unreliable in infants with conjugated hyperbilirubinaemia: Implications for oral prophylaxis of vitamin K deficiency bleeding. *Arch. Dis. Child Fetal Neonatal Ed.* **2003**, *88*, F113–F118. [CrossRef] [PubMed]

87. Heubi, J.E.; Higgins, J.V.; Argao, E.A.; Sierra, R.I.; Specker, B.L. The role of magnesium in the pathogenesis of bone disease in childhood cholestatic liver disease: A preliminary report. *J. Pediatr. Gastroenterol. Nutr.* **1997**, *25*, 301–306. [CrossRef] [PubMed]

88. Cabre, E.; Gonzalez-Huix, F.; Abad-Lacruz, A.; Esteve, M.; Acero, D.; Fernandez-Banares, F.; Xiol, X.; Gassull, M.A. Effect of total enteral nutrition on the short-term outcome of severely malnourished cirrhotics. A randomized controlled trial. *Gastroenterology* **1990**, *98*, 715–720. [CrossRef]

89. Kearns, P.J.; Young, H.; Garcia, G.; Blaschke, T.; O'Hanlon, G.; Rinki, M.; Sucher, K.; Gregory, P. Accelerated improvement of alcoholic liver disease with enteral nutrition. *Gastroenterology* **1992**, *102*, 200–205. [CrossRef]

90. Cabre, E.; Rodriguez-Iglesias, P.; Caballeria, J.; Quer, J.C.; Sanchez-Lombrana, J.L.; Pares, A.; Papo, M.; Planas, R.; Gassull, M.A. Short- and long-term outcome of severe alcohol-induced hepatitis treated with steroids or enteral nutrition: A multicenter randomized trial. *Hepatology* **2000**, *32*, 36–42. [CrossRef] [PubMed]

91. Moreno, L.A.; Gottrand, F.; Hoden, S.; Turck, D.; Loeuille, G.A.; Farriaux, J.P. Improvement of nutritional status in cholestatic children with supplemental nocturnal enteral nutrition. *J. Pediatr. Gastroenterol. Nutr.* **1991**, *12*, 213–216. [CrossRef] [PubMed]

92. Kelly, D.; Tong, C. Neonatal and paediatric infection. In *Viral Hepatitis*, 4th ed.; Wiley Blackwell: Hoboken, NJ, USA, 2012.

93. Fell, J.M.; Reynolds, A.P.; Meadows, N.; Khan, K.; Long, S.G.; Quaghebeur, G.; Taylor, W.J.; Milla, P.J. Manganese toxicity in children receiving long-term parenteral nutrition. *Lancet* **1996**, *347*, 1218–1221. [CrossRef]

94. Huang, C.C.; Chu, N.S.; Lu, C.S.; Wang, J.D.; Tsai, J.L.; Tzeng, J.L.; Wolters, E.C.; Calne, D.B. Chronic manganese intoxication. *Arch. Neurol.* **1989**, *46*, 1104–1106. [CrossRef] [PubMed]

95. Barshes, N.R.; Chang, I.F.; Karpen, S.J.; Carter, B.A.; Goss, J.A. Impact of pretransplant growth retardation in pediatric liver transplantation. *J. Pediatr. Gastroenterol. Nutr.* **2006**, *43*, 89–94. [CrossRef] [PubMed]

96. Rodeck, B.; Melter, M.; Kardorff, R.; Hoyer, P.F.; Ringe, B.; Burdelski, M.; Oldhafer, K.J.; Pichlmayr, R.; Brodehl, J. Liver transplantation in children with chronic end stage liver disease: Factors influencing survival after transplantation. *Transplantation* **1996**, *62*, 1071–1076. [CrossRef] [PubMed]

97. SM F, R.J. Feeding patterns in infants post liver transplant. *J. Pediatr. Gastroenterol.* **2004**, *39*, S94.

98. Bartosh, S.M.; Thomas, S.E.; Sutton, M.M.; Brady, L.M.; Whitington, P.F. Linear growth after pediatric liver transplantation. *J. Pediatr.* **1999**, *135*, 624–631. [CrossRef]

99. Cardona, J.; Houssin, D.; Gauthier, F.; Devictor, D.; Losay, J.; Hadchouel, M.; Bernard, O. Liver transplantation in children with Alagille syndrome—A study of twelve cases. *Transplantation* **1995**, *60*, 339–342. [CrossRef] [PubMed]

100. Kamath, B.M.; Yin, W.; Miller, H.; Anand, R.; Rand, E.B.; Alonso, E.; Bucuvalas, J. Outcomes of liver transplantation for patients with Alagille syndrome: The studies of pediatric liver transplantation experience. *Liver Transpl.* **2012**, *18*, 940–948. [CrossRef] [PubMed]

101. Kelly, D.A. Posttransplant growth failure in children. *Liver Transpl. Surg.* **1997**, *3* (5 Suppl. 1), S32–S39. [PubMed]

102. Van Mourik, I.D.; Beath, S.V.; Brook, G.A.; Cash, A.J.; Mayer, A.D.; Buckels, J.A.; Kelly, D.A. Long-term nutritional and neurodevelopmental outcome of liver transplantation in infants aged less than 12 months. *J. Pediatr. Gastroenterol. Nutr.* **2000**, *30*, 269–275. [CrossRef] [PubMed]

103. Holt, R.I.; Broide, E.; Buchanan, C.R.; Miell, J.P.; Baker, A.J.; Mowat, A.P.; Mieli-Vergani, G. Orthotopic liver transplantation reverses the adverse nutritional changes of end-stage liver disease in children. *Am. J. Clin. Nutr.* **1997**, *65*, 534–542. [PubMed]

104. Amedee-Manesme, O.; Furr, H.C.; Alvarez, F.; Hadchouel, M.; Alagille, D.; Olson, J.A. Biochemical indicators of vitamin A depletion in children with cholestasis. *Hepatology* **1985**, *5*, 1143–1148. [CrossRef] [PubMed]

105. Lapillonne, A.; Hakme, C.; Mamoux, V.; Chambon, M.; Fournier, V.; Chirouze, V.; Lachaux, A. Effects of liver transplantation on long-chain polyunsaturated fatty acid status in infants with biliary atresia. *J. Pediatr. Gastroenterol. Nutr.* **2000**, *30*, 528–532. [CrossRef] [PubMed]
106. Holt, R.I.; Jones, J.S.; Stone, N.M.; Baker, A.J.; Miell, J.P. Sequential changes in insulin-like growth factor I (IGF-I) and IGF-binding proteins in children with end-stage liver disease before and after successful orthotopic liver transplantation. *J. Clin. Endocrinol. Metab.* **1996**, *81*, 160–168. [PubMed]

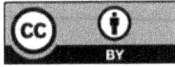

nutrients

MDPI

Article

Sarcopenia Impairs Prognosis of Patients with Hepatocellular Carcinoma: The Role of Liver Functional Reserve and Tumor-Related Factors in Loss of Skeletal Muscle Volume

Kenji Imai *, Koji Takai, Satoshi Watanabe, Tatsunori Hanai, Atsushi Suetsugu, Makoto Shiraki and Masahito Shimizu

Department of Gastroenterology/Internal Medicine, Gifu University Graduate School of Medicine, Gifu 501-1194, Japan; koz@gifu-u.ac.jp (K.T.); ronkalevala777@yahoo.co.jp (S.W.); hanai0606@yahoo.co.jp (T.H.); asue327@yahoo.co.jp (A.S.); mshiraki-gif@umin.ac.jp (M.S.); shimim-gif@umin.ac.jp (M.S.)
* Correspondence: ikenji@gifu-u.ac.jp; Tel.: +81-(58)-230-6308; Fax: +81-(58)-230-6310

Received: 25 August 2017; Accepted: 20 September 2017; Published: 22 September 2017

Abstract: Sarcopenia impairs survival in patients with hepatocellular carcinoma (HCC). This study aimed to clarify the factors that contribute to decreased skeletal muscle volume in patients with HCC. The third lumbar vertebra skeletal muscle index (L3 SMI) in 351 consecutive patients with HCC was calculated to identify sarcopenia. Sarcopenia was defined as an L3 SMI value $\leq 29.0 \text{ cm}^2/\text{m}^2$ for women and $\leq 36.0 \text{ cm}^2/\text{m}^2$ for men. The factors affecting L3 SMI were analyzed by multiple linear regression analysis and tree-based models. Of the 351 HCC patients, 33 were diagnosed as having sarcopenia and showed poor prognosis compared with non-sarcopenia patients ($p = 0.007$). However, this significant difference disappeared after the adjustments for age, sex, Child–Pugh score, maximum tumor size, tumor number, and the degree of portal vein invasion by propensity score matching analysis. Multiple linear regression analysis showed that age ($p = 0.015$) and sex ($p < 0.0001$) were significantly correlated with a decrease in L3 SMI. Tree-based models revealed that sex (female) is the most significant factor that affects L3 SMI. In male patients, L3 SMI was decreased by aging, increased Child–Pugh score (≥ 56 years), and enlarged tumor size (<56 years). Maintaining liver functional reserve and early diagnosis and therapy for HCC are vital to prevent skeletal muscle depletion and improve the prognosis of patients with HCC.

Keywords: hepatocellular carcinoma; skeletal muscle depletion; sarcopenia; prognostic factor

1. Introduction

Hepatocellular carcinoma (HCC) is one of the most common malignancies worldwide. Typically, patients with HCC have a poor clinical course as the prognosis is strongly affected by liver functional reserve and clinical cancer stage [1,2]. The recurrence rate of HCC is extremely high, which is also associated with the poor prognosis [3]. To identify patients with a high mortality risk and to choose the most adequate treatment, a precise prediction of the prognosis of patients with HCC is essential. Thus, several prognostic staging systems, such as Barcelona Clinic Liver Cancer (BCLC) [4], Cancer of the Liver Italian Program (CLIP) [1], and Japan Integrated Staging (JIS) [2], most of which take both clinical cancer stage and liver functional reserve into consideration, have been developed.

Recently, skeletal muscle depletion or sarcopenia, initially defined as the loss of skeletal muscle mass that occurs with aging [5], has garnered attention as a new and promising prognostic factor for various malignancies, including HCC [6–10]. Skeletal muscle volume depletion assessed by computed tomography (CT) predicts poor prognosis of all cancer stages [11], and for sorafenib-treated patients with HCC [12]. Sarcopenia and rapid skeletal muscle depletion are also involved in worse survival in patients with liver cirrhosis [13,14]. These findings strongly suggest that sarcopenia is a significant factor that predicts the prognosis of patients with HCC and liver cirrhosis.

Several pathological conditions, including advanced organ failure, inflammatory disease, malignancy, endocrine disease, sedentary lifestyle, and malnutrition are associated with skeletal muscle depletion [5,15]. In liver disease, the following points can be considered as the main mechanisms of sarcopenia: protein energy malnutrition; imbalance of protein synthesis and breakdown; increased expression of myostatin, a cytokine that strongly suppresses skeletal muscle growth; and increased production of reactive oxygen species and inflammatory cytokines [16]. Therefore, sarcopenia could be a result of various pathological conditions, such as poor liver functional reserve or advanced cancer stages, which in turn affects survival of patients with HCC. However, the precise factors that enhance the progression of sarcopenia and worsen the prognosis of HCC patients have not been evaluated.

The purpose of this study is to identify the factors that contribute to skeletal muscle depletion in HCC patients, especially focusing on liver functional reserve and cancer progression. Based on the results of this study, we will also discuss how to prevent skeletal muscle depletion and improve prognosis in patients with HCC.

2. Materials and Methods

2.1. Patients, Treatment, and Follow-Up Strategy

We evaluated 351 consecutive HCC patients in our hospital between May 2006 and December 2015. HCC nodules were detected using imaging modalities, including dynamic CT, dynamic magnetic resonance imaging (MRI), and abdominal arteriography. HCC was diagnosed based on a typical hypervascular tumor stain on angiography and typical dynamic study findings of enhanced staining in the early phase and attenuation in the delayed phase. The treatment plan in each case was according to the Clinical Practice Guidelines for HCC issued by the Japan Society of Hepatology (JSH) [17]. Patients were thereafter followed on an outpatient basis and had dynamic CT, MRI, or ultrasound every three months after the initial treatment. Recurrent HCC was diagnosed when the typical findings of HCC were observed, and the treatment was still based on the aforementioned guidelines for HCC. Overall survival was defined as the interval from the date of the initial treatment to the date of death or December 2015 for surviving patients. All study participants provided verbal informed consent, which was considered sufficient because this study followed an observational research design that did not require new human biological specimens, and instead relied only on preexisting materials. The study design—including this consent procedure—was approved by the ethics committee of the Gifu University School of Medicine on 7 June 2017 (ethic approval code: 29–26).

2.2. Image Analysis of Skeletal Muscle Volume and Definition of Sarcopenia

Skeletal muscle volume was measured using a CT image that had been taken solely for the purpose of diagnosing HCC prior to the initial treatment. A transverse CT image at the third lumbar vertebra (L3) in the inferior direction was assessed. The muscles in the L3 region—including psoas, erector spinae, quadratus lumborum, transversus abdominis, external and internal obliques, and rectus abdominis—were analyzed using SYNAPSE VINCENT software (version 3.0, Fujifilm Medical, Tokyo, Japan), which enables specific tissue demarcation using Hounsfield unit (HU) thresholds. The muscles were quantified within a range of -29 to $+150$ HU [18], and tissue boundaries were manually corrected as needed. The cross-sectional areas of the muscle (cm^2) at the L3 level computed from each image were normalized by the square of the height (m^2) to obtain the L3 skeletal muscle index (L3 SMI, cm^2/m^2), which was used as an indicator of skeletal muscle volume in previous reports [11,12,16]. Sarcopenia was defined as an L3 SMI value ≤ 29.0 cm^2/m^2 for women and ≤ 36.0 cm^2/m^2 for men, which is according to a previous study [11].

2.3. Statistical Analysis

Overall survival was estimated using the Kaplan–Meier method, and differences between curves were evaluated using the log-rank test. To exclude the effect of possible confounding factors between sarcopenia and non-sarcopenia groups, we performed rigorous adjustments for the following six factors using a propensity score matching analysis: age, sex, Child–Pugh score (CPS), tumor size, tumor number, and the degree of portal vein invasion, which were considered as prognostic factors for HCC patients by previous studies [1,2,4], and showed significant differences between the two groups. The propensity score matching analysis was performed based on the following algorithm: 1:1 optimal match with calipers of width 0.2 of the standard deviation of the logit of the propensity score and no replacement [19]. To identify which of the six factors contributed to decreased L3 SMI, we conducted a multiple linear regression analysis. A tree-based model analysis, which uses the binary recursive partitioning process of the population, was also performed; thus, L3 SMI is similar in patients within each group but different between groups [20,21]. Statistical significance was defined as $p < 0.05$. All statistical analyses were performed using R version 3.3.1 (The R Project for Statistical Computing, Vienna, Austria; http://www.R-project.org/).

3. Results

3.1. Baseline Characteristics and Laboratory Data of Patients

The baseline characteristics and laboratory data of the 351 patients (242 male and 109 female; average age, 70.4 years) are shown in Table 1. The average L3 SMI for all enrolled patients was 43.7 cm^2/m^2, and 33 patients were classified into the sarcopenia group. The average tumor size was 4.2 cm, and 188 patients received curative treatment.

Table 1. Baseline demographic and clinical characteristics.

Variables	Total (n = 351)
Sex (male/female)	242/109
Age (years)	70.4 ± 10.3
Etiology (HBV/HCV/HBV + HCV/others)	43/204/3/101
BMI (kg/m^2)	23.1 ± 3.4
L3 SMI (cm^2/m^2)	43.7 ± 8.6
Sarcopenia (yes/no)	33/318
Child–Pugh score (5/6/7/8/9/10/11)	179/84/52/20/9/6/1
ALB (g/dL)	3.6 ± 0.6
ALT (IU/L)	46.9 ± 44.3
T-Bil (mg/dL)	1.2 ± 1.0
PLT (×10^4/µL)	13.1 ± 7.8
PT (%)	85.3 ± 16.7
FPG (mg/dL)	110.6 ± 34.2
HbA$_{1c}$ (%)	6.0 ± 1.1
AFP (ng/dL)	11,557 ± 73,374
PIVKA-II (mAU/mL)	21,056 ± 125,773
Tumor size (cm)	4.2 ± 3.7
Tumor number (1/≥2)	193/158
Vp (0/1/2/3/4)	289/15/15/15/17
Stage (I/II/III/IV)	79/126/100/46
Curability of initial treatment (yes/no)	188/163
Oral administration of BCAA (yes/no)	153/198
Co-existing diseases (yes/no)	
Renal disease	22/329
Heart disease	45/306
Respiratory disease	16/335
Neurologic disease	22/329
Malignant disease (except HCC)	27/324

Values are presented as average ± standard deviation. HBV, hepatitis B virus; HCV, hepatitis C virus; BMI, body mass index; L3 SMI, third lumbar vertebra skeletal muscle index; ALT, alanine aminotransferase; T-Bil, total bilirubin; PLT, platelet count; PT, prothrombin time; FPG, fasting plasma glucose; AFP, alpha-fetoprotein; PIVKA-II, protein induced by vitamin K absence or antagonists-II; Vp, the degree of portal vein invasion; BCAA, branched-chain amino acids; HCC, hepatocellular carcinoma.

3.2. Comparison of Overall Survival in Sarcopenia and Non-Sarcopenia Groups before and after Adjustments for Possible Confounding Factors

The one-, three-, and five-year overall survival rates of all enrolled patients were 83.0, 61.8, and 42.2%, respectively (Figure 1a). Table 2 shows the clinical characteristics and laboratory data of the sarcopenia (n = 33) and non-sarcopenia (n = 318) groups. Significant differences in sex (male/female = 30/3 vs. 212/106, p = 0.003), body mass index (BMI; kg/m^2, 20.8 vs. 23.3, p < 0.0001), the value of L3 SMI (cm^2/m^2; 30.8 vs. 45.1, p < 0.0001), CPS (5/6/7/8/9/10/11 = 15/7/5/2/0/3/1 vs. 164/77/47/18/9/3/0, p = 0.039), total bilirubin (mg/dL; 1.6 vs. 1.2, p = 0.045), maximum tumor size (cm; 5.6 vs. 4.0, p = 0.020), the degree of portal vein invasion (Vp 0/1/2/3/4 = 24/1/2/2/4 vs. 265/14/13/13/13, p = 0.040), curability of initial treatment (yes/no, 12/21 vs. 175/142, p = 0.039), and prevalence rate of neurologic disease (yes/no, 6/27 vs. 16/302, p = 0.011) were found. Sarcopenia patients died significantly earlier than non-sarcopenia patients (p = 0.007, Figure 1b).

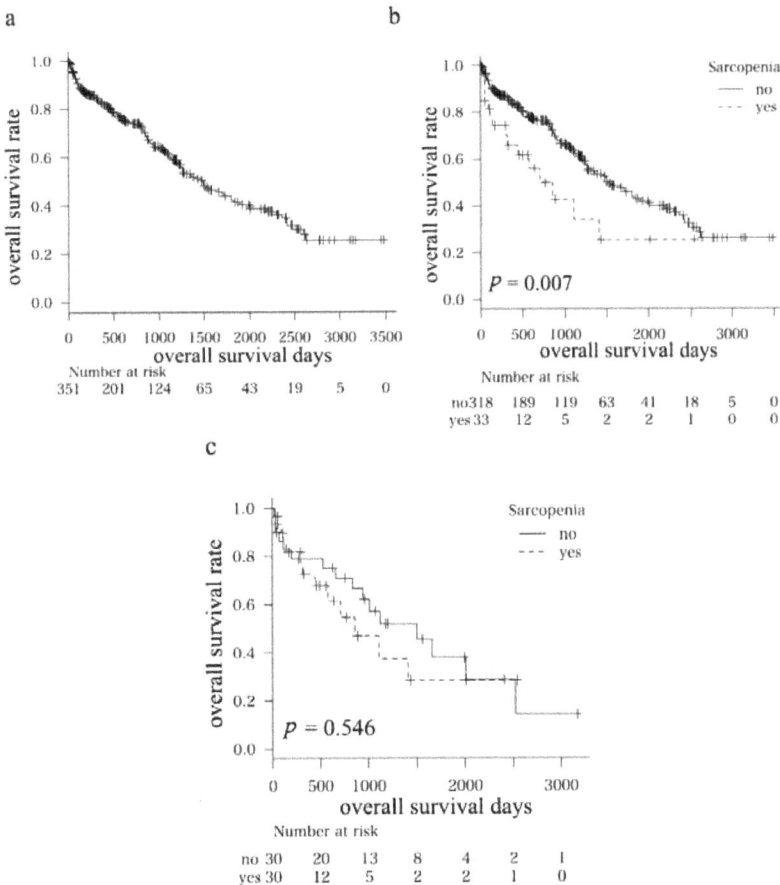

Figure 1. Kaplan–Meier curves for overall survival time in (**a**) all patients; (**b**) subgroups (i.e., sarcopenia and non-sarcopenia groups); and (**c**) subgroups after adjustments for possible confounding factors (age, sex, Child–Pugh score, maximum tumor size, tumor number, and the degree of portal vein invasion) using propensity score matching analysis.

Table 2. Baseline demographic and clinical characteristics of sarcopenia and non-sarcopenia groups.

Variables	Sarcopenia (*n* = 33)	Non-Sarcopenia (*n* = 318)	*p* Value
Sex (male/female)	30/3	212/106	0.003
Age (years)	72.6 ± 1.8	70.2 ± 0.6	0.197
Etiology (HBV/HCV/HBV + HCV/other)	3/22/0/8	40/182/3/93	0.868
BMI (kg/m^2)	20.8 ± 0.6	23.3 ± 0.2	<0.0001
L3 SMI (cm^2/m^2)	30.8 ± 1.3	45.1 ± 0.4	<0.0001
Child–Pugh score (5/6/7/8/9/10/11)	15/7/5/2/0/3/1	164/77/47/18/9/3/0	0.039
ALB (g/dL)	3.5 ± 0.1	3.6 ± 0.03	0.315
ALT (IU/L)	52.2 ± 7.7	46.4 ± 2.5	0.805
T-Bil (mg/dL)	1.6 ± 0.2	1.2 ± 0.06	0.045
PLT (×10^4/µL)	14.5 ± 1.4	13.0 ± 0.4	0.276
PT (%)	89.1 ± 2.9	84.9 ± 0.9	0.176
FPG (mg/dL)	113.3 ± 6.0	110.3 ± 2.0	0.958
HbA$_{1c}$ (%)	6.2 ± 0.2	6.0 ± 0.07	0.356
AFP (ng/dL)	4133 ± 12983	12,319 ± 4158	0.549
PIVKA-II (mAU/mL)	35,910 ± 21,910	19,475 ± 7149	0.476
Tumor size (cm)	5.6 ± 0.6	4.0 ± 0.2	0.020
Tumor number (1/≥2)	20/13	173/145	0.505
Vp (0/1/2/3/4)	24/1/2/2/4	265/14/13/13/13	0.040
Stage (I/II/III/IV)	8/7/12/6	71/117/88/42	0.303
Curability of initial treatment (yes/no)	12/21	176/142	0.039
Oral administration of BCAA (yes/no)	17/16	136/182	0.361
Co-existing diseases (yes/no)			
Renal disease	2/31	20/298	1.000
Heart disease	5/28	40/278	0.593
Respiratory disease	0/33	16/302	0.381
Neurologic disease	6/27	16/302	0.011
Malignant disease (except HCC)	0/33	27/291	0.093

Values are presented as average ± standard deviation. HBV, hepatitis B virus; HCV, hepatitis C virus; BMI, body mass index; L3 SMI, third lumbar vertebra skeletal muscle index; ALT, alanine aminotransferase; T-Bil, total bilirubin; PLT, platelet count; PT, prothrombin time; FPG, fasting plasma glucose; AFP, alpha-fetoprotein; PIVKA-II, protein induced by vitamin K absence or antagonists-II; Vp, the degree of portal vein invasion; BCAA, branched-chain amino acids; HCC, hepatocellular carcinoma.

To clarify the effects of sarcopenia on the prognosis of HCC patients, a propensity score matching analysis was performed after adjusting for liver functional reserve and tumor-related factors. Thirty patients from both sarcopenia and non-sarcopenia groups were chosen (Table 3). No significant differences in all variables except BMI (20.7 vs. 23.2, *p* = 0.002) and L3 SMI (30.5 vs. 46.8, *p* < 0.0001) were found; the adjustments were performed properly. Interestingly, the significant difference in the overall survival between sarcopenia and non-sarcopenia patients observed in the initial analysis (Figure 1b) disappeared after the adjustments for possible confounding factors (*p* = 0.546, Figure 1c).

Table 3. Baseline demographic and clinical characteristics of sarcopenia and non-sarcopenia groups after adjustments for possible confounding factors using propensity score matching analysis.

Variables	Sarcopenia (*n* = 30)	Non-Sarcopenia (*n* = 30)	*p* Value
Sex (male/female)	27/3	28/2	1.000
Age (years)	71.8 ± 9.7	73.0 ± 10.7	0.642
Etiology (HBV/HCV/HBV + HCV/other)	3/21/0/6	3/20/1/6	0.918
BMI (kg/m^2)	20.7 ± 3.0	23.2 ± 2.8	0.002
L3 SMI (cm^2/m^2)	30.5 ± 6.4	46.8 ± 7.4	<0.0001
Child–Pugh score (5/6/7/8/9/10/11)	14/7/5/2/0/1/1	14/9/6/0/1/0/0	0.660
ALB (g/dL)	3.6 ± 0.7	3.6 ± 0.6	0.984
ALT (IU/L)	48.8 ± 57.7	41.8 ± 22.7	0.543
T-Bil (mg/dL)	1.4 ± 1.0	1.0 ± 0.5	0.106
PLT (×10^4/µL)	14.5 ± 13.0	13.4 ± 4.9	0.656
PT (%)	89.8 ± 14.4	87.7 ± 15.5	0.589

Table 3. *Cont.*

Variables	Sarcopenia (*n* = 30)	Non-Sarcopenia (*n* = 30)	*p* Value
FPG (mg/dL)	114.8 ± 40.2	113.6 ± 47.9	0.918
HbA$_{1c}$ (%)	6.3 ± 1.6	5.8 ± 1.2	0.226
AFP (ng/dL)	3531 ± 12,997	1480 ± 4268	0.423
PIVKA-II (mAU/mL)	22,979 ± 89,165	10,893 ± 46,387	0.518
Tumor size (cm)	5.0 ± 3.9	4.4 ± 3.8	0.534
Tumor number (1/≥2)	18/12	18/12	1.000
Vp (0/1/2/3/4)	24/1/2/1/2	22/3/1/2/2	0.852
Stage (I/II/III/IV)	8/7/10/5	7/11/5/7	0.427
Curability of initial treatment (yes/no)	12/18	17/13	0.301

Values are presented as average ± standard deviation. HBV, hepatitis B virus; HCV, hepatitis C virus; BMI, body mass index; L3 SMI, third lumbar vertebra skeletal muscle index; ALT, alanine aminotransferase; T-Bil, total bilirubin; PLT, platelet count; PT, prothrombin time; FPG, fasting plasma glucose; AFP, alpha-fetoprotein; PIVKA-II, protein induced by vitamin K absence or antagonists-II; Vp, the degree of portal vein invasion.

3.3. Significant Factors that Affect L3 SMI Based on Multiple Linear Regression Analysis and Tree-Based Models

Of the six possible confounding factors (age, sex, CPS, tumor size, tumor number, and the degree of portal vein invasion), age (*p* = 0.015) and sex (*p* < 0.0001) were significantly correlated with the value of L3 SMI based on multiple linear regression analysis (Table 4). The following regression equation with an intercept of 46.94 (*p* < 0.0001) was obtained from Equation (1) and (2):

$$\text{L3 SMI (cm}^2/\text{m}^2) = 46.94 - 0.10 \times [\text{Age}] + 5.20 \text{ (for men)} \tag{1}$$

$$\text{L3 SMI (cm}^2/\text{m}^2) = 46.94 - 0.10 \times [\text{Age}] \text{ (for women)} \tag{2}$$

Table 4. Significant factors affecting L3 SMI by multiple linear regression analysis.

Variables	Std. Coefficient	Std. Error	*t* Value	*p* Value
Intercept	46.94	3.06	15.33	<0.0001
Age	−0.10	0.04	−2.44	0.015
Sex (vs. man)	5.20	0.95	5.46	<0.0001

Std. coefficient, standard coefficient; Std. error, standard error.

Furthermore, according to the tree-based models, the most significant factor contributing to the value of L3 SMI was sex; the average L3 SMI in men was 46 cm^2/m^2 and that in women was 40 cm^2/m^2. In men, the most significant factor for decreased L3 SMI was aging; the average L3 SMI in men ≥ 56 and < 56 years old was 45 and 50 cm^2/m^2, respectively. In men ≥ 56 years old, a higher CPS was involved in the loss of skeletal muscle mass; the average L3 SMI with CPS ≥ 9 and < 9 was 38 and 45 cm^2/m^2, respectively. In men < 56 years old, an enlarged tumor size was involved in the loss of skeletal muscle mass; the average L3 SMI with tumor size ≥ 5.7 and < 5.7 cm was 45 and 52 cm^2/m^2, respectively. However, these factors observed in men did not affect the L3 SMI in women. The decision tree for this analysis is shown in Figure 2.

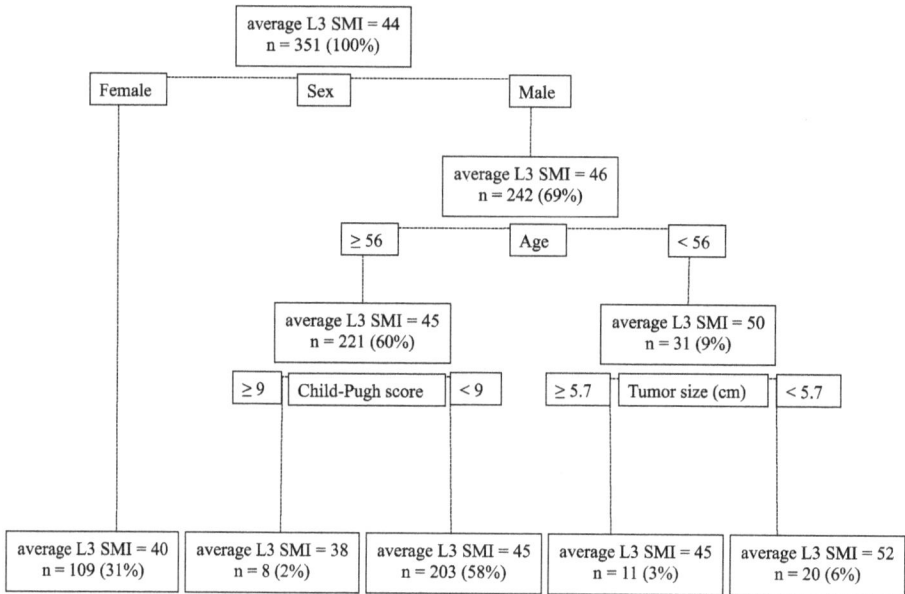

Figure 2. The decision tree for the tree-based models. The differences in L3 SMI between each group become larger with the six factors (age, sex, Child–Pugh score, maximum tumor size, tumor number, and the degree of portal vein invasion).

4. Discussion

The results of this study showed that sarcopenia impairs survival in patients with HCC. These findings are consistent with those of previous studies [6–12]. Thus, skeletal muscle volume measurement using CT, which is commonly used in the clinical setting for HCC, is useful to predict the prognosis of patients with this malignancy.

Here, patients in the sarcopenia group had poorer liver functional reserve, larger tumor size, and more severe portal vein invasion, which significantly contributed to the lower curability of the initial treatment for HCC. Moreover, men, older patients, and those with poorer liver functional reserve and larger tumor size had a lower skeletal muscle volume. Several studies revealed that liver functional reserve and clinical cancer stage are significant prognostic factors for HCC and that, similar to the results in our study, the progression of underlying liver cirrhosis and HCC, in addition to aging, are critically involved in the development of sarcopenia and subsequent poor prognosis of these patients [1,2,4]. The results of the propensity score matching analysis showed that the significant differences in overall survival between the sarcopenia and non-sarcopenia groups disappeared after adjustments for the probable confounding factors associated with the patients' characteristics and tumor factors. This finding may suggest that the sarcopenia group had clinical characteristics—such as old age, poor liver functional reserve, and progressed cancer stage—that affect survival.

Several clinical studies have revealed that sarcopenia might be an independent prognostic factor for HCC [11,12]. In addition, HCC patients with sarcopenia more often have complications with chemotherapy toxicity and this might make the prognosis of the patients more serious [22,23]. On the other hand, skeletal muscle volume in HCC patients was determined, at least in part, by sex, age, CPS, and tumor burden in this study. Based on the findings, it could be said that, at least in men, sarcopenia is a prognostic factor possibly affected by already-known prognostic factors, including liver functional reserve and clinical cancer stage [1,2,4]. Most of the existing prognostic staging systems, such as CLIP and JIS [1,2,4], take liver functional reserve and clinical cancer stage into consideration in predicting prognosis for HCC as accurately as possible. Thus, these findings strongly suggest that maintaining liver functional reserve and early detection and therapy for HCC, which can increase the curability of initial treatment, are effective strategies to improve the prognosis. In addition, reducing the amount of tumor burden and maintaining liver functional reserve, which have been reported repeatedly to improve prognosis for HCC [1,2,4], could be effective measures to prevent skeletal muscle depletion; however, future prospective study is required to evaluate this hypothesis further.

Other possible strategies to prevent skeletal muscle depletion or to increase skeletal muscle mass include nutritional and exercise therapies, both of which have been shown to improve outcomes in patients with liver cirrhosis [24,25]. Oral supplementation with branched chain amino acids is one of the most promising methods [26–28]. Exercise therapy might also be promising in preventing skeletal muscle depletion [29]. Moreover, poor dietary or sedentary lifestyle is considered one of the main causes of sarcopenia [15]; thus, appropriate assessment and modification of lifestyle could be useful to prevent decreased skeletal muscle volume and subsequently to improve the prognosis of patients with HCC and liver cirrhosis. Furthermore, pathological conditions—except liver diseases—that can lead to sarcopenia must also be considered. The aging of HCC patient population is advancing and elderly patients are easily complicated with several diseases which cause sarcopenia. In the present study, the prevalence of patients with neurologic disease, which decreases activities of daily living levels, was significantly high in the sarcopenia group. Therefore, in order to prevent sarcopenia, such patients might especially be recommended to start rehabilitation as early as possible.

In the present study, aging was critically involved in the complication with sarcopenia in men. One of the reasons of this phenomenon might be that decreasing of testosterone caused by aging because this sex hormone is known to promote the growth of skeletal muscle [30]. On the other hand, aging, progression of CPS, and enlargement of tumor size did not have effects on the loss of skeletal muscle volume in women. Because women usually store abundance of fat and generate their energy more preferentially from fat stores than from skeletal muscle stores [31], women might be more resistant to sarcopenia compared to men. In addition to the present study, several clinical trials have defined the optimal cutoff values of skeletal muscle volume which are different between men and women [7,11,32]. These findings may suggest that setting the different cutoff values on every sex is reasonable to evaluate sarcopenia.

This study has some limitations. First, we used our own cutoff values for L3 SMI (i.e., 29.0 cm^2/m^2 for women and 36.0 cm^2/m^2 for men), which are not similar to those of the JSH (i.e., 38.0 cm^2/m^2 for women and 42.0 cm^2/m^2 for men) [16], to determine sarcopenia because the latter could not stratify the risk of mortality for HCC patients. We also did not use the cutoff values reported by the previous reports [7,32], both of which are widely accepted as appropriate values in western countries, because they are not applicable to Japanese HCC patients whose BMIs are small and differ considerably from Western populations. Second, because of the retrospective design of our study, muscle strength such as grip strength and walking speed, which is usually regarded as a diagnostic criterion for sarcopenia [15,16], was not assessed. Future prospective studies that examine the most optimal cutoff values for L3 SMI to diagnose sarcopenia and whether sarcopenia itself worsens the prognosis of patients with HCC should be performed.

5. Conclusions

We demonstrated that L3 SMI, an indicator of skeletal muscle volume, was significantly decreased in female HCC patients. In male patients, L3 SMI was significantly affected by aging, liver functional reserve ($\geq$56 years), and tumor size (<56 years). These findings strongly suggest that more emphasis should be put on maintaining liver functional reserve and reducing tumor burden, both of which are well-reported prognostic factors for HCC [1,2,4], especially in patients with sarcopenia. In conclusion, in addition to the measure for sarcopenia, maintaining liver functional reserve and early detection and curative therapy for HCC are effective ways to improve the prognosis of chronic liver disease patients, especially those with HCC.

Acknowledgments: No funding sources support the preparation of this manuscript.

Author Contributions: Kenji Imai designed the study, analyzed the data, and wrote the manuscript. Koji Takai supervised the treatment for the participants. Satoshi Watanabe, Tatsunori Hanai, Atsushi Suetsugu, and Makoto Shiraki contributed to select the participants and collect the data. Masahito Shimizu mainly reviewed and amended the manuscript. All authors read and approved the final manuscript.

Conflicts of Interest: The authors declare no conflict of interest.

References

1. A new prognostic system for hepatocellular carcinoma: A retrospective study of 435 patients: The cancer of the liver italian program (clip) investigators. *Hepatology* **1998**, *28*, 751–755.

2. Kudo, M.; Chung, H.; Osaki, Y. Prognostic staging system for hepatocellular carcinoma (clip score): Its value and limitations, and a proposal for a new staging system, the japan integrated staging score (jis score). *J. Gastroenterol.* **2003**, *38*, 207–215. [CrossRef] [PubMed]

3. Poon, R.T. Prevention of recurrence after resection of hepatocellular carcinoma: A daunting challenge. *Hepatology* **2011**, *54*, 757–759. [CrossRef] [PubMed]

4. Llovet, J.M.; Bru, C.; Bruix, J. Prognosis of hepatocellular carcinoma: The bclc staging classification. *Semin. Liver Dis.* **1999**, *19*, 329–338. [CrossRef] [PubMed]

5. Rosenberg, I.H. Sarcopenia: Origins and clinical relevance. *J. Nutr.* **1997**, *127*, 990S–991S. [CrossRef] [PubMed]

6. Fujiwara, N.; Nakagawa, H.; Kudo, Y.; Tateishi, R.; Taguri, M.; Watadani, T.; Nakagomi, R.; Kondo, M.; Nakatsuka, T.; Minami, T.; et al. Sarcopenia, intramuscular fat deposition, and visceral adiposity independently predict the outcomes of hepatocellular carcinoma. *J. Hepatol.* **2015**, *63*, 131–140. [CrossRef] [PubMed]

7. Prado, C.M.; Lieffers, J.R.; McCargar, L.J.; Reiman, T.; Sawyer, M.B.; Martin, L.; Baracos, V.E. Prevalence and clinical implications of sarcopenic obesity in patients with solid tumours of the respiratory and gastrointestinal tracts: A population-based study. *Lancet Oncol.* **2008**, *9*, 629–635. [CrossRef]

8. Sabel, M.S.; Lee, J.; Cai, S.; Englesbe, M.J.; Holcombe, S.; Wang, S. Sarcopenia as a prognostic factor among patients with stage iii melanoma. *Ann. Surg. Oncol.* **2011**, *18*, 3579–3585. [CrossRef] [PubMed]

9. Tan, B.H.; Birdsell, L.A.; Martin, L.; Baracos, V.E.; Fearon, K.C. Sarcopenia in an overweight or obese patient is an adverse prognostic factor in pancreatic cancer. *Clin. Cancer Res. Off. J. Am. Assoc. Cancer Res.* **2009**, *15*, 6973–6979. [CrossRef] [PubMed]

10. Van Vledder, M.G.; Levolger, S.; Ayez, N.; Verhoef, C.; Tran, T.C.; Ijzermans, J.N. Body composition and outcome in patients undergoing resection of colorectal liver metastases. *Br. J. Surg.* **2012**, *99*, 550–557. [CrossRef] [PubMed]

11. Iritani, S.; Imai, K.; Takai, K.; Hanai, T.; Ideta, T.; Miyazaki, T.; Suetsugu, A.; Shiraki, M.; Shimizu, M.; Moriwaki, H. Skeletal muscle depletion is an independent prognostic factor for hepatocellular carcinoma. *J. Gastroenterol.* **2015**, *50*, 323–332. [CrossRef] [PubMed]

12. Imai, K.; Takai, K.; Hanai, T.; Ideta, T.; Miyazaki, T.; Kochi, T.; Suetsugu, A.; Shiraki, M.; Shimizu, M. Skeletal muscle depletion predicts the prognosis of patients with hepatocellular carcinoma treated with sorafenib. *Int. J. Mol. Sci.* **2015**, *16*, 9612–9624. [CrossRef] [PubMed]

13. Hanai, T.; Shiraki, M.; Nishimura, K.; Ohnishi, S.; Imai, K.; Suetsugu, A.; Takai, K.; Shimizu, M.; Moriwaki, H. Sarcopenia impairs prognosis of patients with liver cirrhosis. *Nutrition* **2015**, *31*, 193–199. [CrossRef] [PubMed]

14. Hanai, T.; Shiraki, M.; Ohnishi, S.; Miyazaki, T.; Ideta, T.; Kochi, T.; Imai, K.; Suetsugu, A.; Takai, K.; Moriwaki, H.; et al. Rapid skeletal muscle wasting predicts worse survival in patients with liver cirrhosis. *Hepatol. Res.* **2016**, *46*, 743–751. [CrossRef] [PubMed]

15. Cruz-Jentoft, A.J.; Baeyens, J.P.; Bauer, J.M.; Boirie, Y.; Cederholm, T.; Landi, F.; Martin, F.C.; Michel, J.P.; Rolland, Y.; Schneider, S.M.; et al. Sarcopenia: European consensus on definition and diagnosis: Report of the european working group on sarcopenia in older people. *Age Ageing* **2010**, *39*, 412–423. [CrossRef] [PubMed]

16. Nishikawa, H.; Shiraki, M.; Hiramatsu, A.; Moriya, K.; Hino, K.; Nishiguchi, S. Japan society of hepatology guidelines for sarcopenia in liver disease (1st edition): Recommendation from the working group for creation of sarcopenia assessment criteria. *Hepatol. Res.* **2016**, *46*, 951–963. [CrossRef] [PubMed]

17. Clinical practice guidelines for hepatocellular carcinoma—The Japan society of hepatology 2009 update. *Hepatol. Res. Off. J. Jpn. Soc. Hepatol.* **2010**, *40*, 2–144.

18. Mitsiopoulos, N.; Baumgartner, R.N.; Heymsfield, S.B.; Lyons, W.; Gallagher, D.; Ross, R. Cadaver validation of skeletal muscle measurement by magnetic resonance imaging and computerized tomography. *J. Appl. Physiol.* **1998**, *85*, 115–122. [PubMed]

19. Austin, P.C. Propensity-score matching in the cardiovascular surgery literature from 2004 to 2006: A systematic review and suggestions for improvement. *J. Thorac. Cardiovasc. Surg.* **2007**, *134*, 1128–1135. [CrossRef] [PubMed]

20. Pociot, F.; Karlsen, A.E.; Pedersen, C.B.; Aalund, M.; Nerup, J.; European Consortium for I.G.S. Novel analytical methods applied to type 1 diabetes genome-scan data. *Am. J. Hum. Genet.* **2004**, *74*, 647–660. [CrossRef] [PubMed]

21. Banerjee, M.; Muenz, D.G.; Chang, J.T.; Papaleontiou, M.; Haymart, M.R. Tree-based model for thyroid cancer prognostication. *J. Clin. Endocrinol. Metab.* **2014**, *99*, 3737–3745. [CrossRef] [PubMed]

22. Mir, O.; Coriat, R.; Blanchet, B.; Durand, J.P.; Boudou-Rouquette, P.; Michels, J.; Ropert, S.; Vidal, M.; Pol, S.; Chaussade, S.; et al. Sarcopenia predicts early dose-limiting toxicities and pharmacokinetics of sorafenib in patients with hepatocellular carcinoma. *PLoS ONE* **2012**, *7*, e37563. [CrossRef] [PubMed]

23. Prado, C.M.; Antoun, S.; Sawyer, M.B.; Baracos, V.E. Two faces of drug therapy in cancer: Drug-related lean tissue loss and its adverse consequences to survival and toxicity. *Curr. Opin. Clin. Nutr. Metab. Care* **2011**, *14*, 250–254. [CrossRef] [PubMed]

24. Jones, J.C.; Coombes, J.S.; Macdonald, G.A. Exercise capacity and muscle strength in patients with cirrhosis. *Liver Transplant.* **2012**, *18*, 146–151. [CrossRef] [PubMed]

25. Plauth, M.; Cabre, E.; Riggio, O.; Assis-Camilo, M.; Pirlich, M.; Kondrup, J.; Ferenci, P.; Holm, E.; Vom Dahl, S.; Muller, M.J.; et al. Espen guidelines on enteral nutrition: Liver disease. *Clin. Nutr.* **2006**, *25*, 285–294. [CrossRef] [PubMed]

26. Marchesini, G.; Bianchi, G.; Merli, M.; Amodio, P.; Panella, C.; Loguercio, C.; Rossi Fanelli, F.; Abbiati, R. Nutritional supplementation with branched-chain amino acids in advanced cirrhosis: A double-blind, randomized trial. *Gastroenterology* **2003**, *124*, 1792–1801. [CrossRef]

27. Moriwaki, H.; Shiraki, M.; Fukushima, H.; Shimizu, M.; Iwasa, J.; Naiki, T.; Nagaki, M. Long-term outcome of branched-chain amino acid treatment in patients with liver cirrhosis. *Hepatol. Res.* **2008**, *38*, S102–S106. [CrossRef] [PubMed]

28. Muto, Y.; Sato, S.; Watanabe, A.; Moriwaki, H.; Suzuki, K.; Kato, A.; Kato, M.; Nakamura, T.; Higuchi, K.; Nishiguchi, S.; et al. Effects of oral branched-chain amino acid granules on event-free survival in patients with liver cirrhosis. *Clin. Gastroenterol. Hepatol.* **2005**, *3*, 705–713. [CrossRef]

29. Vincent, H.K.; Raiser, S.N.; Vincent, K.R. The aging musculoskeletal system and obesity-related considerations with exercise. *Ageing Res. Rev.* **2012**, *11*, 361–373. [CrossRef] [PubMed]

30. Grossmann, M.; Hoermann, R.; Gani, L.; Chan, I.; Cheung, A.; Gow, P.J.; Li, A.; Zajac, J.D.; Angus, P. Low testosterone levels as an independent predictor of mortality in men with chronic liver disease. *Clin. Endocrinol.* **2012**, *77*, 323–328. [CrossRef] [PubMed]

31. Riggio, O.; Angeloni, S.; Ciuffa, L.; Nicolini, G.; Attili, A.F.; Albanese, C.; Merli, M. Malnutrition is not related to alterations in energy balance in patients with stable liver cirrhosis. *Clin. Nutr.* **2003**, *22*, 553–559. [CrossRef]

32. Montano-Loza, A.J.; Meza-Junco, J.; Prado, C.M.; Lieffers, J.R.; Baracos, V.E.; Bain, V.G.; Sawyer, M.B. Muscle wasting is associated with mortality in patients with cirrhosis. *Clin. Gastroenterol. Hepatol.* **2012**, *10*, 166–173, 173.e1. [CrossRef] [PubMed]

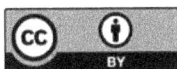

nutrients

MDPI

Article

Comparison of Prognostic Impact between the Child-Pugh Score and Skeletal Muscle Mass for Patients with Liver Cirrhosis

Hiroki Nishikawa, Hirayuki Enomoto *, Akio Ishii, Yoshinori Iwata, Yuho Miyamoto, Noriko Ishii, Yukihisa Yuri, Kunihiro Hasegawa, Chikage Nakano, Takashi Nishimura, Kazunori Yoh, Nobuhiro Aizawa, Yoshiyuki Sakai, Naoto Ikeda, Tomoyuki Takashima, Ryo Takata, Hiroko Iijima and Shuhei Nishiguchi

Department of Hepatobiliary and Pancreatic disease, Department of Internal Medicine, Hyogo College of Medicine, 1-1, Mukogawacho, Nishinomiyashi, Hyogo 663-8501, Japan; nishikawa_6392@yahoo.co.jp (H.N.); akio0010@yahoo.co.jp (A.I.); yo-iwata@hyo-med.ac.jp (Y.I.); yuho.0818.1989@gmail.com (Y.M.); ishinori1985@yahoo.co.jp (N.I.); gyma27ijo04td@gmail.com (Y.Y.); hiro.red1230@gmail.com (K.H.); chikage@hyo-med.ac.jp (C.N.); tk-nishimura@hyo-med.ac.jp (T.N.); mm2wintwin@ybb.ne.jp (K.Y.); nobu23hiro@yahoo.co.jp (N.A.); sakai429@hyo-med.ac.jp (Y.S.); nikeneko@hyo-med.ac.jp (N.I.); tomo0204@yahoo.co.jp (T.T.); chano_chano_rt@yahoo.co.jp (R.T.); hiroko-i@hyo-med.ac.jp (H.I.); nishiguc@hyo-med.ac.jp (S.N.)
* Correspondence: enomoto@hyo-med.ac.jp; Tel.: +81-798-45-6111; Fax: +81-798-45-6608

Received: 13 May 2017; Accepted: 9 June 2017; Published: 12 June 2017

Abstract: Aims: To investigate the influence of skeletal muscle mass index (SMI) as determined by bioimpedance analysis (BIA) (appendicular skeletal muscle mass/(height)^2) on survival by comparing the Child-Pugh score in patients with liver cirrhosis (LC, n = 383, average age = 65.2 years). Patients and methods: In terms of comparison of the effects of SMI and other markers on survival, we used time-dependent receiver operating characteristics (ROC) analysis. Results: The average SMI for male was 7.4 cm^2/m^2 whereas that for female was 6.0 cm^2/m^2 (p < 0.0001). As for the Child-Pugh score, five points were in the majority, both in males (51.7%, (106/205)) and females (44.9%, (80/178)). For both genders, the survival curve was well stratified according to SMI (p < 0.0001 for males and p = 0.0056 for females). In the multivariate analysis for survival, SMI and Child-Pugh scores were found to be significant both in males and females. In time-dependent ROC analyses, all area under the ROCs (AUROCs) for SMI in each time point were higher than those for Child-Pugh scores in males, while in females AUROCs for Child-Pugh scores at each time point were higher than those for SMI. Conclusion: SMI using BIA can be helpful for predicting outcomes, at least in male LC patients.

Keywords: liver cirrhosis; bioimpedance analysis; skeletal muscle mass index; Child-Pugh score; prognosis

---

1. Introduction

The liver is the pivotal organ for metabolism and it metabolizes carbohydrates, lipids, and proteins, which are the so-called "three major nutrients" [1–4]. Liver cirrhosis (LC) is an end-stage form in liver diseases and LC is characterized by several metabolic or nutritional disorders and portal hypertension-related complications such as ascites or varices, all of which can lead to dismal clinical outcome [1–4]. Over the past two or three decades, numerous clinical and biochemical predictors have been proposed in an effort to more accurately predict the prognosis in LC patients and evaluate their short and long-term survival correctly [5–9]. The Child-Pugh scoring system and the Model for End-stage Liver Disease (MELD) scoring system are two major prognostic scoring systems in LC patients [5–9]. In particular, the MELD score is calculated by three easily available and reproducible laboratory tests and is useful for predicting outcomes for patients undergoing liver transplantation (LT) [5]. In our country, LT is not common due to the shortage of transplanted liver and the Child-Pugh scoring system has been preferably used for assessing prognosis in LC patients.

Sarcopenia is a clinical entity as determined by skeletal muscle mass loss and decline of muscle strength and this clinical entity has recently drawn much attention among clinicians owing to its significant deleterious impact on outcomes [10–16]. LC can be associated with secondary sarcopenia because of protein metabolic disorder and/or energy metabolic disorder [11,14,15]. Skeletal muscle mass loss can be linked to poorer clinical outcomes in LC patients, hepatocellular carcinoma (HCC) patients, or patients with other malignancies [17–26]. Skeletal muscle mass can be assessed by computed tomography (CT), magnetic resonance imaging (MRI), dual energy X-ray absorptiometry and bioimpedance analysis (BIA), which are consistent and accurate assessment modalities [14,15,17,19,27,28]. Among these modalities, BIA is particularly attractive since it can noninvasively determine body composition analysis in LC patients [14,15,17,19,27,28].

However, which of two prognostic markers (i.e., the Child-Pugh scoring system and skeletal muscle mass) has stronger influence on clinical outcomes in patients with LC remains unclear. Addressing these questions may be clinically of significance. The aim of this study was to investigate the influence of skeletal muscle mass as determined by data in BIA on survival compared with the Child-Pugh score in patients with LC.

2. Patients and Methods

2.1. Patients

The current study was a single center retrospective study. Between October 2005 and October 2015, a total of 529 LC individuals with BIA data available were admitted at the Division of Hepatobiliary and Pancreatic disease, Department of Internal Medicine, Hyogo College of Medicine, Hyogo, Japan. In our department, BIA (Inbody 720, Tokyo, Japan) was routinely performed in the resting and standing position principally on an outpatient basis for patients who consented to nutritional evaluation. In this analysis, skeletal muscle mass was evaluated using BIA data. Of these patients, patients with severe ascites (n = 24) were excluded from this study as body weight, body mass index (BMI), and skeletal muscle mass index (SMI) using BIA may be overestimated in these patients [29,30]. Twenty-three subjects had been lost to follow-up within one year after performing BIA and they were excluded from this analysis for avoiding bias. In the remaining 482 subjects, 99 had HCC on radiological findings at baseline and they were also excluded because presence of HCC can affect the interpretation of BIA data. A total of 383 subjects were therefore analyzed in the current study. Follow-up observation after BIA included periodical blood tests, radiological assessments by ultrasonography (US), CT, or MRI in order to detect HCC incidence every 3–6 months. There was no patient who underwent LT during observation period. LC was diagnosed using pathological findings, radiological findings such as US, CT, or MRI and/or laboratory data including liver fibrosis markers [31–33]. In patients with lower serum albumin level (less than 3.5 g/dL), liver supporting therapies including branched-chain amino acid (BCAA) treatment or late evening snack with BCAA enriched snacks were in consideration [4,34,35]. In patients with hepatitis virus-related LC, antiviral treatments including direct acting antivirals, interferon-based regimens or nucleoside analogues therapy were also in consideration [4,34]. SMI was calculated as reported elsewhere [28]. Briefly, SMI was defined as "appendicular skeletal muscle mass/(height (m))^2" [28]. We retrospectively investigated the influence of SMI on survival in males and females, as compared with Child-Pugh scores, which was well established prognostic marker [7–9]. In terms of the comparison of the effects of SMI and other markers on survival, we used time-dependent receiver operating characteristics (ROC) analysis [36]. We also investigated parameters associated with overall survival (OS) in the univariate and multivariate analyses. HCC diagnosis and treatment choices for HCC were as reported elsewhere [37,38].

The ethical committee meeting in Hyogo College of Medicine acknowledged the current study protocol and this study strictly followed all regulations of the Declaration of Helsinki.

2.2. Statistical Analyses

Categorical parameters were compared by Fisher's exact test. Continuous parameters were compared by unpaired *t*-test, Mann-Whitney *U* test, or Kruskal-Wallis test, as applicable. In continuous parameters, ROC curve analysis for survival was conducted for the purpose of setting the optimal cutoff point that is linked to maximal sum of specificity and sensitivity and we classified continuous parameters into two groups using these cutoff points, which was then treated as dichotomous covariates in the univariate analysis. Survival curve was created by using the Kaplan-Meier method and compared in the log-rank test. Parameters with *p* value < 0.05 in the univariate analysis were finally subjected to the multivariate analysis in the Cox proportional hazards model. OS was defined as the time interval from the date of performing BIA until death from any cause or the last follow-up visit. Additionally, we analyzed time-dependent ROC curves of SMI, Child-Pugh scores, and variables which revealed to be significant in the multivariate analysis for survival, and compared between area under the ROCs (AUROCs) for above parameters in each time point (two-, three-, four-, five-, six-, and seven-years) [36].

Data are shown as the average ± standard deviation (SD) unless otherwise mentioned. Statistical significance was set at *p* < 0.05. Statistical analysis was performed with the JMP 11 (SAS Institute Inc., Cary, NC, USA).

3. Results

3.1. Baseline Characteristics

The baseline characteristics of the analyzed subjects (*n* = 383) are presented in Table 1. They included 205 males and 178 females with an average ± SD age of 65.2 ± 10.3 years. The median follow-up periods were 3.2 years (range: 0.2–10.7 years). The average ± SD value in SMI for male was 7.4 ± 0.9 cm^2/m^2 whereas that for female was 6.0 ± 0.7 cm^2/m^2 (*p* < 0.0001). According to the Asian Working Group for Sarcopenia criteria (AWGS), the cut-off values for SMI are 7.0 kg/m^2 for male and 5.7 kg/m^2 for female. [28] The proportion of decreased SMI (D-SMI: less than each cutoff value as defined by AWGS criteria) in male was 36.1% (74/205) and that in female was 34.8% (62/178). A total of 136 patients (35.5%) had D-SMI. As for Child-Pugh scores, five points was in the majority, both in males (51.7%, (106/205)) and females (44.9%, (80/178)). In males, SMI significantly correlated with age (overall significance, *p* < 0.0001), while in females it did not (overall significance, *p* = 0.1921) (Figure 1A,B). In both males and females, SMI significantly correlated with BMI (*p* values, both <0.0001) (Figure 1C,D). In both males (*p* = 0.3716) and females (*p* = 0.1330), SMI did not significantly correlate with the Child-Pugh classification (Figure 1E,F).

3.2. Cumulative OS Rates for the Entire Cohort, Male and Female According to SMI

For the entire cohort (*n* = 383), the one-, three-, and five-year cumulative OS rates were 92.7%, 82.4%, and 59.2%, respectively, in patients with D-SMI, and 97.2%, 92.2%, and 84.4%, respectively, in patients without D-SMI (*p* < 0.0001) (Figure 2). For males (*n* = 205), the one-, three-, and five-year cumulative OS rates were 91.9%, 78.0%, and 53.6%, respectively, in patients with D-SMI, and 96.2%, 92.0%, and 84.7%, respectively, in patients without D-SMI (*p* < 0.0001) (Figure 3A). For females (*n* = 178), the one-, three-, and five-year cumulative OS rates were 93.6%, 87.7%, and 66.1%, respectively, in patients with D-SMI, and 98.3%, 92.4%, and 83.8%, respectively, in patients without D-SMI (*p* = 0.0056) (Figure 3B).

Table 1. Baseline characteristics (n = 383).

Variables	Number or Average ± SD	Male (n = 205)	Female (n = 178)	p Value (Male vs. Female)
Age (years)	65.2 ± 10.3	64.1 ± 10.8	66.4 ± 9.5	0.0403
Body mass index (kg/m^2)	23.3 ± 3.9	23.4 ± 3.8	23.2 ± 4.0	0.6028
Skeletal muscle mass index (cm^2/m^2)	6.7 ± 1.1	7.4 ± 0.9	6.0 ± 0.7	<0.0001
Causes of liver disease Hepatitis B/Hepatitis C/others	32/235/116	22/122/61	10/113/55	0.2043
Child-Pugh scores, 5/6/7/8/9/10/11	186/93/58/28/13/3/2	106/42/31/15/6/3/2	80/51/27/13/7/0/0	0.2587
Total bilirubin (mg/dL)	1.3 ± 1.1	1.3 ± 1.3	1.2 ± 0.7	0.2319
Serum albumin (g/dL)	3.7 ± 0.53	3.7 ± 0.54	3.6 ± 0.51	0.3897
Prothrombin time (%)	77.0 ± 13.8	77.5 ± 13.4	76.4 ± 14.2	0.4532
Platelets (×10^4/mm^3)	10.6 ± 5.5	10.5 ± 5.3	10.7 ± 5.7	0.8093
Serum sodium (mmol/L)	139.7 ± 2.5	139.3 ± 2.5	140.2 ± 2.6	0.0004
Serum creatinine (mg/dL)	0.74 ± 0.51	0.84 ± 0.65	0.62 ± 0.22	<0.0001
Total cholesterol (mg/dL)	154.0 ± 36.8	152.8 ± 35.4	155.2 ± 38.4	0.5250
Triglyceride (mg/dL)	90.5 ± 45.1	95.5 ± 53.0	84.8 ± 33.0	0.2144
AST (IU/L)	49.3 ± 34.8	49.4 ± 32.3	49.2 ± 37.5	0.9417
ALT (IU/L)	42.6 ± 38.9	43.9 ± 34.2	41.0 ± 43.7	0.0951
Fasting blood glucose (mg/dL)	110.9 ± 34.7	114.8 ± 39.9	106.4 ± 27.0	0.0101
Ascites, yes/no	44/339	25/180	19/159	0.7484

Data are expressed as number or average ± standard deviation (SD). AST: aspartate aminotransferase; ALT: alanine aminotransferase.

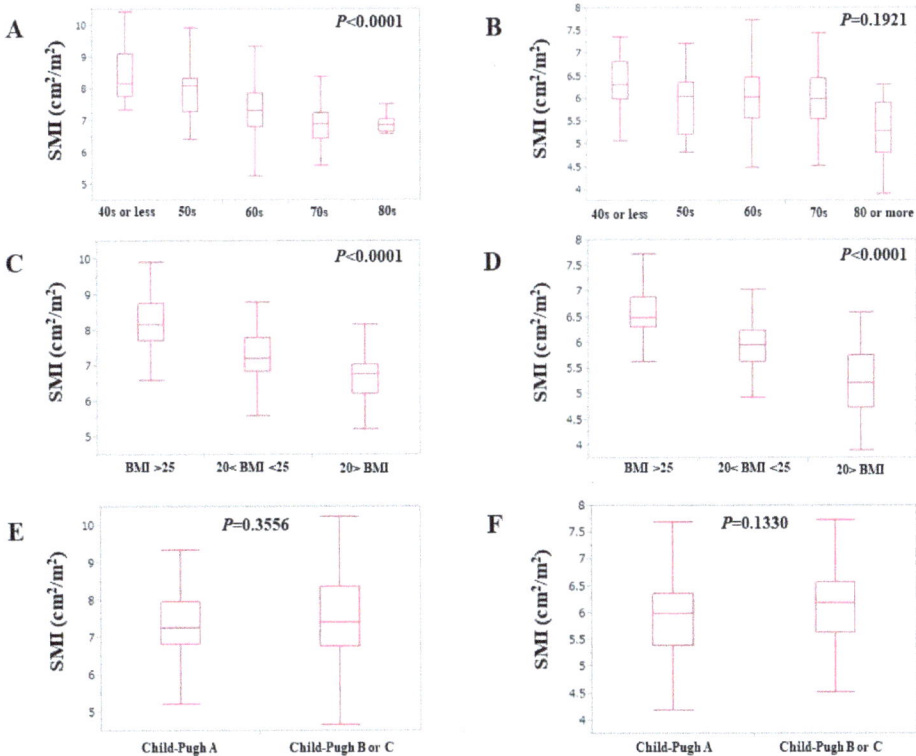

Figure 1. (**A,B**) Relationship between SMI and age in males (**A**) and females (**B**). (**C,D**) Relationship between SMI and BMI in males (**C**) and females (**D**). (**E,F**) Relationship between SMI and Child-Pugh classification in males (**E**) and females (**F**). SMI: skeletal muscle mass index; BMI: body mass index.

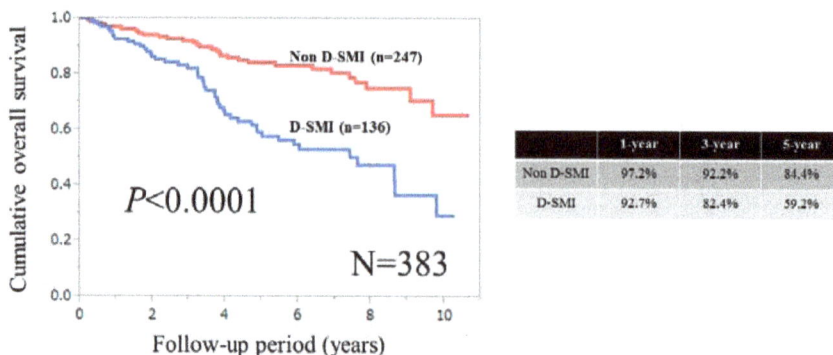

Figure 2. Cumulative overall survival for the entire cohort (*n* = 383). The one-, three-, and five-year cumulative OS rates were 92.7%, 82.4% and 59.2%, respectively, in patients with decreased SMI (D-SMI), and 97.2%, 92.2% and 84.4%, respectively, in patients without D-SMI ($p < 0.0001$). D-SMI was defined according to the Asian Working Group for Sarcopenia criteria. The cut-off values for SMI are 7.0 kg/m^2 for males and 5.7 kg/m^2 for females. SMI: skeletal muscle mass index; D-SMI: decreased SMI.

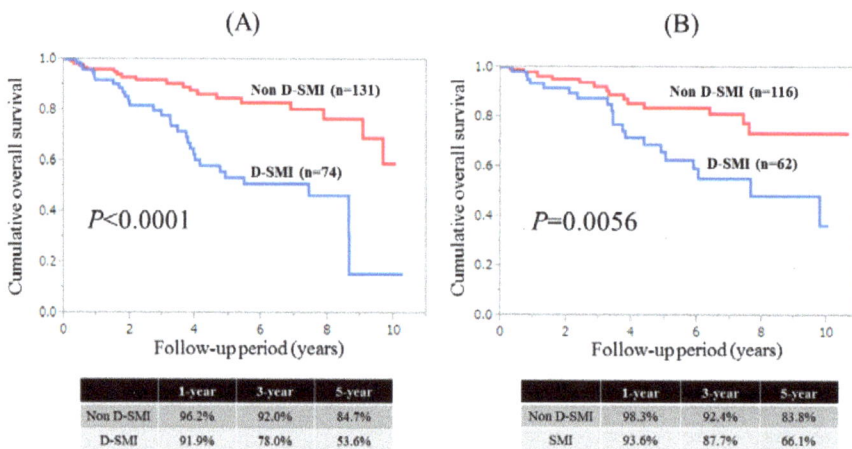

Figure 3. Cumulative overall survival for males (**A**) *n* = 205 and for females (**B**) *n* = 178 in patients with and without D-SMI. SMI: skeletal muscle mass index; D-SMI: decreased SMI.

Using ROC analysis for survival, the optimal cut-off point for SMI was 7.0 cm^2/m^2 in males (AUROC = 0.672, sensitivity = 64.6%, specificity = 69.4%) and 5.4 cm^2/m^2 in females (AUROC = 0.658, sensitivity = 45.7%, specificity = 83.9%). When the cut-off value of 5.4 cm^2/m^2 was adapted to our female patients (cut-off value for female in WAGS; 5.7 cm^2/m^2), similar results were obtained. That is, patients with D-SMI had significantly poorer survival rates than those without D-SMI ($p = 0.0076$).

3.3. Causes for Death for Males and Females

In male, during the observation period, 48 patients (23.4%) died. The causes for death were liver failure in 28 patients, HCC progression in 10 patients and miscellaneous causes in 10 patients. In female, during the observation period, 35 patients (19.7%) died. The causes for death were liver failure in 28 patients, HCC progression in four patients and miscellaneous causes in three patients.

3.4. Univariate and Multivariate Analyses of Parameters Contributing to OS for Males

Univariate analysis identified the following factors as significantly associated with OS for males: age ($p = 0.0041$); SMI ($p < 0.0001$); Child-Pugh score ($p = 0.0252$); aspartate aminotransferase ($p = 0.0150$); alanine aminotransferase (ALT) ($p = 0.0407$); serum albumin ($p = 0.0011$); serum sodium ($p = 0.0133$); serum creatinine ($p = 0.0088$); and BMI ($p = 0.0041$) (Table 2a). Since the Child-Pugh score includes serum albumin, it was not entered into the multivariate analysis, and since age and BMI significantly correlated with SMI, they were also excluded in the multivariate analysis to avoid the effect of collinearity. The hazard ratios (HRs) and 95% confidence intervals (CIs) calculated by using multivariate analysis for the six significant variables ($p < 0.05$) in the univariate analysis are presented in Table 2b. SMI ($p = 0.0005$) and Child-Pugh score ($p = 0.0424$) were found to be significant predictors related to OS in the multivariate analysis (Table 2b).

Table 2. (a) Univariate analyses of factors linked to overall survival for males ($n = 205$). (b) Multivariate analyses of factors linked to overall survival for male.

(a)		
Variables	Number of Each Category	Univariate *p* Value
Age (years) $\geq$ 70, yes/no	91/114	0.0041
Cause of liver diseases, B/C/others	22/122/61	0.2746
SMI $\geq$ 7.0 cm^2/m^2, yes/no	127/78	<0.0001
Child-Pugh score $\geq$ 6, yes/no	99/106	0.0252
AST $\geq$ 29 IU/L, yes/no	146/59	0.0150
ALT $\geq$ 47 IU/L, yes/no	63/142	0.0407
Serum albumin $\geq$ 3.7 g/dL, yes/no	113/92	0.0011
Total bilirubin $\geq$ 2.0 mg/dL, yes/no	29/176	0.1539
Prothrombin time $\geq$ 77.1%, yes/no	111/94	0.4521
Platelet count $\geq$ 9.4 $\times$ 10^4/mm^3, yes/no	101/104	0.2360
Total cholesterol $\geq$ 124 mg/dL, yes/no	165/40	0.2398
Triglyceride $\geq$ 56 mg/dL, yes/no	170/35	0.0649
Serum sodium $\geq$ 138 mmol/L, yes/no	166/39	0.0133
Fasting blood glucose $\geq$ 97 mg/dL, yes/no	145/60	0.4942
Serum creatinine $\geq$ 0.78 mg/dL, yes/no	84/121	0.0088
Body mass index $\geq$ 23.4 kg/m^2, yes/no	91/114	0.0041
Ascites, yes/no	25/180	0.0712

(b)			
Variables	Multivariate Analysis		
	Hazard Ratio	95% CI	*p* Value
SMI (per one cm^2/m^2)	0.571	0.416–0.777	0.0005
AST (per one IU/L)	1.005	0.987–1.022	0.5683
ALT (per one IU/L)	0.990	0.972–1.008	0.3002
Child-Pugh score (per one point)	1.270	1.020–1.520	0.0424
Serum sodium (per one mmol/L)	0.912	0.807–1.033	0.1481
Serum creatinine (per one mg/dL)	1.104	0.769–1.397	0.4914

CI: confidence interval; SMI: skeletal muscle mass index; AST: aspartate aminotransferase; ALT: alanine aminotransferase.

3.5. Univariate and Multivariate Analyses of Parameters Contributing to OS for Females

Univariate analysis identified the following parameters as significantly associated with OS for females: age ($p = 0.0214$); SMI ($p = 0.0076$); Child-Pugh score ($p = 0.0009$); ALT ($p = 0.0104$); serum albumin ($p = 0.0003$); prothrombin time (PT) ($p = 0.0355$); platelet count ($p = 0.0333$); triglyceride ($p = 0.0011$); serum creatinine ($p = 0.0137$); BMI ($p = 0.0270$) and presence of ascites ($p < 0.0001$) (Table 3a). As the Child-Pugh score includes serum albumin, PT, and ascites, they were not entered into the multivariate analysis, and because BMI significantly correlated with SMI, it was also excluded in the multivariate analysis to avoid the effect of collinearity. The HRs and 95% CIs calculated by using multivariate analysis for the seven significant variables ($p < 0.05$) in the univariate analysis are presented in Table 3b. SMI ($p = 0.0016$) and Child-Pugh scores ($p < 0.0001$) were found to be significant predictors related to OS in the multivariate analysis (Table 3b).

Table 3. (**a**) Univariate analyses of factors linked to overall survival for female ($n = 178$). (**b**) Multivariate analyses of factors linked to overall survival for female.

(a)

Variables	Number of Each Category	Univariate p value
Age (years) $\geq$ 77, yes/no	22/156	0.0214
Cause of liver diseases, B/C/others	10/113/55	0.5037
SMI $\geq$ 5.4 cm^2/m^2, yes/no	139/39	0.0076
Child-Pugh score $\geq$ 6, yes/no	98/80	0.0009
AST $\geq$ 80 IU/L, yes/no	20/158	0.0544
ALT $\geq$ 58 IU/L, yes/no	32/146	0.0104
Serum albumin $\geq$ 3.4 g/dL, yes/no	117/61	0.0003
Total bilirubin $\geq$ 2.3 mg/dL, yes/no	10/168	0.7607
Prothrombin time $\geq$ 73.7%, yes/no	103/75	0.0355
Platelet count $\geq$ 9.7 $\times 10^4$/mm^3, yes/no	92/86	0.0333
Total cholesterol $\geq$ 176 mg/dL, yes/no	49/129	0.0558
Triglyceride $\geq$ 72 mg/dL, yes/no	108/70	0.0011
Serum sodium $\geq$ 139 mmol/L, yes/no	143/35	0.4064
Fasting blood glucose $\geq$ 89 mg/dL, yes/no	142/36	0.2428
Serum creatinine $\geq$ 0.63 mg/dL, yes/no	66/112	0.0137
Body mass index $\geq$ 23.4 kg/m^2, yes/no	78/100	0.0270
Ascites, yes/no	19/159	<0.0001

(b)

Variables	Multivariate Analysis		
	Hazard ratio	95% CI	p Value
Age (per one year)	1.018	0.977–1.063	0.3998
SMI (per one cm^2/m^2)	0.450	0.270–0.731	0.0016
ALT (per one IU/L)	0.987	0.967–1.107	0.0506
Platelet count (per one $\times 10^4$/mm^3)	0.919	0.828–1.008	0.0943
Child-Pugh score (per one point)	1.938	1.400–2.690	<0.0001
Triglyceride (per one mg/dL)	0.998	0.983–1.011	0.7760
Serum creatinine (per one mg/dL)	2.546	0.413–10.860	0.2545

CI: confidence interval; SMI: skeletal muscle mass index; AST: aspartate aminotransferase; ALT: alanine aminotransferase.

3.6. Time-Dependent ROC Analyses for OS in Males

Results for time-dependent ROC analyses at two-, three-, four-, five-, six-, and seven-years of SMI and the Child-Pugh scores for males are shown in Figure 4A. All AUROCs for SMI at each time point were higher than those for Child-Pugh scores, denoting that SMI had consistently superior predictive ability for OS over Child-Pugh scores.

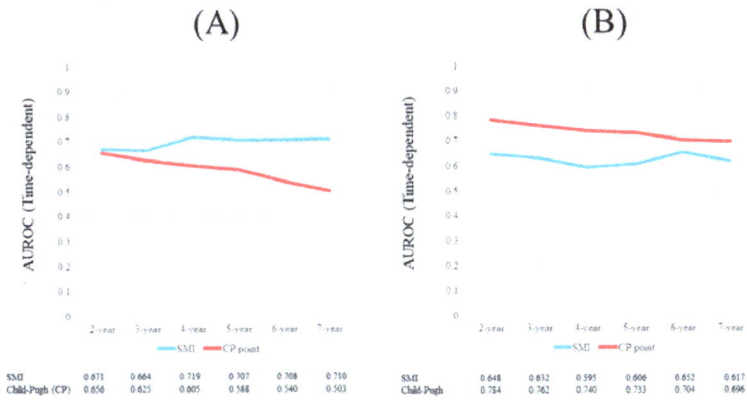

SMI	0.671	0.664	0.719	0.707	0.708	0.710
Child-Pugh (CP)	0.656	0.625	0.605	0.588	0.540	0.503

SMI	0.648	0.632	0.595	0.606	0.652	0.617
Child-Pugh	0.754	0.762	0.740	0.733	0.704	0.696

Figure 4. (**A**) Results for time-dependent ROC analyses at two-, three, four-, five-, six-, and seven-years of SMI and Child-Pugh scores for males; (**B**) Results for time-dependent ROC analyses at two-, three-, four-, five-, six-, and seven-years of SMI and Child-Pugh scores for females. ROC; receiver operating characteristics, AUROC; area under the ROC, SMI; skeletal muscle mass index, CP; Child-Pugh.

3.7. Time-Dependent ROC Analyses for OS in Females

Results for time-dependent ROC analyses at two-, three-, four-, five-, six-, and seven-years of SMI and Child-Pugh score for female were shown in Figure 4B. All AUROCs for Child-Pugh scores at each time point were higher than those for SMI, denoting that Child-Pugh scores had consistently superior predictive ability for OS over SMI.

3.8. Time-Dependent ROC Analyses for OS in Male Patients with Child-Pugh A

Results for time-dependent ROC analyses at two-, three-, four-, and five-years of SMI and Child-Pugh scores for male Child-Pugh A patients ($n = 148$) are shown in Figure 5A. All AUROCs for SMI in each time point were higher than those for Child-Pugh scores, denoting that SMI had consistently superior predictive ability for OS over Child-Pugh scores.

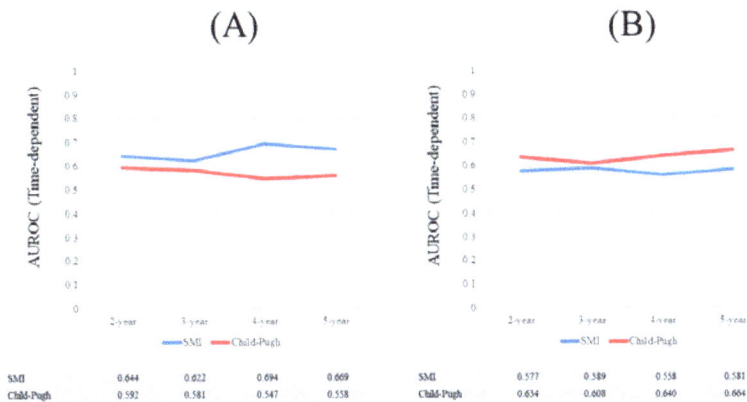

SMI	0.644	0.622	0.694	0.609
Child-Pugh	0.592	0.581	0.547	0.558

SMI	0.577	0.589	0.558	0.581
Child-Pugh	0.634	0.608	0.640	0.664

Figure 5. (**A**) Results for time-dependent ROC analyses at two-, three-, four-, and five-years of SMI and Child-Pugh scores for male Child-Pugh A patients; (**B**) Results for time-dependent ROC analyses at two-, three-, four-, and five-years of SMI and Child-Pugh scores for female Child-Pugh A patients. ROC; receiver operating characteristics, AUROC; area under the ROC, SMI; skeletal muscle mass index.

3.9. Time-Dependent ROC Analyses for OS in Female Patients with Child-Pugh A

Results for time-dependent ROC analyses at two-, three-, four-, and five-years of SMI and Child-Pugh scores for female Child-Pugh A patients (n = 131) are shown in Figure 5B. All AUROCs for Child-Pugh score in each time point were higher than those for SMI, denoting that Child-Pugh scores had consistently superior predictive ability for OS over SMI.

3.10. Time-Dependent ROC Analyses for OS in Male Patients with Child-Pugh B or C

Results for time-dependent ROC analyses at two-, three-, four-, and five-years of SMI and Child-Pugh scores for male Child-Pugh B or C patients (n = 57) are shown in Figure 6A. All AUROCs for SMI at each time point were higher than those for Child-Pugh scores, denoting that SMI had consistently superior predictive ability for OS over Child-Pugh scores.

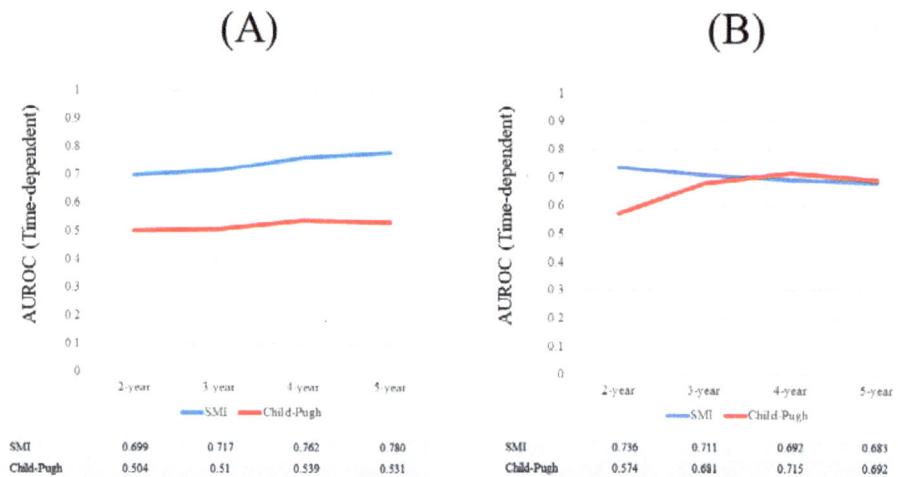

	2-year	3-year	4-year	5-year
SMI	0.699	0.717	0.762	0.780
Child-Pugh	0.504	0.51	0.539	0.531

	2-year	3-year	4-year	5-year
SMI	0.736	0.711	0.692	0.683
Child-Pugh	0.574	0.681	0.715	0.692

Figure 6. (**A**) Results for time-dependent ROC analyses at two-, three-, four-, and five-years of SMI and Child-Pugh score for male Child-Pugh B or C patients; (**B**) Results for time-dependent ROC analyses at two-, three-, four-, and five-years of SMI and Child-Pugh scores for female Child-Pugh B or C patients. ROC; receiver operating characteristics, AUROC; area under the ROC, SMI; skeletal muscle mass index.

3.11. Time-Dependent ROC Analyses for OS in Female Patients with Child-Pugh B or C

Results for time-dependent ROC analyses at two-, three-, four-, and five-years of SMI and Child-Pugh scores for female Child-Pugh B or C patients (n = 47) are shown in Figure 6B. At four- and five-years, Child-Pugh scores had higher AUROC than SMI.

4. Discussion

To the best of our knowledge, this is the first comparative study in SMI and Child-Pugh scores on clinical outcomes in LC patients. The Child-Pugh scoring system is a well-established prognostic system in LC patients [5–9]. While, SMI in LC has been currently attracting much attention owing to its well predictive performance [14–17,19,27,28]. Investigation into the influence of SMI on outcomes in LC patients is pivotal and, particularly, clarifying which of these two markers has stronger predictive impact for LC is clinically essential in light of creating a novel prognostic system in LC patients. We, therefore, conducted this comparative analysis to address this question. Since skeletal muscle mass significantly can differ between male and female, we analyzed and discussed separately in males and females.

In our results, for males, SMI and Child-Pugh scores were revealed to be significant for OS in the multivariate analysis, and all AUROCs for SMI at each time point were higher than those for Child-Pugh scores. Additionally, in subgroup analyses for male patients with Child-Pugh A or Child-Pugh B or C, SMI had consistently higher AUROCs than the Child-Pugh score. For females, similar results were obtained in the multivariate analysis, however, all AUROCs for Child-Pugh scores at each time point were higher than those for SMI. These results denote that SMI as a predictor can perform well as compared with Child-Pugh score at least in male LC patients. Our current results may provide new information and shed some lights for the better comprehension of prognosis in LC patients. The significant difference in baseline characteristics in such as SMI, age, serum sodium, and serum creatinine between males and females can explain the different results according to gender. In particular, aging can be a significant predictor in LC patients [14,39,40]. Our country is an aging country [39,40]. The reasons for results in time-dependent ROC analysis in females may be attributed to our results that SMI did not significantly correlate with age in females.

In view of our current results, some interventional therapies, including BCAA therapy, testosterone therapy, or exercise, can be considered especially in male LC patients with lower skeletal muscle mass for ameliorating prognosis [13,35,41–43]. However, firm recommendations for LC patients are not currently available. As for cut-off value for BIA, AWGS recommends 2SDs below the average muscle mass of young adults (7.0 cm^2/m^2 for male and 5.7 cm^2/m^2 for female) [28]. In our outcome based ROC analysis, the optimal cut-off points for survival were 7.0 cm^2/m^2 for males and 5.4 cm^2/m^2 for females, which were quite similar to recommendations in AWGS and their recommendations were well validated in our analysis. From the viewpoint of outcome-based analysis, our results may be worthy of reporting.

As described above, it is of note that SMI significantly correlated with age in males, but not in females. In general, changes in muscle mass occur with aging and muscle mass loss is a common condition which is recognized as a part of aging [44]. However, our results showed that the rates of muscle mass decline can vary according to gender, suggesting that factors other than aging, such as diet intake and lifestyle, may influence the maintenance of healthy muscle mass [45]. On the other hand, although the liver transplantation allocation system utilizes MELD score to prioritize organs to the most ill subjects, MELD scores do not perform better than Child-Pugh scores in non-transplant settings. In other words, MELD scores can perform well in decompensated LC rather than compensated LC [8]. Due to the high proportion of patients with Child-Pugh A in our cohort, we did not include MELD scores in the analysis.

Several limitations must be acknowledged in our current analysis. First, this study is a single-center retrospective observational study utilizing data for BIA and parameters reflecting muscle function such as hang grip strength or walking speed were not assessed in this analysis. In future studies, both skeletal muscle mass and muscle function should be evaluated in outcome based analyses. Second, patients with severe ascites were excluded from our analysis because SMI can be overestimated in these patients. Thus, the number of Child-Pugh C patients was rather small and our results cannot be adapted to such patients. Body composition analyses using BIA can be challenging in LC patients with severe ascites. Finally, various treatments for underlying liver diseases were performed during follow-up period in each patient, potentially creating bias. However, our study results denoted that SMI had higher predictive ability, at least in male LC patients. Results in time-dependent ROC analysis support our assertion for the predictive superiority of SMI over Child-Pugh scores in males.

In conclusion, SMI can be accessible for predicting outcomes, at least in male LC patients. Some interventions for male patients with lower SMI may be recommended.

Acknowledgments: The authors would like to thank all medical staff in our hospital for data collection. Financial support is none.

Author Contributions: Hiroki Nishikawa and Hirayuki Enomoto analyzed the data and wrote the paper. Shuhei Nishiguchi supervised this work. The other remaining authors collected data.

Conflicts of Interest: The authors declare no conflict of interest.

Abbreviations

LC: liver cirrhosis; MELD: Model for End-stage Liver Disease; LT: liver transplantation; HCC: hepatocellular carcinoma; CT: computed tomography; MRI: magnetic resonance imaging; BIA: bioimpedance analysis; SMI: skeletal muscle mass index; BMI: body mass index; US: ultrasonography; BCAA: branched-chain amino acid; ROC: receiver operating characteristic curve; OS: overall survival; AUROC: area under the receiver operating characteristic curve; SD: standard deviation; AWGS: Asian Working Group for Sarcopenia criteria; D-SMI: decreased SMI; ALT: alanine aminotransferase; HR: hazard ratios; CI: confidence interval.

References

1. Cheung, K.; Lee, S.S.; Raman, M. Prevalence and mechanisms of malnutrition in patients with advanced liver disease, and nutrition management strategies. *Clin. Gastroenterol. Hepatol.* **2012**, *10*, 117–125. [CrossRef] [PubMed]
2. Charlton, M.R. Branched-chain amino acid enriched supplements as therapy for liver disease. *J. Nutr.* **2006**, *136* (Suppl. 1), 295S–298S. [CrossRef]
3. Kawaguchi, T.; Izumi, N.; Charlton, M.R.; Sata, M. Branched-chain amino acids as pharmacological nutrients in chronic liver disease. *Hepatology* **2011**, *54*, 1063–1070. [CrossRef] [PubMed]
4. Fukui, H.; Saito, H.; Ueno, Y.; Uto, H.; Obara, K.; Sakaida, I.; Shibuya, A.; Seike, M.; Nagoshi, S.; Segawa, M.; et al. Evidence-based clinical practice guidelines for liver cirrhosis 2015. *J. Gastroenterol.* **2016**, *51*, 629–650. [CrossRef] [PubMed]
5. Kamath, P.S.; Wiesner, R.H.; Malinchoc, M.; Kremers, W.; Therneau, T.M.; Kosberg, C.L.; D'Amico, G.; Dickson, E.R.; Kim, W.R. A model to predict survival in patients with end-stage liver disease. *Hepatology* **2001**, *33*, 464–470. [CrossRef] [PubMed]
6. Kim, W.R.; Biggins, S.W.; Kremers, W.K.; Wiesner, R.H.; Kamath, P.S.; Benson, J.T.; Edwards, E.; Therneau, T.M. Hyponatremia and mortality among patients on the liver-transplant waiting list. *N. Engl. J. Med.* **2008**, *359*, 1018–1026. [CrossRef] [PubMed]
7. D'Amico, G.; Garcia-Tsao, G.; Pagliaro, L. Natural history and prognostic indicators of survival in cirrhosis: A systematic review of 118 studies. *J. Hepatol.* **2006**, *44*, 217–231. [CrossRef] [PubMed]
8. Cholongitas, E.; Papatheodoridis, G.V.; Vangeli, M.; Terreni, N.; Patch, D.; Burroughs, A.K. Systematic review: The model for end-stage liver disease—Should it replace Child-Pugh's classification for assessing prognosis in cirrhosis? *Aliment. Pharmacol. Ther.* **2005**, *22*, 1079–1089. [CrossRef] [PubMed]
9. Botta, F.; Giannini, E.; Romagnoli, P.; Fasoli, A.; Malfatti, F.; Chiarbonello, B.; Testa, E.; Risso, D.; Colla, G.; Testa, R. MELD scoring system is useful for predicting prognosis in patients with liver cirrhosis and is correlated with residual liver function: A European study. *Gut* **2003**, *52*, 134–139. [CrossRef] [PubMed]
10. Periyalwar, P.; Dasarathy, S. Malnutrition in cirrhosis: Contribution and consequences of sarcopenia on metabolic and clinical responses. *Clin. Liver Dis.* **2012**, *16*, 95–131. [CrossRef] [PubMed]
11. Cruz-Jentoft, A.J.; Landi, F.; Schneider, S.M.; Zúñiga, C.; Arai, H.; Boirie, Y.; Chen, L.K.; Fielding, R.A.; Martin, F.C.; Michel, J.P.; et al. Prevalence of and interventions for sarcopenia in ageing adults: A systematic review. Report of the International Sarcopenia Initiative (EWGSOP and IWGS). *Age Ageing* **2014**, *43*, 748–759. [CrossRef] [PubMed]
12. Sinclair, M.; Gow, P.J.; Grossmann, M.; Angus, P.W. Review article: Sarcopenia in cirrhosis—Aetiology, implications and potential therapeutic interventions. *Aliment. Pharmacol. Ther.* **2016**, *43*, 765–777. [CrossRef] [PubMed]
13. Hanai, T.; Shiraki, M.; Nishimura, K.; Ohnishi, S.; Imai, K.; Suetsugu, A.; Takai, K.; Shimizu, M.; Moriwaki, H. Sarcopenia impairs prognosis of patients with liver cirrhosis. *Nutrition* **2015**, *31*, 193–199. [CrossRef] [PubMed]
14. Nishikawa, H.; Shiraki, M.; Hiramatsu, A.; Moriya, K.; Hino, K.; Nishiguchi, S. JSH guidelines for sarcopenia in liver disease (first edition): Recommendation from the working group for creation of sarcopenia assessment criteria in the JSH. *Hepatol. Res.* **2016**, *46*, 951–963. [CrossRef] [PubMed]
15. Santilli, V.; Bernetti, A.; Mangone, M.; Paoloni, M. Clinical definition of sarcopenia. *Clin. Cases Miner. Bone Metab.* **2014**, *11*, 177–180. [CrossRef] [PubMed]
16. Nardelli, S.; Lattanzi, B.; Torrisi, S.; Greco, F.; Farcomeni, A.; Gioia, S.; Merli, M.; Riggio, O. Sarcopenia is Risk Factor for Development of Hepatic Encephalopathy After Transjugular Intrahepatic Portosystemic Shunt Placement. *Clin. Gastroenterol. Hepatol.* **2017**, *15*, 934–936. [CrossRef] [PubMed]

17. Itoh, S.; Shirabe, K.; Matsumoto, Y.; Yoshiya, S.; Muto, J.; Harimoto, N.; Yamashita, Y.; Ikegami, T.; Yoshizumi, T.; Nishie, A.; et al. Effect of body composition on outcomes after hepatic resection for hepatocellular carcinoma. *Ann. Surg. Oncol.* **2014**, *21*, 3063–3068. [CrossRef] [PubMed]
18. Carrara, G.; Pecorelli, N.; De Cobelli, F.; Cristel, G.; Damascelli, A.; Beretta, L.; Braga, M. Preoperative sarcopenia determinants in pancreatic cancer patients. *Clin. Nutr.* **2016**. [CrossRef] [PubMed]
19. Fujiwara, N.; Nakagawa, H.; Kudo, Y.; Tateishi, R.; Taguri, M.; Watadani, T.; Nakagomi, R.; Kondo, M.; Nakatsuka, T.; Minami, T.; et al. Sarcopenia, intramuscular fat deposition, and visceral adiposity independently predict the outcomes of hepatocellular carcinoma. *J. Hepatol.* **2015**, *63*, 131–140. [CrossRef] [PubMed]
20. Zhuang, C.L.; Huang, D.D.; Pang, W.Y.; Zhou, C.J.; Wang, S.L.; Lou, N.; Ma, L.L.; Yu, Z.; Shen, X. Sarcopenia is an Independent Predictor of Severe Postoperative Complications and Long-Term Survival after Radical Gastrectomy for Gastric Cancer: Analysis from a Large-Scale Cohort. *Medicine* **2016**, *95*, e3164. [CrossRef] [PubMed]
21. Harimoto, N.; Shirabe, K.; Yamashita, Y.I.; Ikegami, T.; Yoshizumi, T.; Soejima, Y.; Ikeda, T.; Maehara, Y.; Nishie, A.; Yamanaka, T. Sarcopenia as a predictor of prognosis in patients following hepatectomy for hepatocellular carcinoma. *Br. J. Surg.* **2013**, *100*, 1523–1530. [CrossRef] [PubMed]
22. Antoun, S.; Borget, I.; Lanoy, E. Impact of sarcopenia on the prognosis and treatment toxicities in patients diagnosed with cancer. *Curr. Opin. Support Palliat. Care* **2013**, *7*, 383–389. [CrossRef] [PubMed]
23. Iritani, S.; Imai, K.; Takai, K.; Hanai, T.; Ideta, T.; Miyazaki, T.; Suetsugu, A.; Shiraki, M.; Shimizu, M.; Moriwaki, H. Skeletal muscle depletion is an independent prognostic factor for hepatocellular carcinoma. *J. Gastroenterol.* **2015**, *50*, 323–332. [CrossRef] [PubMed]
24. Kamachi, S.; Mizuta, T.; Otsuka, T.; Nakashita, S.; Ide, Y.; Miyoshi, A.; Kitahara, K.; Eguchi, Y.; Ozaki, I.; Anzai, K. Sarcopenia is a risk factor for the recurrence of hepatocellular carcinoma after curative treatment. *Hepatol. Res.* **2016**, *46*, 201–208. [CrossRef] [PubMed]
25. Suzuki, Y.; Okamoto, T.; Fujishita, T.; Katsura, M.; Akamine, T.; Takamori, S.; Morodomi, Y.; Tagawa, T.; Shoji, F.; Maehara, Y. Clinical implications of sarcopenia in patients undergoing complete resection for early non-small cell lung cancer. *Lung Cancer* **2016**, *101*, 92–97. [CrossRef] [PubMed]
26. Harimoto, N.; Yoshizumi, T.; Shimokawa, M.; Sakata, K.; Kimura, K.; Itoh, S.; Ikegami, T.; Ikeda, T.; Shirabe, K.; Maehara, Y. Sarcopenia is a poor prognostic factor following hepatic resection in patients 70 years of age and older with hepatocellular carcinoma. *Hepatol. Res.* **2016**, *46*, 1247–1255. [CrossRef] [PubMed]
27. Hamaguchi, Y.; Kaido, T.; Okumura, S.; Kobayashi, A.; Hammad, A.; Tamai, Y.; Inagaki, N.; Uemoto, S. Proposal for new diagnostic criteria for low skeletal muscle mass based on computed tomography imaging in Asian adults. *Nutrition* **2016**, *32*, 1200–1205. [CrossRef] [PubMed]
28. Chen, L.K.; Liu, L.K.; Woo, J.; Assantachai, P.; Auyeung, T.W.; Bahyah, K.S.; Chou, M.Y.; Chen, L.Y.; Hsu, P.S.; Krairit, O.; et al. Sarcopenia in Asia: Consensus Report of the Asian Working Group for Sarcopenia. *J. Am. Med. Dir. Assoc.* **2014**, *15*, 95–101. [CrossRef] [PubMed]
29. Dasarathy, S. Consilience in sarcopenia of cirrhosis. *J. Cachexia Sarcopenia Muscle* **2012**, *3*, 225–237. [CrossRef] [PubMed]
30. Montano-Loza, A.J. Clinical relevance of sarcopenia in patients with cirrhosis. *World J. Gastroenterol.* **2014**, *20*, 8061–8071. [CrossRef] [PubMed]
31. Kudo, M.; Zheng, R.Q.; Kim, S.R.; Okabe, Y.; Osaki, Y.; Iijima, H.; Itani, T.; Kasugai, H.; Kanematsu, M.; Ito, K.; et al. Diagnostic accuracy of imaging for liver cirrhosis compared to histologically proven liver cirrhosis. A multicenter collaborative study. *Intervirology* **2008**, *51*, 17–26. [CrossRef] [PubMed]
32. Zarski, J.P.; Sturm, N.; Guechot, J.; Paris, A.; Zafrani, E.S.; Asselah, T.; Boisson, R.C.; Bosson, J.L.; Guyader, D.; Renversez, J.C.; et al. Comparison of nine blood tests and transient elastography for liver fibrosis in chronic hepatitis C: The ANRS HCEP-23 study. *J. Hepatol.* **2012**, *56*, 55–62. [CrossRef] [PubMed]
33. Tsochatzis, E.A.; Gurusamy, K.S.; Ntaoula, S.; Cholongitas, E.; Davidson, B.R.; Burroughs, A.K. Elastography for the diagnosis of severity of fibrosis in chronic liver disease: A meta-analysis of diagnostic accuracy. *J. Hepatol.* **2011**, *54*, 650–659. [CrossRef] [PubMed]
34. Kumada, H.; Okanoue, T.; Onji, M.; Moriwaki, H.; Izumi, N.; Tanaka, E.; Chayama, K.; Sakisaka, S.; Takehara, T.; Oketani, M.; et al. Guidelines for the treatment of chronic hepatitis and cirrhosis due to hepatitis C virus infection for the fiscal year 2008 in Japan. *Hepatol. Res.* **2010**, *40*, 8–13. [CrossRef] [PubMed]

35. Kappus, M.R.; Mendoza, M.S.; Nguyen, D.; Medici, V.; McClave, S.A. Sarcopenia in Patients with Chronic Liver Disease: Can It Be Altered by Diet and Exercise? *Curr. Gastroenterol. Rep.* **2016**, *18*, 43. [CrossRef] [PubMed]
36. Heagerty, P.J.; Zheng, Y. Survival model predictive accuracy and ROC curves. *Biometrics* **2005**, *61*, 92–105. [CrossRef] [PubMed]
37. European Association for the Study of the Liver; European Organisation for Research and Treatment of Cancer. EASL-EORTC Clinical Practice guidelines: Management of hepatocellular carcinoma. *J. Hepatol.* **2012**, *56*, 908–943.
38. Kudo, M.; Izumi, N.; Kokudo, N.; Matsui, O.; Sakamoto, M.; Nakashima, O.; Kojiro, M.; Makuuchi, M.; HCC Expert Panel of Japan Society of Hepatology. Management of hepatocellular carcinoma in Japan: Consensus-Based Clinical Practice Guidelines proposed by the Japan Society of Hepatology (JSH) 2010 updated version. *Dig Dis.* **2011**, *29*, 339–364. [CrossRef] [PubMed]
39. Asahina, Y.; Tsuchiya, K.; Tamaki, N.; Hirayama, I.; Tanaka, T.; Sato, M.; Yasui, Y.; Hosokawa, T.; Ueda, K.; Kuzuya, T.; et al. Effect of aging on risk for hepatocellular carcinoma in chronic hepatitis C virus infection. *Hepatology* **2010**, *52*, 518–527. [CrossRef] [PubMed]
40. Osaki, Y.; Nishikawa, H. Treatment for hepatocellular carcinoma in Japan over the last three decades: Our experience and published work review. *Hepatol Res.* **2015**, *45*, 59–74. [CrossRef] [PubMed]
41. Davuluri, G.; Krokowski, D.; Guan, B.J.; Kumar, A.; Thapaliya, S.; Singh, D.; Hatzoglou, M.; Dasarathy, S. Metabolic adaptation of skeletal muscle to hyperammonemia drives the beneficial effects of l-leucine in cirrhosis. *J. Hepatol.* **2016**, *65*, 929–937. [CrossRef] [PubMed]
42. Sinclair, M.; Grossmann, M.; Hoermann, R.; Angus, P.W.; Gow, P.J. Testosterone therapy increases muscle mass in men with cirrhosis and low testosterone: A randomised controlled trial. *J. Hepatol.* **2016**, *65*, 906–913. [CrossRef] [PubMed]
43. Dasarathy, S. Cause and management of muscle wasting in chronic liver disease. *Curr. Opin. Gastroenterol.* **2016**, *32*, 159–165. [CrossRef] [PubMed]
44. St-Onge, M.P. Relationship between body composition changes and changes in physical function and metabolic risk factors in aging. *Curr. Opin. Clin. Nutr. Metab. Care* **2005**, *8*, 523–528. [PubMed]
45. Syddall, H.; Evandrou, M.; Cooper, C.; Sayer, A.A. Social inequalities in grip strength, physical function, and falls among community dwelling older men and women: Findings from the Hertfordshire Cohort Study. *J. Aging Health* **2009**, *21*, 913–939. [CrossRef] [PubMed]

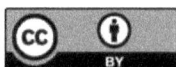

nutrients

MDPI

Article

Impact of Virtual Touch Quantification in Acoustic Radiation Force Impulse for Skeletal Muscle Mass Loss in Chronic Liver Diseases

Hiroki Nishikawa, Takashi Nishimura, Hirayuki Enomoto *, Yoshinori Iwata, Akio Ishii, Yuho Miyamoto, Noriko Ishii, Yukihisa Yuri, Ryo Takata, Kunihiro Hasegawa, Chikage Nakano, Kazunori Yoh, Nobuhiro Aizawa, Yoshiyuki Sakai, Naoto Ikeda, Tomoyuki Takashima, Shuhei Nishiguchi and Hiroko Iijima

Division of Hepatobiliary and Pancreatic disease, Department of Internal Medicine, Hyogo College of Medicine, Hyogo 6638501, Japan; nishikawa_6392@yahoo.co.jp (H.N.); tk-nishimura@hyo-med.ac.jp (T.N.); yo-iwata@hyo-med.ac.jp (Y.I.); akio0010@yahoo.co.jp (A.I.); yuho.0818.1989@gmail.com (Y.M.); ishinori1985@yahoo.co.jp (N.I.); gyma27ijo04td@gmail.com (Y.Y.); chano_chano_rt@yahoo.co.jp (R.T.); hiro.red1230@gmail.com (K.H.); chikage@hyo-med.ac.jp (C.N.); mm2wintwin@ybb.ne.jp (K.Y.); nobu23hiro@yahoo.co.jp (N.A.); sakai429@hyo-med.ac.jp (Y.S.); nikeneko@hyo-med.ac.jp (N.I.); tomo0204@yahoo.co.jp (T.T.); nishiguc@hyo-med.ac.jp (S.N.); hiroko-i@hyo-med.ac.jp (H.I.)
* Correspondence: enomoto@hyo-med.ac.jp; Tel.: +81-798-45-6111; Fax: +81-798-45-6608

Received: 2 June 2017; Accepted: 14 June 2017; Published: 16 June 2017

Abstract: Background and aims: We sought to clarify the relationship between virtual touch quantification (VTQ) in acoustic radiation force impulse and skeletal muscle mass as assessed by bio-electronic impedance analysis in patients with chronic liver diseases (CLDs, n = 468, 222 males and 246 females, median age = 62 years). Patients and methods: Decreased skeletal muscle index (D-SMI) was defined as skeletal muscle index (SMI) <7.0 kg/m^2 for males and as SMI <5.7 kg/m^2 for females, according to the recommendations in current Japanese guidelines. We examined the correlation between SMI and VTQ levels and investigated factors linked to D-SMI in the univariate and multivariate analyses. The area under the receiver operating curve (AUROC) for the presence of D-SMI was also calculated. Results: In patients with D-SMI, the median VTQ level was 1.64 meters/second (m/s) (range, 0.93–4.32 m/s), while in patients without D-SMI, the median VTQ level was 1.11 m/s (range, 0.67–4.09 m/s) (p < 0.0001). In the multivariate analysis, higher VTQ was found to be an independent predictor linked to the presence of D-SMI (p < 0.0001). In receiver operating characteristic analysis, body mass index had the highest AUROC (0.805), followed by age (0.721) and VTQ (0.706). Conclusion: VTQ levels can be useful for predicting D-SMI in patients with CLDs.

Keywords: virtual touch quantification; skeletal muscle mass; bio-electronic impedance analysis; liver fibrosis marker; predictive ability

---

1. Introduction

The severity of liver fibrosis in patients with chronic liver diseases (CLDs) is the major determinant of long-term clinical outcomes, driving both the development of liver-related complications and mortality [1–4]. Thus, evaluating the degree of liver fibrosis correctly plays a pivotal role for the control of disease progression and for creating treatment strategies and evaluating the prognosis for CLD patients [5,6]. High diagnostic accuracy, easy accessibility, and the possibility for follow-up examinations can lead to the implementation of non-invasive diagnostic methods into daily clinical practice.

Acoustic radiation force impulse (ARFI), which is a technology designed to measure shear wave-front at multiple sites to estimate tissue stiffness, is a novel ultrasound-based radiological technique for non-invasively assessing the degree of tissue stiffness [7–10]. This modality can evaluate the degree of liver fibrosis easily and accurately in the clinical settings [10,11]. ARFI elastography has two modes which involve qualitative response and quantitative response for virtual touch quantification (VTQ), and it measures transverse shear wave velocity values in meters/second (m/s). The shear wave velocity reflects tissue stiffness through a simple method: the stiffer the tissue, the higher shear wave velocity [7–11]. A recent meta-analysis demonstrated that ARFI elastography was a good method for evaluating the degree of liver fibrosis and had similar predictive value to transient elastography for significant fibrosis and liver cirrhosis (LC) [12]. Another recent study reported that spleen stiffness measured by ARFI imaging can predict clinical outcomes for LC patients with high accuracy [13]. On the other hand, several serum liver fibrosis markers for predicting the degree of liver fibrosis have been proposed and validated as well as radiological modalities for assessing liver fibrosis [12,14–16]. Of these, FIB-4 index and aspartate aminotransferase (AST) to platelet ratio index (APRI) have been the most widely utilized liver fibrosis markers in CLD patients [16–21].

On the other hand, skeletal muscle is regarded as having a role in maintaining energy metabolism and nutritional status, and the depletion of skeletal muscle mass may be a considerable impairment circumstance [22–25]. Skeletal muscle mass loss can be affected by aging, while LC is occasionally associated with this muscular disorder [22,23]. In our previous investigation, the percentage of skeletal muscle mass loss as determined by bio-electronic impedance analysis (BIA) in LC subjects was significantly higher than that in subjects with chronic hepatitis without LC [26]. Other studies have claimed the significant role of muscle mass assessment in LC patients as a helpful marker for reflecting malnutrition and liver function and for predicting clinical outcomes [26–30]. Recently, sarcopenic obesity, which is the coexistence of sarcopenia as defined by low muscle mass and muscle strength and obesity, has been treated with much caution due to its close linkage to clinical outcomes in CLD patients [31,32].

Considering these reports, the speculation that liver fibrosis marker level is associated with the development of skeletal muscle loss in patients with CLDs may be true. Several reports showing that the proportion of decreased skeletal muscle mass (D-SMI) demonstrated a linear increment with liver fibrosis progression in non-alcoholic fatty liver disease (NAFLD) or non-alcoholic steatohepatitis (NASH) patients support our hypothesis [33–35]. However, an extensive literature search has not shown the relationship between skeletal muscle mass and the liver fibrosis markers in CLD patients, and these clinical questions should be fully addressed. In this study, we sought to clarify the relationship between radiological or serum liver fibrosis markers (VTQ, FIB-4 index, APRI, and platelet count) and skeletal muscle mass, as well as to investigate factors linked to the decrease in skeletal muscle mass in CLD patients.

2. Patients and Methods

2.1. Patients

In this retrospective study, we analyzed 549 patients with CLD who were admitted to the Division of Hepatobiliary and Pancreatic disease, Department of Internal Medicine, Hyogo College of Medicine, Hyogo, Japan between October 2008 and May 2014, and were assessed using BIA to diagnose decreased skeletal muscle mass. All CLD patients who agreed to nutritional evaluation were included. Next, patients without data for VTQ ($n = 48$), those with advanced malignancies which potentially affect the development of muscle mass loss ($n = 16$), and those with severe ascites ($n = 17$) were excluded. Patients with severe ascites were excluded because body weight and body mass index (BMI) may be overestimated in these patients, and skeletal muscle index (SMI) may also be overestimated by BIA [26]. Several edematous patients with advanced cirrhosis (Child-Pugh B or C), hypoalbuminemia, and severe ascites were thus excluded from the current analysis. A total of 468 CLD patients were therefore analyzed. In this study, 447 patients underwent liver biopsy. For patients without liver biopsy data ($n = 21$), LC was determined by radiological findings such as deformity of the liver surface and presence of varices. We assessed skeletal muscle mass by employing SMI using BIA at baseline. SMI indicates appendicular skeletal muscle mass divided by height squared (cm^2/m^2). D-SMI was defined as SMI <7.0 kg/m^2 for males and as SMI <5.7 kg/m^2 for females, according to the recommendations in current Japanese guidelines [26]. We examined the correlation between SMI and liver fibrosis markers (VTQ, FIB-4 index, APRI, and platelet count) and investigated factors linked to D-SMI in the univariate and multivariate analyses.

APRI score was calculated as reported elsewhere: AST level/upper limit of normal level for AST/platelet count ($\times 10^9/L$) $\times$ 100 [17–20]. The FIB-4 index was calculated as reported elsewhere: age (years) $\times$ AST (IU/L) /platelet count ($\times 10^9/L$) $\times \sqrt{}$alanine aminotransferase (ALT) (IU/L) [19–21]. Our protocols for liver biopsy were detailed in our previous study, and the degrees of liver fibrosis and inflammation were determined as reported elsewhere [36]. The ethics committee meeting of Hyogo college of medicine acknowledged this study protocol (approval number: 2117, approval date: 1 March 2016). And our study protocol conformed to all of the regulations of the Declaration of Helsinki.

2.2. Measurement for VTQ

We have routinely used a Siemens ACUSON S2000/3000 (Mochida Siemens Medical Systems, Tokyo, Japan) for VTQ measurement. The method for VTQ measurement by ARFI was conducted as reported elsewhere [10]. Briefly, using intercostal approach by one experienced sonologist, the examination for VTQ measurement was performed on the right lobe of the liver with a measurement depth of 2–3 cm below the liver surface. When successful acquisitions for VTQ data six times at different sites in the liver were obtained on each subject, the median value of these was calculated and data were presented in m/s [10].

2.3. Statistical Analysis

For quantitative parameters, the statistical analysis between groups was performed using Student's *t* test, Mann-Whitney U-test, Kruskal-Wallis test, Fisher's exact test, or Spearman's rank correlation coefficient r_s as appropriate. Parameters with *p* value < 0.05 in the univariate analysis were entered into the multivariate analysis utilizing the logistic regression analysis. In the multivariate analyses, significant variables in the univariate analyses were changed to dichotomous covariates using each median value. Receiver operating characteristic curve (ROC) analysis for the presence of D-SMI was performed for calculating the area under the ROC (AUROC) in baseline quantitative variables. *p* values of less than 0.05 were considered to suggest significance. Data are presented as median values (range) unless otherwise mentioned. Statistical analysis was performed with the JMP 11 (SAS Institute Inc., Cary, NC, USA).

3. Results

3.1. Baseline Characteristics

The baseline characteristics of the analyzed subjects (*n* = 468) are shown in Table 1. There are 222 males and 246 females with the median (range) age of 62 (18–90) years. In terms of liver fibrosis stages, F4 was observed in 178 patients, F3 in 73, F2 in 73, F1 in 114, F0 in 9, and not tested in 21. Patients predominantly presented with hepatitis C virus (HCV) infection (57.1%, 267/468). The median (range) SMI for males and females were 7.35 (4.66–11.05) cm^2/m^2 and 5.86 (3.50–8.10) cm^2/m^2, respectively. In this analysis, there were 76 male patients with D-SMI (33.3%) and 99 female patients with D-SMI (40.2%) (*p* = 0.1823). VTQ ranged from 0.67 m/s to 4.32 m/s (median, 1.34 m/s). FIB-4 index ranged from 0.12 to 2.61 (median, 1.03). APRI ranged from 0.09 to 7.58 (median, 0.83). In males, a significant inverse correlation between VTQ and SMI was found ($r_s = -0.4276, p < 0.0001$). Similarly, in females, a significant inverse correlation between VTQ and SMI was found ($r_s = -0.2384, p = 0.0002$) (Figure 1A,B).

Table 1. Baseline characteristics ($n = 468$).

Variables	Number or Median (Range)
Age (years)	62 (18–90)
Gender, male/female	222/246
SMI (cm^2/m^2), male	7.35 (4.66–11.05)
SMI (cm^2/m^2), female	5.86 (3.50–8.10)
BMI (kg/m^2)	22.26 (13.05–41.94)
Cause of liver disease, B/C/B and C/alcoholic/others	47/267/4/17/133
AST (IU/L)	36 (12–182)
ALT (IU/L)	35 (7–268)
Serum albumin (g/dL)	3.9 (2.6–5.1)
Total bilirubin (mg/dL)	0.9 (0.2–5.1)
Prothrombin time (%)	89.8 (43.3–133.6)
Platelet count ($\times 10^4$/mm^3)	14.9 (2.1–50.4)
Total cholesterol (mg/dL)	167 (82–448)
Triglyceride (mg/dL)	91 (27–572)
Fasting blood glucose (mg/dL)	99 (70–298)
Serum creatinine (mg/dL)	0.67 (0.32–7.69)
BTR	5.58 (1.63–11.86)
Serum ammonia (µg/dL)	31 (5–137)
C reactive protein (mg/dL)	0.1 (0–2.4)
VTQ (m/s)	1.34 (0.67–4.32)
FIB-4 index	1.03 (0.12–2.61)
APRI	0.83 (0.09–7.58)
F stage, 0/1/2/3/4/NT	9/114/73/73/178/21

SMI: skeletal muscle index; BMI: body mass index; AST: aspartate aminotransferase; ALT: alanine aminotransferase; BTR: branched-chain amino acid to tyrosine ratio; VTQ: virtual touch quantification; APRI: AST to platelet ratio index; NT: not tested.

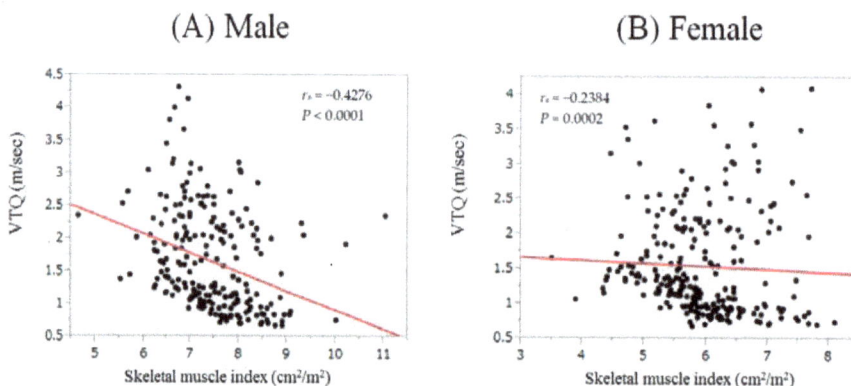

Figure 1. (**A**) Correlation between virtual touch quantification (VTQ) and skeletal muscle index (SMI) in males. Significant inverse correlation between VTQ and SMI was found ($r_s = -0.4276$, $p < 0.0001$); (**B**) Correlation between VTQ and SMI in females. Significant inverse correlation between VTQ and SMI was found ($r_s = -0.2384$, $p = 0.0002$).

3.2. VTQ Level according to The Degree of Liver Fibrosis

For the entire cohort (excluding 21 patients with missing data for liver histology, $n = 447$), the stepwise increase of VTQ level was found according to the severity of liver fibrosis (overall significance, $p < 0.0001$). (Figure 2A) Similarly, for patients with HCV (excluding patients with missing data for liver histology, $n = 246$), the stepwise increase of VTQ level was also found according to the severity of liver fibrosis (overall significance, $p < 0.0001$) (Figure 2B).

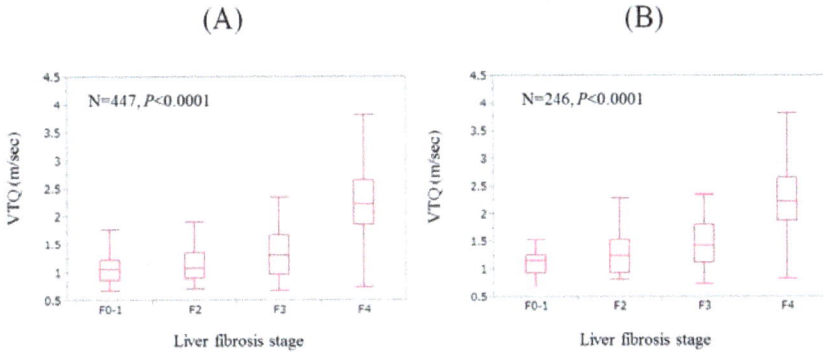

Figure 2. (**A**) VTQ level according to liver fibrosis stage for the entire cohort (excluding 21 patients with missing data for liver histology, $n = 447$). The stepwise increase of VTQ level was found according to the severity of liver fibrosis (overall significance, $p < 0.0001$); (**B**) VTQ level according to liver fibrosis stage for patients with hepatitis C virus (HCV) (excluding patients with missing data for liver histology, $n = 246$). The stepwise increase of VTQ level was found according to the severity of liver fibrosis (overall significance, $p < 0.0001$).

3.3. VTQ Level in Patients with and without D-SMI

In patients with D-SMI, the median VTQ level was 1.64 m/s (range, 0.93–4.32 m/s), while in patients without D-SMI, the median VTQ level was 1.11 m/s (range, 0.67–4.09 m/s) ($p < 0.0001$) (Figure 3A).

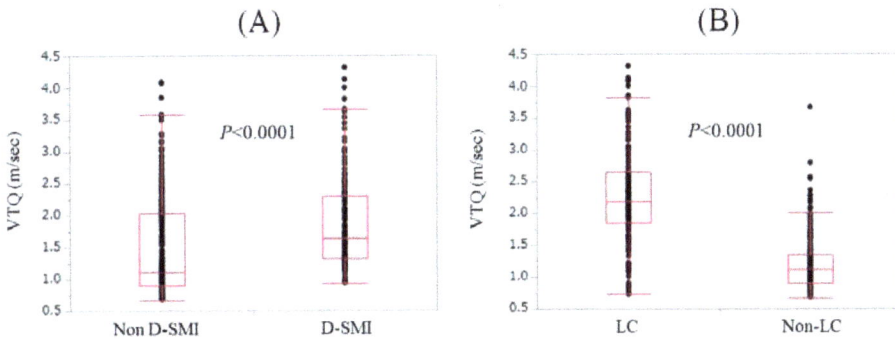

Figure 3. (**A**) VTQ level in patients with and without decreased skeletal muscle mass (D-SMI). In patients with D-SMI, the median VTQ level was 1.64 m/s (range, 0.93–4.32 m/s), while in patients without D-SMI, the median VTQ level was 1.11 m/s (range, 0.67–4.09 m/s) ($p < 0.0001$); (**B**) VTQ level according to liver cirrhosis (LC) status. In patients with LC, the median VTQ level was 2.18 m/s (range, 0.73–4.32 m/s), while in patients without LC, the median VTQ level was 1.11 m/s (range, 0.67–3.67 m/s) ($p < 0.0001$).

3.4. VTQ Level according to LC Status

In patients with LC, the median VTQ level was 2.18 m/s (range, 0.73–4.32 m/s), while in patients without LC, the median VTQ level was 1.11 m/s (range, 0.67–3.67 m/s) ($p < 0.0001$) (Figure 3B).

3.5. ROC Analysis for the Presence of D-SMI

Results for ROC analyses (AUROC, optimal cutoff point, sensitivity, and specificity) for the presence of D-SMI are presented in Table 2. BMI had the highest AUROC (0.805), followed by age (AUROC = 0.721), VTQ (AUROC = 0.706), and serum albumin (AUROC = 0.698).

Table 2. ROC analysis for decreased skeletal muscle index.

	AUROC	Cutoff Value	Sensitivity (%)	Specificity (%)
Age	0.721	62	72.57	62.80
Body mass index	0.805	22.78	85.14	61.77
AST	0.469	57.0	78.87	24.91
ALT	0.532	72.0	89.14	18.77
Serum albumin	0.698	4.0	85.14	54.27
Total bilirubin	0.535	0.80	53.4	54.95
Prothrombin time	0.504	85.7	68.57	38.91
Platelet count	0.579	17.8	76.00	41.64
Total cholesterol	0.521	192	76.57	31.06
Triglyceride	0.576	102	72.57	46.42
Fasting blood glucose	0.466	127	12.0	91.13
Serum creatinine	0.476	0.89	18.29	88.05
BTR	0.563	5.93	68.57	47.78
Serum ammonia	0.478	64	94.51	12.0
C reactive protein	0.548	0	53.71	57.68
VTQ	0.706	1.12	94.86	50.51
FIB-4 index	0.635	0.772	84.57	37.2
APRI	0.564	0.716	64.57	51.54

AUROC: area under the receiver operating curve; AST: aspartate aminotransferase; ALT: alanine aminotransferase; BTR: branched-chain amino acid to tyrosine ratio; VTQ: virtual touch quantification; APRI: AST to platelet ratio index.

3.6. Relationship between VTQ and Baseline Variables

Age (r_s = 0.4418, $p < 0.0001$), AST (r_s = 0.3315, $p < 0.0001$), total bilirubin (r_s = 0.1994, $p < 0.0001$), serum ammonia (r_s = 0.3191, $P < 0.0001$), FIB-4 index (r_s = 0.2122, $p = 0.0001$), and APRI (r_s = 0.6011, $p < 0.0001$) had significantly positive correlations with VTQ level. SMI in males (r_s = −0.4276, $p < 0.0001$), SMI in females (r_s = −0.2384, $p = 0.0002$), serum albumin (r_s = −0.5538, $p < 0.0001$), prothrombin time (r_s = −0.5504, $p < 0.0001$), platelet count (r_s = −0.6152, $p < 0.0001$), total cholesterol (r_s = −0.3941, $p < 0.0001$), triglyceride (r_s = −0.2075, $p < 0.0001$), and branched-chain amino acid to tyrosine ratio (BTR) (r_s = −0.6061, $p < 0.0001$) had significant inverse correlations with VTQ level (Table 3).

3.7. Univariate and Multivariate Analyses of Factors Contributing to The Presence of D-SMI

Significant variables linked to the presence of D-SMI in the univariate analyses are: age ($p < 0.0001$); BMI ($p < 0.0001$); serum albumin ($p < 0.0001$); platelet count ($p = 0.0044$); BTR ($p = 0.0219$); VTQ ($p < 0.0001$); FIB-4 index ($p < 0.0001$); and APRI ($p = 0.0204$) (Table 4). The odds ratios (ORs) and 95% confidence intervals calculated by using multivariate analysis for the eight significant parameters ($p < 0.05$) in the univariate analysis are presented in Table 5. BMI ($p < 0.0001$), age ($p < 0.0001$), serum albumin ($p < 0.0001$), BTR ($p = 0.0031$), VTQ ($p < 0.0001$), and FIB-4 index ($p = 0.0425$) were found to be independent predictors associated with the presence of D-SMI (Table 5).

Table 3. Relationship between VTQ level and baseline data.

	r_s	*p* Value
Age	0.4418	<0.0001
SMI, male	−0.4276	<0.0001
SMI, female	−0.2384	0.0002
Body mass index	−0.0746	0.1071
AST	0.3315	<0.0001
ALT	0.0121	0.7947
Serum albumin	−0.5538	<0.0001
Total bilirubin	0.1994	<0.0001
Prothrombin time	−0.5504	<0.0001
Platelet count	−0.6152	<0.0001
Total cholesterol	−0.3941	<0.0001
Triglyceride	−0.2075	<0.0001
Fasting blood glucose	0.0731	0.1140
Serum creatinine	0.0679	0.1427
BTR	−0.6061	<0.0001
Serum ammonia	0.3191	<0.0001
C reactive protein	0.0559	0.2277
FIB-4 index	0.2122	<0.0001
APRI	0.6011	<0.0001

VTQ: virtual touch quantification; SMI: skeletal muscle index; AST: aspartate aminotransferase; ALT: alanine aminotransferase; BTR: branched-chain amino acid to tyrosine ratio; APRI: AST to platelet ratio index.

Table 4. Comparison of baseline characteristics between patients with D-SMI (n = 185) and those without D-SMI (n = 304).

	Decreased Skeletal Muscle Mass (D-SMI) (n = 175)	Non D-SMI (n = 293)	*p* Value
Age (years)	67 (25–90)	58 (18–81)	<0.0001
Gender, male/female	76/99	146/147	0.1823
Cause of liver disease B/C/B and C/Alcohol/Others	15/113/2/6/39	32/154/2/11/94	0.0988
BMI (kg/m^2)	20.28 (13.05–31.14)	23.78 (17.21–41.94)	<0.0001
Serum albumin (g/dL)	3.7 (2.6–4.9)	4.1 (2.7–5.1)	<0.0001
Total bilirubin (mg/dL)	0.8 (0.3–5.1)	0.9 (0.2–4.7)	0.2045
Prothrombin time (%)	89.4 (55.5–123)	90.0 (43.3–133.6)	0.8143
Platelet count ($\times 10^4$/mm^3)	13.7 (3.3–40.8)	15.7 (2.1–50.4)	0.0044
AST (IU/L)	38 (13–125)	35 (12–182)	0.2571
ALT (IU/L)	34 (7–268)	36 (8–247)	0.2449
Total cholesterol (mg/dL)	166 (85–292)	167 (82–448)	0.3264
Triglyceride	85 (27–554)	97 (29–572)	0.1026
Fasting blood glucose	96 (70–298)	101 (73–249)	0.2169
BTR	5.33 (1.63–11.86)	5.83 (1.79–10.46)	0.0219
Serum creatinine (mg/dL)	0.65 (0.32–7.67)	0.68 (0.35–6.5)	0.3808
Serum ammonia	31 (10–105)	30 (5–137)	0.4519
C reactive protein	0 (0–2.3)	0.1 (0–2.4)	0.5844
VTQ	1.64 (0.93–4.32)	1.11 (0.67–4.09)	<0.0001
FIB-4 index	1.15 (0.36–2.61)	0.96 (0.12–2.60)	<0.0001
APRI	0.97 (0.20–4.23)	0.70 (0.09–7.58)	0.0204

SMI: skeletal muscle index; BMI: body mass index; AST: aspartate aminotransferase; ALT: alanine aminotransferase; BTR: branched-chain amino acid to tyrosine ratio; VTQ: virtual touch quantification; APRI: AST to platelet ratio index.

Table 5. Multivariate analyses of factors linked to the presence of D-SMI.

Variables	Multivariate Analysis		
	OR	95% CI	*p* Value
BMI (per one kg/m^2)	1.712	1.523–1.925	<0.0001
Age (per one year)	0.922	0.895–0.953	<0.0001
Platelet count (per one $\times 10^4$/mm^3)	1.017	0.969–1.068	0.5003
Serum albumin (per one g/dL)	4.832	2.148–10.872	<0.0001
BTR (per one)	1.374	1.107–1.704	0.0031
VTQ (per one m/s)	0.278	0.167–0.462	<0.0001
FIB-4 index (per one)	0.625	0.384–0.955	0.0425
APRI (per one)	0.455	0.189–1.095	0.0735

OR: Odds ratio; CI: confidence interval; BMI: body mass index; BTR: branched-chain amino acid to tyrosine ratio; VTQ: virtual touch quantification; APRI: AST to platelet ratio index.

4. Discussion and Conclusions

Radiological and serum liver fibrosis markers are useful markers and have been preferably used in the clinical settings for their non-invasiveness and easy availability [7–11,13]. Indeed, the stepwise increase of VTQ level according to the severity of liver fibrosis was found in our data. However, there have been no available data for the relationship between skeletal muscle mass and VTQ level in CLD patients. Because skeletal muscle mass in CLDs has been drawing much caution due to its prognostic significance, addressing this problem may be clinically essential [23,26,28–30]. We therefore conducted the current analysis. To the best of our knowledge, this is the first report linking skeletal muscle loss with liver damage in CLDs in a Japanese population using data for VTQ.

In our results, a significant inverse correlation between SMI and VTQ level in both males and females, and a significant difference of VTQ level between patients with and without D-SMI were found. Additionally, AUROC of VTQ for D-SMI was 0.706, and higher VTQ levels were revealed to be significantly associated with the development of D-SMI in the multivariate analysis ($p < 0.0001$). These results denote that VTQ level can be helpful for not only assessing the degree of liver fibrosis, but also for predicting D-SMI. A recent Korean study ($n = 309$) demonstrated that significant stratification was found in terms of the proportion of sarcopenia as evaluated by the appendicular skeletal muscle mass divided by body weight among subjects with normal livers, those with NAFLD, and those with NASH, which were in line with our current data [35].

Although LC-related muscle mass loss is defined as secondary sarcopenia as well as chronic inflammatory diseases and advanced malignancies, aging can cause D-SMI in CLDs at least in part [24,26]. The significant positive correlation between age and VTQ level ($r_s = 0.4418$, $p < 0.0001$) may be associated with our current results. The fact that FIB-4 index includes age may also well explain the statistical significance of FIB-4 index for predicting D-SMI in the multivariate analysis. As a greater number of Japanese CLD patients have been aging in recent years, this is a critical problem.

BTR had the second strongest correlation with VTQ level ($r_s = -0.6061$) and was revealed to be an independent predictor for the development of D-SMI ($p = 0.0031$). The liver is a central organ for the metabolism of three major classes of molecules: fats, proteins, and carbohydrates [37,38]. Deterioration in liver functional reserve can be accompanied by numerous nutritional disorders, and BTR reflects the nutritional state [39,40]. Poor nutritional status can cause muscle mass depletion. Branched-chain amino acid granules are promising for ameliorating muscle mass depletion [28]. In a sense, VTQ level may be helpful for assessing nutritional state in CLD patients. It is also of note that VTQ level had significant positive correlation with serum ammonia level ($r_s = 0.3191$, $p < 0.0001$). Elevated serum ammonia levels lead to the suppression of protein synthesis in the muscle [6,23,26].

In our results, lower BMI had strong impact on D-SMI, while in the Korean national study with large NAFLD cohort ($n = 2761$), the proportion of sarcopenia using dual-energy X-ray absorptiometry was prominent in obese patients [34]. The average BMIs in our study and their study were 22.8 kg/m^2

and 25.8 kg/m^2, respectively. In our cohort, 109 patients (23.3%) had BMI >25 kg/m^2 and only five patients (1.1%) had BMI >35 kg/m^2. The distribution of BMI in baseline characteristics between these studies may lead to such different results. The incidence of sarcopenic obesity has been increasing and the relation between muscle mass and BMI should be further examined in future studies [31,32].

We acknowledge several weak points to our study. First, this is a retrospective single center Japanese study. Thus, whether our data can be applied to other ethnic backgrounds remains unclear. Second, in this cross-sectional study, we are unable to interpret any causal relationship; in other words, an in-depth mechanism for the independent association between D-SMI and liver fibrosis was not clarified in our study. Third, liver biopsy has a significant limitation for sampling errors in evaluating the severity of liver fibrosis. Finally, patients with severe ascites who are expected to have D-SMI with higher rates were excluded from our analysis, potentially leading to bias. Caution should therefore be exercised when interpreting our results. However, our current results presented that VTQ can be useful for predicting D-SMI in CLD patients. In our previous investigation, we reported that a predictive model involving VTQ level is promising for assessing the risk of liver carcinogenesis [10]. Thus, we anticipate that VTQ involves various clinical significances for CLD patients.

In conclusion, VTQ level can provide useful insights for predicting D-SMI in patients with CLDs.

Acknowledgments: The authors would like to thank all medical staff in our nutritional guidance room and ultrasound center for data collection.

Author Contributions: Hiroki Nishikawa, Takashi Nishimura and Hirayuki Enomoto analyzed data and wrote the paper. Hiroko Iijima supervised this study. Other remaining authors collected data.

Conflicts of Interest: The authors declare no conflict of interest.

Abbreviations

CLDs: chronic liver diseases; ARFI: acoustic radiation force impulse; VTQ: virtual touch quantification; m/s: meters/second; LC: liver cirrhosis; AST: aspartate aminotransferase; BIA: bio-electronic impedance analysis; APRI: AST to platelet ratio index; NAFLD: non-alcoholic fatty liver disease; NASH: non-alcoholic steatohepatitis; BMI: body mass index; SMI: skeletal muscle mass; D-SMI: decreased skeletal muscle mass; ALT: alanine aminotransferase; ROC: receiver operating characteristic curve; AUROC: area under the ROC; HCV: hepatitis C virus; BTR: branched-chain amino acid to tyrosine ratio; ORs: odds ratios.

References

1. Van der Meer, A.J.; Berenguer, M. Reversion of disease manifestations after HCV eradication. *J. Hepatol.* **2016**, *65*, 95–108. [CrossRef] [PubMed]
2. Karanjia, R.N.; Crossey, M.M.; Cox, I.J.; Fye, H.K.; Njie, R.; Goldin, R.D.; Taylor-Robinson, S.D. Hepatic steatosis and fibrosis: Non-invasive assessment. *World J. Gastroenterol.* **2016**, *22*, 9880–9897. [CrossRef] [PubMed]
3. Friedrich-Rust, M.; Poynard, T.; Castera, L. Critical comparison of elastography methods to assess chronic liver disease. *Nat. Rev. Gastroenterol. Hepatol.* **2016**, *13*, 402–411. [CrossRef] [PubMed]
4. Westbrook, R.H.; Dusheiko, G. Natural history of hepatitis C. *J. Hepatol.* **2014**, *61*, 58–68. [CrossRef] [PubMed]
5. Yu, M.L. Hepatitis C Treatment from "Response-guided" to "Resource-guided" therapy in the transition era from IFN-containing to IFN-free regimens. *J. Gastroenterol. Hepatol.* **2017**. [CrossRef] [PubMed]
6. Majumdar, A.; Kitson, M.T.; Roberts, S.K. Systematic review: Current concepts and challenges for the direct-acting antiviral era in hepatitis C cirrhosis. *Aliment. Pharmacol. Ther.* **2016**, *43*, 1276–1292. [CrossRef] [PubMed]
7. Lupsor, M.; Badea, R.; Stefanescu, H.; Sparchez, Z.; Branda, H.; Serban, A.; Maniu, A. Performance of a new elastographic method (ARFI technology) compared to unidimensional transient elastography in the noninvasive assessment of chronic hepatitis C. Preliminary results. *J. Gastrointestin. Liver Dis.* **2009**, *18*, 303–310. [PubMed]
8. Takahashi, H.; Ono, N.; Eguchi, Y.; Eguchi, T.; Kitajima, Y.; Kawaguchi, Y.; Nakashita, S.; Ozaki, I.; Mizuta, T.; Toda, S.; et al. Evaluation of acoustic radiation force impulse elastography for fibrosis staging of chronic liver disease: A pilot study. *Liver Int.* **2010**, *30*, 538–545. [CrossRef] [PubMed]

9.   Friedrich-Rust, M.; Wunder, K.; Kriener, S.; Sotoudeh, F.; Richter, S.; Bojunga, J.; Herrmann, E.; Poynard, T.; Dietrich, C.F.; Vermehren, J.; et al. Liver fibrosis in viral hepatitis: Noninvasive assessment with acoustic radiation force impulse imaging versus transient elastography. *Radiology* **2009**, *252*, 595–604. [CrossRef] [PubMed]

10.   Aoki, T.; Iijima, H.; Tada, T.; Kumada, T.; Nishimura, T.; Nakano, C.; Kishino, K.; Shimono, Y; Yoh, K.; Takata, R.; et al. Prediction of development of hepatocellular carcinoma using a new scoring system involving virtual touch quantification in patients with chronic liver diseases. *J. Gastroenterol.* **2017**, *52*, 104–112. [CrossRef] [PubMed]

11.   Friedrich-Rust, M.; Nierhoff, J.; Lupsor, M.; Sporea, I.; Fierbinteanu-Braticevici, C.; Strobel, D.; Takahashi, H.; Yoneda, M.; Suda, T.; Zeuzem, S.; et al. Performance of acoustic radiation force impulse imaging for the staging of liver fibrosis: A pooled meta-analysis. *J. Viral Hepat.* **2012**, *19*, 212–219. [CrossRef] [PubMed]

12.   Bota, S.; Herkner, H.; Sporea, I.; Salzl, P.; Sirli, R.; Neghina, A.M.; Peck-Radosavljevic, M. Meta-analysis: ARFI elastography versus transient elastography for the evaluation of liver fibrosis. *Liver Int.* **2013**, *33*, 1138–1147. [CrossRef] [PubMed]

13.   Takuma, Y.; Morimoto, Y.; Takabatake, H.; Toshikuni, N.; Tomokuni, J.; Sahara, A.; Matsueda, K.; Yamamoto, H. Measurement of spleen stiffness with acoustic radiation force impulse imaging predicts mortality and hepatic decompensation in patients with liver cirrhosis. *Clin. Gastroenterol. Hepatol.* **2016**. [CrossRef] [PubMed]

14.   Lurie, Y.; Webb, M.; Cytter-Kuint, R.; Shteingart, S.; Lederkremer, G.Z. Non-invasive diagnosis of liver fibrosis and cirrhosis. *World J. Gastroenterol.* **2015**, *21*, 11567–11583. [CrossRef] [PubMed]

15.   De Lucca Schiavon, L.; Narciso-Schiavon, J.L.; de Carvalho-Filho, R.J. Non-invasive diagnosis of liver fibrosis in chronic hepatitis C. *World J. Gastroenterol.* **2014**, *20*, 2854–2866. [CrossRef] [PubMed]

16.   Castera, L.; Forns, X.; Alberti, A. Non-invasive evaluation of liver fibrosis using transient elastography. *J. Hepatol.* **2008**, *48*, 835–847. [CrossRef] [PubMed]

17.   Lin, Z.H.; Xin, Y.N.; Dong, Q.J.; Wang, Q.; Jiang, X.J.; Zhan, S.H.; Sun, Y.; Xuan, S.Y. Performance of the aspartate aminotransferase-to-platelet ratio index for the staging of hepatitis C-related fibrosis: An updated meta-analysis. *Hepatology* **2011**, *53*, 726–736. [CrossRef] [PubMed]

18.   Nishikawa, H.; Nishijima, N.; Enomoto, H.; Sakamoto, A.; Nasu, A.; Komekado, H.; Nishimura, T.; Kita, R.; Kimura, T.; Iijima, H.; et al. Comparison of FIB-4 index and aspartate aminotransferase to platelet ratio index on carcinogenesis in chronic hepatitis B treated with entecavir. *J. Cancer* **2017**, *8*, 152–161. [CrossRef] [PubMed]

19.   Xiao, G.; Yang, J.; Yan, L. Comparison of diagnostic accuracy of aspartate aminotransferase to platelet ratio index and fibrosis-4 index for detecting liver fibrosis in adult patients with chronic hepatitis B virus infection: A systemic review and meta-analysis. *Hepatology* **2015**, *61*, 292–302. [CrossRef] [PubMed]

20.   Kim, W.R.; Berg, T.; Asselah, T.; Flisiak, R.; Fung, S.; Gordon, S.C.; Janssen, H.L.A.; Lampertico, P.; Lau, D.; Bornstein, J.D.; et al. Evaluation of APRI and FIB-4 scoring systems for non-invasive assessment of hepatic fibrosis in chronic hepatitis B patients. *J. Hepatol.* **2016**, *64*, 773–780. [CrossRef] [PubMed]

21.   Houot, M.; Ngo, Y.; Munteanu, M.; Marque, S.; Poynard, T. Systematic review with meta-analysis: Direct comparisons of biomarkers for the diagnosis of fibrosis in chronic hepatitis C and B. *Aliment. Pharmacol. Ther.* **2016**, *43*, 16–29. [CrossRef] [PubMed]

22.   Cruz-Jentoft, A.J.; Baeyens, J.P.; Bauer, J.M.; Boirie, Y.; Cederholm, T.; Landi, F.; Martin, F.C.; Michel, J.P.; Rolland, Y.; Schneider, S.M.; et al. Sarcopenia: European consensus on definition and diagnosis: Report of the European Working Group on Sarcopenia in older people. *Age Ageing* **2010**, *39*, 412–423. [CrossRef] [PubMed]

23.   Dasarathy, S. Consilience in sarcopenia of cirrhosis. *J. Cachexia Sarcopenia Muscle* **2012**, *3*, 225–237. [CrossRef] [PubMed]

24.   Dasarathy, S.; Merli, M. Sarcopenia from mechanism to diagnosis and treatment in liver disease. *J. Hepatol.* **2016**, *65*, 1232–1244. [CrossRef] [PubMed]

25.   Sinclair, M.; Gow, P.J.; Grossmann, M.; Angus, P.W. Review article: Sarcopenia in cirrhosis-aetiology, implications and potential therapeutic interventions. *Aliment. Pharmacol. Ther.* **2016**, *43*, 765–777. [CrossRef] [PubMed]

26. Nishikawa, H.; Shiraki, M.; Hiramatsu, A.; Moriya, K.; Hino, K.; Nishiguchi, S. Japan Society of Hepatology guidelines for sarcopenia in liver disease: Recommendation from the working group for creation of sarcopenia assessment criteria. *Hepatol. Res.* **2016**, *46*, 951–963. [CrossRef] [PubMed]

27. Carey, E.J.; Lai, J.C.; Wang, C.W.; Dasarathy, S.; Lobach, I.; Montano-Loza, A.J.; Dunn, M.A. A multi-center study to define sarcopenia in patients with end-stage liver disease. *Liver Transpl.* **2017**. [CrossRef] [PubMed]

28. Hanai, T.; Shiraki, M.; Nishimura, K.; Ohnishi, S.; Imai, K.; Suetsugu, A.; Takai, K.; Shimizu, M.; Moriwaki, H. Sarcopenia impairs prognosis of patients with liver cirrhosis. *Nutrition* **2015**, *31*, 193–199. [CrossRef] [PubMed]

29. Durand, F.; Buyse, S.; Francoz, C.; Laouénan, C.; Bruno, O.; Belghiti, J.; Moreau, R.; Vilgrain, V.; Valla, D. Prognostic value of muscle atrophy in cirrhosis using psoas muscle thickness on computed tomography. *J. Hepatol.* **2014**, *60*, 1151–1157. [CrossRef] [PubMed]

30. Hanai, T.; Shiraki, M.; Watanabe, S.; Kochi, T.; Imai, K.; Suetsugu, A.; Takai, K.; Moriwaki, H.; Shimizu, M. Sarcopenia predicts minimal hepatic encephalopathy in patients with liver cirrhosis. *Hepatol. Res.* **2017**. [CrossRef] [PubMed]

31. Itoh, S.; Yoshizumi, T.; Kimura, K.; Okabe, H.; Harimoto, N.; Ikegami, T.; Uchiyama, H.; Shirabe, K.; Nishie, A.; Maehara, Y. Effect of sarcopenic obesity on outcomes of living-donor liver transplantation for hepatocellular carcinoma. *Anticancer Res.* **2016**, *36*, 3029–3034. [PubMed]

32. Hara, N.; Iwasa, M.; Sugimoto, R.; Mifuji-Moroka, R.; Yoshikawa, K.; Terasaka, E.; Hattori, A.; Ishidome, M.; Kobayashi, Y.; Hasegawa, H.; et al. Sarcopenia and sarcopenic obesity are prognostic factors for overall survival in patients with cirrhosis. *Intern. Med.* **2016**, *55*, 863–870. [CrossRef] [PubMed]

33. Petta, S.; Ciminnisi, S.; Di Marco, V.; Cabibi, D.; Cammà, C.; Licata, A.; Marchesini, G.; Craxì, A. Sarcopenia is associated with severe liver fibrosis in patients with non-alcoholic fatty liver disease. *Aliment. Pharmacol. Ther.* **2017**, *45*, 510–518. [CrossRef] [PubMed]

34. Lee, Y.H.; Kim, S.U.; Song, K.; Park, J.Y.; Kim, D.Y.; Ahn, S.H.; Lee, B.W.; Kang, E.S.; Cha, B.S.; Han, K.H. Sarcopenia is associated with significant liver fibrosis independently of obesity and insulin resistance in nonalcoholic fatty liver disease: Nationwide surveys (KNHANES 2008–2011). *Hepatology* **2016**, *63*, 776–786. [CrossRef] [PubMed]

35. Koo, B.K.; Kim, D.; Joo, S.K.; Kim, J.H.; Chang, M.S.; Kim, B.G.; Lee, K.L.; Kim, W. Sarcopenia is an independent risk factor for non-alcoholic steatohepatitis and significant fibrosis. *J. Hepatol.* **2017**, *66*, 123–131. [CrossRef] [PubMed]

36. Bedossa, P. Intraobserver and interobserver variations in liver biopsy interpretation in patients with chronic hepatitis C. *Hepatology* **1994**, *20*, 15–20.

37. Charlton, M.R. Branched-chain amino acid enriched supplements as therapy for liver disease. *J. Nutr.* **2006**, *136*, 295–298. [CrossRef]

38. Kawaguchi, T.; Izumi, N.; Charlton, M.R.; Sata, M. Branched-chain amino acids as pharmacological nutrients in chronic liver disease. *Hepatology* **2011**, *54*, 1063–1070. [CrossRef] [PubMed]

39. Alberino, F.; Gatta, A.; Amodio, P.; Merkel, C.; Di Pascoli, L.; Boffo, G.; Caregaro, L. Nutrition and survival in patients with liver cirrhosis. *Nutrition* **2001**, *17*, 445–450. [CrossRef]

40. Suzuki, K.; Suzuki, K.; Koizumi, K.; Ichimura, H.; Oka, S.; Takada, H.; Kuwayama, H. Measurement of serum branched-chain amino acids to tyrosine ratio level is useful in a prediction of a change of serum albumin level in chronic liver disease. *Hepatol. Res.* **2008**, *38*, 267–272. [CrossRef] [PubMed]

nutrients

Article

Predictors Associated with Increase in Skeletal Muscle Mass after Sustained Virological Response in Chronic Hepatitis C Treated with Direct Acting Antivirals

Kazunori Yoh, Hiroki Nishikawa, Hirayuki Enomoto *, Akio Ishii, Yoshinori Iwata,
Yuho Miyamoto, Noriko Ishii, Yukihisa Yuri, Kunihiro Hasegawa, Chikage Nakano,
Takashi Nishimura, Nobuhiro Aizawa, Yoshiyuki Sakai, Naoto Ikeda, Tomoyuki Takashima,
Ryo Takata, Hiroko Iijima and Shuhei Nishiguchi

Division of Hepatobiliary and Pancreatic Disease, Department of Internal Medicine, Hyogo College of Medicine,
Hyogo 663-8501, Japan; mm2wintwin@ybb.ne.jp (K.Y.); hi-nishikawa@hyo-med.ac.jp (H.N.);
akio0010@yahoo.co.jp (A.I.); yo-iwata@hyo-med.ac.jp (Y.I.); yuho.0818.1989@gmail.com (Y.M.);
ishinori1985@yahoo.co.jp (N.I.); gyma27ijo04td@gmail.com (Y.Y.); hiro.red1230@gmail.com (K.H.);
chikage@hyo-med.ac.jp (C.N.); tk-nishimura@hyo-med.ac.jp (T.N.); nobu23hiro@yahoo.co.jp (N.A.);
sakai429@hyo-med.ac.jp (Y.S.); nikeneko@hyo-med.ac.jp (N.I.); tomo0204@yahoo.co.jp (T.T.);
chano_chano_rt@yahoo.co.jp (R.T.); hiroko-i@hyo-med.ac.jp (H.I.); nishiguc@hyo-med.ac.jp (S.N.)
* Correspondence: enomoto@hyo-med.ac.jp; Tel.: +81-798-45-6111; Fax: +81-798-456-608

Received: 10 September 2017; Accepted: 12 October 2017; Published: 18 October 2017

Abstract: Aims: We aimed to examine changes in skeletal muscle mass in chronic hepatitis C (CHC) patients undergoing interferon (IFN)-free direct acting antivirals (DAAs) therapy who achieved sustained virological response (SVR). Patients and methods: A total of 69 CHC patients treated with DAAs were analyzed. We compared the changes in skeletal muscle index (SMI) using bio-impedance analysis at baseline and SMI at SVR. SMI was calculated as the sum of skeletal muscle mass in upper and lower extremities divided by height squared (cm^2/m^2). Further, we identified pretreatment parameters contributing to the increased SMI at SVR. Results: SMI in males at baseline ranged from 6.73 to 9.08 cm^2/m^2 (median, 7.65 cm^2/m^2), while that in females ranged from 4.45 to 7.27 cm^2/m^2 (median, 5.81 cm^2/m^2). At SVR, 36 patients (52.2%) had increased SMI as compared with baseline. In the univariate analysis, age ($p = 0.0392$), hyaluronic acid ($p = 0.0143$), and branched-chain amino acid to tyrosine ratio (BTR) ($p = 0.0024$) were significant pretreatment factors linked to increased SMI at SVR. In the multivariate analysis, only BTR was an independent predictor linked to the increased SMI at SVR ($p = 0.0488$). Conclusion: Pretreatment BTR level can be helpful for predicting increased SMI after SVR in CHC patients undergoing IFN-free DAAs therapy.

Keywords: chronic hepatitis C; direct acting antiviral; sustained virological response; skeletal muscle mass

---

1. Introduction

The ultimate goal of treatment for chronic hepatitis C (CHC) is to eliminate the hepatitis C virus (HCV) and thereby to suppress the liver disease progression and the liver carcinogenesis [1–3]. In cases with sustained virological response (SVR), the incidence of disease progression or carcinogenesis has been reported to be markedly decreased [1,2,4,5]. CHC therapy has dramatically changed with the recent accessibility of direct acting antivirals (DAAs). Protease inhibitors including telaprevir, simeprevir, or vaniprevir containing pegylated-interferon (Peg-IFN)α2a or Peg-IFNα2b and ribavirin (RBV) combination therapy (IFN-based triple therapy) have demonstrated higher SVR rates [6]. Further, IFN-free DAAs therapies such as daclatasvir (DCV)/asunaprevir (ASV), sofosbuvir (SOF)/RBV, ledipasvir (LDV)/SOF, LDV/SOF/RBV, and SOF/velpatasvir have also demonstrated excellent SVR rates [4,5,7,8]. Recently, almost all CHC patients have been able to eradicate HCV in a comfortable manner [3].

On the other hand, skeletal muscle loss (SML) has been shown to be an adverse predictor in patients with liver diseases and has drawn much caution among clinicians because of its linkage to clinical outcomes [9–11]. Skeletal muscle mass is maintained by a balance between protein synthesis and protein breakdown, and muscle mass loss can occur due to an increment in proteolysis or a reduction in protein synthesis, or both disorders [12–14]. There have been compelling evidences to show that SML is one of the major complications in liver cirrhosis (LC) due to the LC-related double metabolic burdens (i.e., protein metabolic and energy metabolic disorders) [11,12,15–25]. Thus, for CHC patients treated with antiviral therapies, maintaining skeletal muscle mass is crucial. However, to the best of our knowledge, there have been no available data with regard to changes in skeletal muscle mass for CHC patients with SVR who underwent IFN-free DAAs therapy. Further, identifying pretreatment factors linked to the improvement in skeletal muscle mass may be pivotal for creating nutritional strategies in CHC patients after SVR.

The aims of the current study were therefore to examine changes in skeletal muscle mass in CHC patients undergoing IFN-free DAAs therapy who achieved SVR and to identify pretreatment predictors that are associated with the improvement in skeletal muscle mass.

2. Patients and Methods

2.1. Patients and Skeletal Muscle Mass Measurement

This study was a single center retrospective study. All study participants were CHC patients with data for skeletal muscle mass at baseline and SVR. Patients without those data were excluded from the current analysis.

For all analyzed subjects, skeletal muscle mass was assessed using bio-impedance analysis (BIA, Inbody720, Takumi Ltd., Aichi, Japan) in the standing position. BIA is a device which can measure the body fat mass, body water mass, and body muscle mass using differences in frequency [11].

Our current study participants were CHC patients treated with IFN-free DAAs therapy (DCV/ASV, SOF/LDV, SOF/LDV/RBV, SOF/RBV, or others) who were admitted at the Division of Hepatobiliary and Pancreatic disease, Department of Internal Medicine, Hyogo College of Medicine, Hyogo, Japan between August 2013 and August 2015. All patients achieved SVR and had available data for BIA. In this analysis, SVR was defined as the disappearance of serum HCV-RNA at a time point more than 12 weeks after the completion of each DAA therapy. In principal, BIA was routinely performed at baseline and at SVR 24 (24 weeks after the completion of DAAs therapy). All patients had no ascites on radiologic findings. Skeletal muscle index (SMI) was defined as the sum of skeletal muscle mass in the upper and lower extremities divided by height squared (cm^2/m^2), using data from BIA [11]. We compared the changes in SMI at baseline and SMI at SVR. Patients with increased SMI were defined as those with an SMI at SVR that was more than the SMI at baseline. Further, we identified pretreatment parameters contributing to the increased SMI using univariate and multivariate analyses. Included pretreatment parameters (potentially relevant factors with the development of SML in view of current published articles) are listed in Table 1 [9,11–14]. The ethical committee meeting at Hyogo College of Medicine approved our current study protocol and this study strictly followed all provisions of the Declaration of Helsinki.

Table 1. Baseline data (*n* = 69).

Variables	Number or Median (Range)
Age (years)	63 (25–83)
Gender, male/female	31/38
Body mass index (kg/m^2)	22.1 (15.7–32.8)
Skeletal muscle index (cm^2/m^2), male	7.65 (6.73–9.08)
Skeletal muscle index (cm^2/m^2), female	5.81 (4.45–7.27)
Total bilirubin (mg/dL)	0.8 (0.3–3.0)
Serum albumin (g/dL)	4.1 (2.8–4.9)
Prothrombin time (%)	83.4 (61.1–119.4)
Platelets ($\times 10^4$/mm^3)	15.5 (3.3–27.8)
Serum sodium (mmol/L)	140 (129–144)
eGFR (mL/min/1.73 m^2)	84 (33–142)
Total cholesterol (mg/dL)	159 (110–234)
Triglyceride (mg/dL)	88 (33–779)
AST (IU/L)	37 (15–140)
ALT (IU/L)	37 (11–155)
Fasting blood glucose (mg/dL)	94 (74–187)
HbA1c (NSGP)	5.5 (4.1–9.7)
BTR	4.94 (2.13–9.09)
Alpha-fetoprotein (ng/mL)	4.2 (1.3–224.9)
Hyaluronic acid (ng/mL)	103 (9–699)
FIB-4 index	2.46 (0.66–20.04)
HCV genotype, 1/2	55/14
HCV viral load (log IU/L)	6.2 (5.0–7.7)

Data are expressed as number or median (range). eGFR; estimated glomerular filtration rate, AST; aspartate aminotransferase, ALT; alanine aminotransferase, NGSP; National Glycohemoglobin Standardization Program, BTR; branched-chain amino acid to tyrosine ratio, HCV; hepatitis C virus.

2.2. Statistical Analysis

First, the distribution of each parameter (normal or not) was assessed by the Shapiro-Wilk test. Categorical variables were compared by Fisher's exact test. Continuous variables were compared by unpaired *t*-test, paired *t*-test, or Mann-Whitney *U* test as applicable. For predicting increased SMI, candidate variables were identified by univariate analysis; variables with $p < 0.10$ were analyzed by a multivariate logistic regression analysis. Data are presented as median value (range) unless otherwise mentioned. Statistical significance was set at $p < 0.05$. Statistical analysis was performed with JMP 11 (SAS Institute Inc., Cary, NC, USA).

3. Results

3.1. Baseline Characteristics

Baseline characteristics in the present study are shown in Table 1. Our study cohort (*n* = 69; 55 in HCV genotype 1 and 14 in genotype 2) included 31 males and 38 females with a median (range) age of 63 (25–83) years. SMI in males at baseline ranged from 6.73 to 9.08 cm^2/m^2 (median, 7.65 cm^2/m^2), while SMI in females at baseline ranged from 4.45 to 7.27 cm^2/m^2 (median, 5.81 cm^2/m^2). According to current guidelines, the proportion of low SMI in males (<7.0 cm^2/m^2) was 22.6% (7/31) and that in females (<5.7 cm^2/m^2) was 44.7% (17/38) [11]. For the entire cohort, SMI had normal distribution.

3.2. Changes in SMI for the Entire Cohort (n = 69)

The median SMI for the entire cohort at baseline was 6.62 cm^2/m^2 (range, 4.45–9.08 cm^2/m^2), while the median SMI for the entire cohort at SVR was 6.51 cm^2/m^2 (range, 4.55–9.30 cm^2/m^2). ($p = 0.6352$, Figure 1A) The proportion of increased SMI at SVR compared with the SMI at baseline was 52.2% (36/69, 19 males and 17 females).

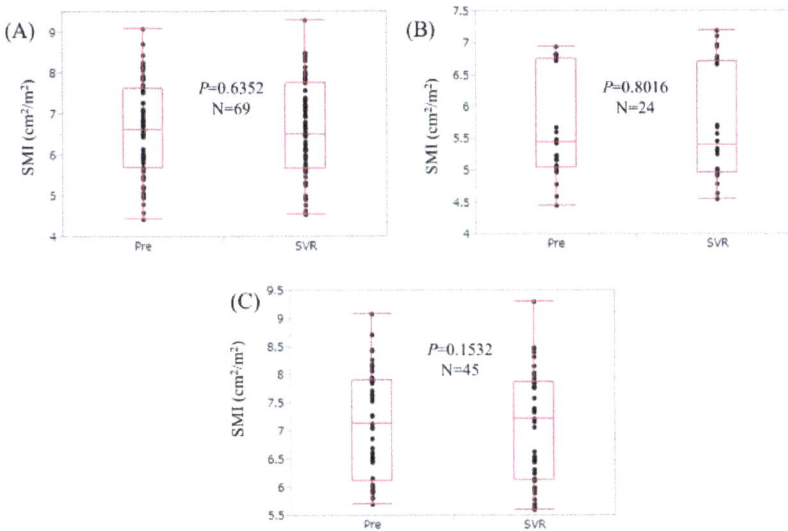

Figure 1. Changes in skeletal muscle index (SMI) during interferon (IFN)-free direct acting antivirals (DAAs) therapy at pretreatment and sustained virological response (SVR). (**A**) For the entire cohort ($n = 69$); (**B**) For patients with low muscle mass at baseline ($n = 24$, as defined by current guidelines [11]); (**C**) For patients without low muscle mass at baseline ($n = 45$, as defined by current guidelines [11]).

3.3. Changes in SMI for Patients with Low Muscle Mass (Low SMI) at Baseline (n = 24)

The median SMI for patients with low muscle mass (low SMI) at baseline was 5.44 cm^2/m^2 (range, 4.45–6.95 cm^2/m^2), while the median SMI for those patients at SVR was 5.40 cm^2/m^2 (range, 4.55–7.20 cm^2/m^2) ($p = 0.8016$, Figure 1B).

3.4. Changes in SMI for Patients without Low Muscle Mass (Low SMI) at Baseline (n = 45)

The median SMI for patients without low muscle mass (low SMI) at baseline was 7.13 cm^2/m^2 (range, 5.70–9.08 cm^2/m^2), while the median SMI for those patients at SVR was 7.22 cm^2/m^2 (range, 5.59–9.30 cm^2/m^2) ($p = 0.1532$, Figure 1C).

3.5. Changes in SMI According to Baseline FIB-4 Index

We compared changes in SMI according to FIB-4 index. Patients with baseline FIB-4 index ≥ 2.46 (the median value in our cohort) were defined as the high FIB-4 index group ($n = 34$), while those with baseline FIB-4 index <2.46 were defined as the low FIB-4 index group ($n = 35$). In the high FIB-4 index group, SMI at SVR did not significantly increase as compared with baseline levels ($p = 0.9812$). In the low FIB-4 index group, SMI at SVR tended to significantly increase as compared with baseline levels ($p = 0.0879$) (Figure 2).

(A) High FIB-4 index group (B) Low FIB-4 index group

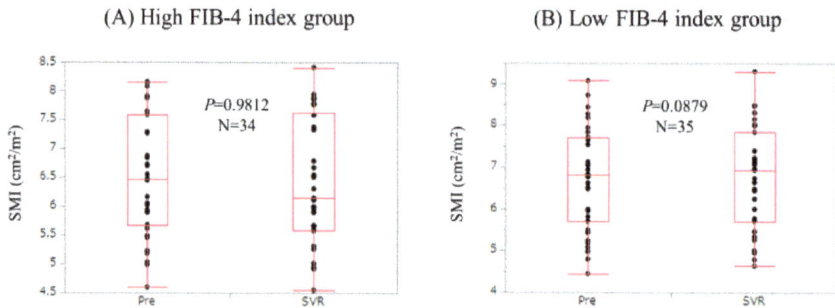

Figure 2. Changes in SMI according to baseline FIB-4 index. (**A**) Patients with baseline FIB-4 index $\geq$2.46 (the median value in our cohort) were defined as the high FIB-4 index group ($n = 34$). SMI at SVR did not significantly increase as compared with baseline levels ($p = 0.9812$); (**B**) Patients with baseline FIB-4 index <2.46 were defined as the low FIB-4 index group ($n = 35$). SMI at SVR tended to significantly increase as compared with baseline levels ($p = 0.0879$).

3.6. Changes in SMI According to HCV Serotype

In the HCV serotype 1 group ($n = 55$), SMI at SVR did not significantly increase as compared with baseline levels ($p = 0.5777$). In the HCV serotype 2 group ($n = 14$), SMI at SVR tended to significantly decrease as compared with baseline levels ($p = 0.0708$) (Figure 3).

(A) HCV serotype 1 (B) HCV serotype 2

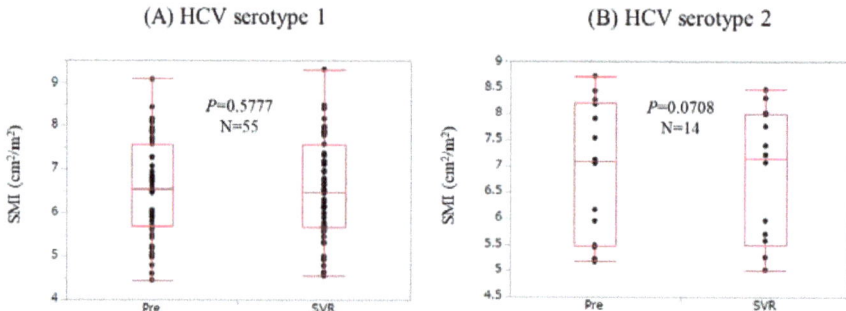

Figure 3. Changes in SMI according to HCV serotype. (**A**) In the HCV serotype 1 group ($n = 55$), SMI at SVR did not significantly increase as compared with baseline levels ($p = 0.5777$); (**B**) In the HCV serotype 2 group ($n = 14$), SMI at SVR tended to significantly decrease as compared with baseline levels ($p = 0.0708$).

3.7. Changes in SMI According to HCV Viral Load

We compared changes in SMI according to baseline HCV viral load. Patients with baseline HCV viral load >6.2 log IU/mL (the median value in our cohort) were defined as the high HCV viral load group ($n = 34$), while those with baseline HCV viral load $\leq$6.2 log IU/mL were defined as the low HCV viral load ($n = 35$). In the high HCV viral load group, SMI at SVR did not significantly increase as compared with baseline levels ($p = 0.3797$). In the low HCV viral load group, SMI at SVR did not significantly increase as compared with baseline levels ($p = 0.1772$) (Figure 4).

(A) HCV high viral load (>6.2 Log IU/ml)   (B) HCV low viral load (≤6.2 Log IU/ml)

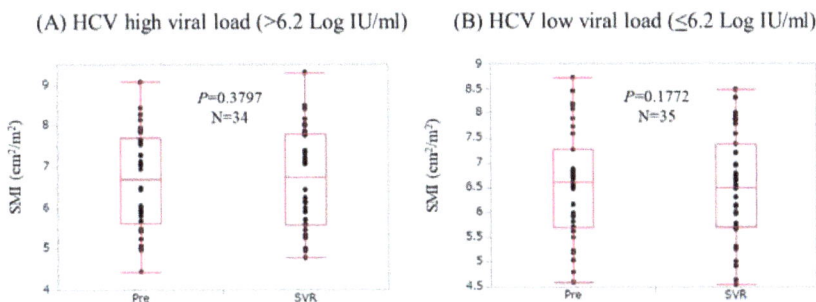

Figure 4. Changes in SMI according to HCV viral load. Patients with baseline HCV viral load >6.2 log IU/mL (the median value in our cohort) were defined as the high HCV viral load group (n = 34), while those with baseline HCV viral load ≤6.2 log IU/mL were defined as the low HCV viral load (n = 35). (**A**) In the high HCV viral load group, SMI at SVR did not significantly increase as compared with baseline levels (p = 0.3797); (**B**) In the low HCV viral load group, SMI at SVR did not significantly increase as compared with baseline levels (p = 0.1772).

3.8. Changes in SMI According to Age

We compared changes in SMI according to age. Patients with the age of >63 years (the median value in our cohort) were defined as the elderly group (n = 34), while those with the age of ≤63 years were defined as the non-elderly group (n = 35). In the elderly group, SMI at SVR did not significantly increase as compared with baseline levels (p = 0.1662). In the non-elderly group, SMI at SVR did not significantly increase as compared with baseline levels (p = 0.5105) (Figure 5).

(A) Elderly group (>63 years)   (B) Non-elderly group (≤63 years)

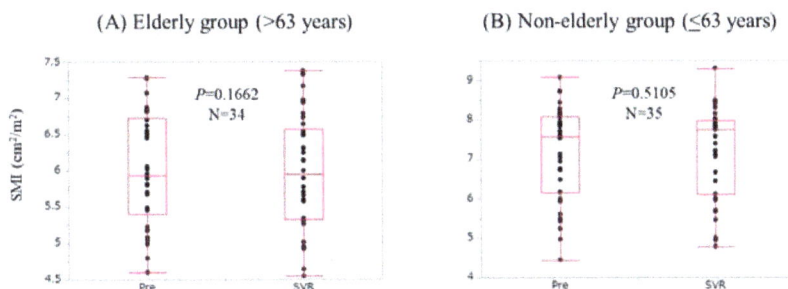

Figure 5. Changes in SMI according age. Patients with the age of >63 years (the median value in our cohort) were defined as the elderly group (n = 34), while those with the age of ≤63 years were defined as the non-elderly group (n = 35). (**A**) In the elderly group, SMI at SVR did not significantly increase as compared with baseline levels (p = 0.1662); (**B**) In the non-elderly group, SMI at SVR did not significantly increase as compared with baseline levels (p = 0.5105).

3.9. Comparison of Baseline Characteristics Between Patients with and without Increased SMI

Comparison of baseline characteristics between patients with increased SMI (n = 36) and without increased SMI (n = 33) is shown in Table 2. Age (p = 0.0392) and hyaluronic acid level (p = 0.0143) in the increased SMI group were significantly lower than those in the non-increased SMI group. Branched-chain amino acid to tyrosine ratio (BTR) in the increased SMI group was significantly higher than those in the non-increased SMI group (p = 0.0024). FIB-4 index in the increased SMI group tended to be significantly lower than that in the non-increased SMI group (p = 0.0656).

Table 2. Comparison of baseline characteristics between patients with increased SMI (I-SMI, $n = 36$) and without I-SMI ($n = 33$).

Variables	I-SMI ($n = 36$)	Non-I-SMI ($n = 33$)	p Value
Age (years)	59 (25–78)	65 (39–83)	0.0392
Gender, male/female	18/18	13/20	0.4693
Serum albumin (g/dL)	4.1 (3.3–4.9)	4.1 (2.8–4.6)	0.6883
Total bilirubin (mg/dL)	0.8 (0.3–2.5)	0.7 (0.4–3.0)	0.3416
Prothrombin time (%)	84.05 (67–108.4)	82.8 (61.1–119.4)	0.4161
Platelet count ($\times 10^4$/mm^3)	17.35 (3.6–25.3)	14.2 (3.3–27.8)	0.3433
AST (IU/L)	29.5 (15–140)	45 (19–120)	0.2735
ALT (IU/L)	36.5 (11–155)	39 (13–104)	0.4971
Serum sodium (mmol/L)	140 (129–144)	141 (135–143)	0.7724
Total cholesterol (mg/dL)	158 (110–228)	159 (126–234)	0.5347
Triglyceride (mg/dL)	92 (33–174)	88 (45–779)	0.9091
Fasting blood glucose (mg/dL)	93 (74–187)	96 (85–130)	0.1224
eGFR (mL/min/1.73 m^2)	85 (33–141)	82 (36–142)	0.8803
HbA1c (NSGP)	5.5 (4.7–9.7)	5.5 (4.1–7.0)	0.4911
Body mass index (kg/m^2)	21.95 (15.7–30.8)	22.5 (17.4–32.8)	0.3988
BTR	5.16 (3.01–9.09)	4.19 (2.13–8.36)	0.0024
Hyaluronic acid (ng/mL)	80 (9–437)	156 (17–699)	0.0143
FIB-4 index	1.94 (0.66–20.04)	3.53 (0.96–15.29)	0.0656
Alpha-fetoprotein (ng/mL)	3.1 (1.9–224.9)	7.3 (1.3–183.3)	0.4694
HCV genotype, 1/2	31/5	24/9	0.2331
HCV-RNA (log IU/L)	6.3 (5.1–7.2)	6.2 (5.0–7.7)	0.9380

AST; aspartate aminotransferase, ALT; alanine aminotransferase, eGFR; estimated glomerular filtration rate, NGSP; National Glycohemoglobin Standardization Program, BTR; branched chain amino acid to tyrosine ratio, HCV; hepatitis C virus. Patients with I-SMI indicate those with an SMI at SVR the was more than the SMI at baseline.

3.10. Multivariate Analyses of Factors Linked to the Presence of Increased SMI

Multivariate analysis for the above four factors with $p < 0.10$ (i.e., age, hyaluronic acid, FIB-4 index, and BTR) showed that only BTR was a significant prognostic pretreatment factor linked to the presence of increased SMI ($p = 0.0488$). (Table 3) Odds ratios and 95% confidence intervals are demonstrated in Table 3.

Table 3. Multivariate analysis of factors contributing to the increased SMI.

Variables	Multivariate Analysis	
	OR (95% CI)	p Value
Age (per one year)	1.029 (0.977–1.089)	0.2797
Hyaluronic acid (per one ng/mL)	1.002 (0.998–1.006)	0.3794
BTR (per one)	0.648 (0.398–0.998)	0.0488
FIB-4 index (per one)	0.996 (0.832–1.221)	0.9688

OR; Odds ratio, CI; confidence interval, BTR; branched-chain amino acid to tyrosine ratio.

4. Discussion

Liver disease patients are aging in our country and SML is also associated with aging [11]. In other words, SML in liver disease patients can occur, irrespective of the degree of liver fibrosis stage. CHC therapy has dramatically improved due to the introduction of DAAs [1,4]. As described earlier, SML can be an adverse predictor in patients with liver diseases, although there are limited clinical data showing that skeletal muscle mass improvement can lead to favorable clinical outcomes in CHC patients, and reversing skeletal muscle mass loss is a priority field for therapeutic strategies in these patients [9–13]. In view of these backgrounds, addressing clinical queries to which factors are associated with the improvement of skeletal muscle mass after SVR may be a point of focus, and our current results may therefore be worthy of reporting.

In the multivariate analysis, only pretreatment BTR value was an independent predictor linked to increased SMI. BTR has also been shown to decrease in cirrhotic patients. Furthermore, BTR is widely used in Japan as an easily measurable indicator of amino acid imbalance and it is also closely related to protein synthesis in the muscle [9,26]. In addition, in our previous study, we demonstrated that lower BTR was associated with decreased skeletal muscle mass in patients with chronic liver diseases, which is in agreement with our current data [27]. In a sense, measuring BTR can lead to creating strategies for nutritional intervention from the view point of skeletal muscle mass. In patients with well-preserved protein synthesis ability, as reflected by a higher BTR level, HCV eradication may lead to the acceleration of protein synthesis in the muscle; this is a major finding in the current study. On the contrary, considering our current results, patients with LC status are expected to have poor improvement in skeletal muscle mass even after HCV eradication. Patients with a higher baseline FIB-4 index had poor improvement in skeletal muscle mass at SVR in our results, and this observation can support our hypothesis. In such patients, some interventions including exercise may be recommended [9,12,13]. In compensated LC patients, walking 5000 or more steps per day may be ideal [28]. On the other hand, it is of note that the proportion of low SMI in males was rather lower than that in females (22.6% vs. 44.7%). Significant differences in baseline characteristics between males and females (age; $p < 0.0001$, FIB-4 index; $p = 0.0196$, BTR; $p = 0.0292$, data not shown) may account for our current results.

It is of interest that in the HCV serotype 2 group, SMI at SVR tended to significantly decrease as compared with baseline levels ($p = 0.0708$). One possible reason for these results is that in HCV serotype 2 patients, RBV was used in most cases. RBV-related anemia may cause muscle mass decrease.

Whether SMI increment presents a good prognosis in chronic liver disease patients has yet to be clarified. On the other hand, previous investigators reported that a higher BTR was a favorable predictor for LC patients [29]. In our results, higher BTR was associated with SMI increment. In view of this, SMI increment in CHC patients can result in a good prognosis. However, further studies will be required to confirm these results.

Our study had the drawbacks of a small sample size for analysis, and how these short-term outcomes translate into long-term outcomes has yet to be determined. In addition, several important variables that could influence the outcome were overlooked (diet, exercise, and other pharmacological therapies), as they were not included in the current analysis. The causal relationship between BTR and skeletal muscle mass should also be elucidated. Thus, further well-designed and larger studies with longer observation periods will be needed in the future. However, our results denote that pretreatment BTR level is a useful predictor for improvement in skeletal muscle mass after SVR in CHC patients treated with DAAs.

5. Conclusions

In conclusion, pretreatment BTR levels can be helpful for predicting increased SMI after SVR in CHC patients undergoing IFN-free DAAs therapy.

Acknowledgments: The authors would like to thank all medical staff in our hospital for data collection.

Author Contributions: K.Y., H.N., S.N. and H.E. conceived and designed the experiments; K.Y., H.N. and H.E. performed the experiments; K.Y., H.N. and H.E. analyzed the data; A.I., Y.I., Y.M., N.I., Y.Y., K.H., C.N., T.N., N.A., Y.S., N.I., T.T., R.T. and H.I. contributed reagents/materials/analysis tools; K.Y., H.N. and H.E. wrote the paper.

Conflicts of Interest: In the current study, the authors declare that they have no conflicts of interest.

Abbreviations

CHC	chronic hepatitis C
HCV	hepatitis C virus
SVR	sustained virological response
DAA	direct acting antiviral
SMV	Simeprevir
Peg-IFN	pegylated interferon
RBV	Ribavirin
DCV	Daclatasvir
ASV	Asunaprevir
SOF	Sofosbuvir
LDV	Ledipasvir
SML	skeletal muscle loss
LC	liver cirrhosis
BIA	bio-impedance analysis
SMI	skeletal muscle index
BTR	branched-chain amino acid to tyrosine ratio

References

1. Wang, L.S.; D'Souza, L.S.; Jacobson, I.M. Hepatitis C—A clinical review. *J. Med. Virol.* **2016**, *88*, 1844–1855. [CrossRef] [PubMed]
2. Van der Meer, A.J.; Berenguer, M. Reversion of disease manifestations after HCV eradication. *J. Hepatol.* **2016**, *65*, S95–S108. [CrossRef] [PubMed]
3. Majumdar, A.; Kitson, M.T.; Roberts, S.K. Systematic review: Current concepts and challenges for the direct-acting antiviral era in hepatitis C cirrhosis. *Aliment. Pharmacol. Ther.* **2016**, *43*, 1276–1292. [CrossRef] [PubMed]
4. Gutierrez, J.A.; Lawitz, E.J.; Poordad, F. Interferon-free, direct-acting antiviral therapy for chronic hepatitis C. *J. Viral Hepat.* **2015**, *22*, 861–870. [CrossRef] [PubMed]
5. Jacobson, I.M. The HCV treatment revolution continues: Resistance considerations, pangenotypic efficacy, and advances in challenging populations. *Gastroenterol. Hepatol.* **2016**, *12*, 1–11.
6. Welch, N.M.; Jensen, D.M. Pegylated interferon based therapy with second-wave direct-acting antivirals in genotype 1 chronic hepatitis C. *Liver Int.* **2015**, *35*, 11–17. [CrossRef] [PubMed]
7. Terrault, N.A.; Zeuzem, S.; Di Bisceglie, A.M.; Lim, J.K.; Pockros, P.J.; Frazier, L.M.; Kuo, A.; Lok, A.S.; Shiffman, M.L.; Ben Ari, Z. Effectiveness of ledipasvir-sofosbuvir combination in patients with hepatitis C virus infection and factors associated with sustained virologic response. *Gastroenterology* **2016**, *151*, 1131–1140. [CrossRef] [PubMed]
8. Mir, F.; Kahveci, A.S.; Ibdah, J.A.; Tahan, V. Sofosbuvir/velpatasvir regimen promises an effective pan-genotypic hepatitis C virus cure. *Drug Des. Dev. Ther.* **2017**, *11*, 497–502. [CrossRef] [PubMed]
9. Sinclair, M.; Gow, P.J.; Grossmann, M.; Angus, P.W. Review article: Sarcopenia in cirrhosis-aetiology, implications and potential therapeutic interventions. *Aliment. Pharmacol. Ther.* **2016**, *43*, 765–777. [CrossRef] [PubMed]
10. Petta, S.; Ciminnisi, S.; Di Marco, V.; Cabibi, D.; Cammà, C.; Licata, A.; Marchesini, G.; Craxì, A. Sarcopenia is associated with severe liver fibrosis in patients with non-alcoholic fatty liver disease. *Aliment. Pharmacol. Ther.* **2016**, *45*, 510–518. [CrossRef] [PubMed]
11. Nishikawa, H.; Shiraki, M.; Hiramatsu, A.; Moriya, K.; Hino, K.; Nishiguchi, S. Japan Society of Hepatology guidelines for sarcopenia in liver disease (1st edition): Recommendation from the working group for creation of sarcopenia assessment criteria. *Hepatol. Res.* **2016**, *46*, 951–963. [CrossRef] [PubMed]
12. Dasarathy, S.; Merli, M. Sarcopenia from mechanism to diagnosis and treatment in liver disease. *J. Hepatol.* **2016**, *65*, 1232–1244. [CrossRef] [PubMed]
13. Dasarathy, S. Consilience in sarcopenia of cirrhosis. *J. Cachexia Sarcopenia Muscle* **2012**, *3*, 225–237. [CrossRef] [PubMed]

14. Santilli, V.; Bernetti, A.; Mangone, M.; Paoloni, M. Clinical definition of sarcopenia. *Clin. Cases Miner. Bone Metab.* **2014**, *11*, 177–180. [CrossRef] [PubMed]

15. Cruz-Jentoft, A.J.; Landi, F.; Schneider, S.M.; Zúñiga, C.; Arai, H.; Boirie, Y.; Chen, L.K.; Fielding, R.A.; Martin, F.C.; Michel, J.P. Prevalence of and interventions for sarcopenia in ageing adults: A systematic review. Report of the international sarcopenia initiative (EWGSOP and IWGS). *Age Ageing* **2014**, *43*, 748–759. [CrossRef] [PubMed]

16. Hanai, T.; Shiraki, M.; Nishimura, K.; Ohnishi, S.; Imai, K.; Suetsugu, A.; Takai, K.; Shimizu, M.; Moriwaki, H. Sarcopenia impairs prognosis of patients with liver cirrhosis. *Nutrition* **2015**, *31*, 193–199. [CrossRef] [PubMed]

17. Nardelli, S.; Lattanzi, B.; Torrisi, S.; Greco, F.; Farcomeni, A.; Gioia, S.; Merli, M.; Riggio, O. Sarcopenia is risk factor for development of hepatic encephalopathy after transjugular intrahepatic portosysthemic shunt placement. *Clin. Gastroenterol. Hepatol.* **2017**, *15*, 934–936. [CrossRef] [PubMed]

18. Kalafateli, M.; Mantzoukis, K.; Choi Yau, Y.; Mohammad, A.O.; Arora, S.; Rodrigues, S.; de Vos, M.; Papadimitriou, K.; Thorburn, D.; O'Beirnr, J. Malnutrition and sarcopenia predict post-liver transplantation outcomes independently of the Model for End-stage Liver Disease score. *J. Cachexia Sarcopenia Muscle* **2017**, *8*, 113–121. [CrossRef] [PubMed]

19. Chen, L.K.; Liu, L.K.; Woo, J.; Assantachai, P.; Auyeung, T.W.; Bahyah, K.S.; Chou, M.Y.; Chen, L.Y.; Hsu, P.S.; Krairit, O.; et al. Sarcopenia in Asia: Consensus report of the Asian Working Group for Sarcopenia. *J. Am. Med. Dir. Assoc.* **2014**, *15*, 95–101. [CrossRef] [PubMed]

20. Hiraoka, A.; Michitaka, K.; Ueki, H.; Kaneto, M.; Aibiki, T.; Okudaira, T.; Kawakami, T.; Yamago, H.; Suga, Y.; Tomida, H.; et al. Sarcopenia and two types of presarcopenia in Japanese patients with chronic liver disease. *Eur. J. Gastroenterol. Hepatol.* **2016**, *28*, 940–947. [CrossRef] [PubMed]

21. Dos Santos, L.; Cyrino, E.S.; Antunes, M.; Santos, D.A.; Sardinha, L.B. Sarcopenia and physical independence in older adults: The independent and synergic role of muscle mass and muscle function. *J. Cachexia Sarcopenia Muscle* **2017**, *8*, 245–250. [CrossRef] [PubMed]

22. Kalyani, R.R.; Corriere, M.; Ferrucci, L. Age-related and disease-related muscle loss: The effect of diabetes, obesity, and other diseases. *Lancet Diabetes Endocrinol.* **2014**, *2*, 819–829. [CrossRef]

23. Kaido, T.; Tamai, Y.; Hamaguchi, Y.; Okumura, S.; Kobayashi, A.; Shirai, H.; Yagi, S.; Kamo, N.; Hammad, A.; Inagaki, N.; et al. Effects of pretransplant sarcopenia and sequential changes in sarcopenic parameters after living donor liver transplantation. *Nutrition* **2017**, *33*, 195–198. [CrossRef] [PubMed]

24. Merli, M.; Giusto, M.; Lucidi, C.; Giannelli, V.; Pentassuglio, I.; Di Gregorio, V.; Lattanzi, B.; Riggio, O. Muscle depletion increases the risk of overt and minimal hepatic encephalopathy: Results of a prospective study. *Metab. Brain Dis.* **2013**, *28*, 281–284. [CrossRef] [PubMed]

25. Kalafateli, M.; Konstantakis, C.; Thomopoulos, K.; Triantos, C. Impact of muscle wasting on survival in patients with liver cirrhosis. *World J. Gastroenterol.* **2015**, *21*, 7357–7361. [CrossRef] [PubMed]

26. Suzuki, K.; Suzuki, K.; Koizumi, K.; Ichimura, H.; Oka, S.; Takada, H.; Kuwayama, H. Measurement of serum branched-chain amino acids to tyrosine ratio level is useful in a prediction of a change of serum albumin level in chronic liver disease. *Hepatol. Res.* **2008**, *38*, 267–272. [CrossRef] [PubMed]

27. Nishikawa, H.; Enomoto, H.; Ishii, A.; Iwata, Y.; Miyamoto, Y.; Ishii, N.; Yuri, Y.; Takata, R.; Hasegawa, K.; Nakano, C.; et al. Development of a simple predictive model for decreased skeletal muscle mass in patients with compensated chronic liver disease. *Hepatol. Res.* **2017**. [CrossRef] [PubMed]

28. Hayashi, F.; Matsumoto, Y.; Momoki, C.; Yuikawa, M.; Okada, G.; Hamakawa, E.; Kawamura, E.; Hagihara, A.; Toyama, M.; Fujii, H.; et al. Physical inactivity and insufficient dietary intake are associated with the frequency of sarcopenia in patients with compensated viral liver cirrhosis. *Hepatol. Res.* **2013**, *43*, 1264–1275. [CrossRef] [PubMed]

29. Nishikawa, H.; Osaki, Y. Clinical significance of therapy using branched-chain amino acid granules in patients with liver cirrhosis and hepatocellular carcinoma. *Hepatol. Res.* **2014**, *44*, 149–158. [CrossRef] [PubMed]

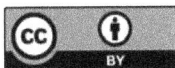

nutrients

MDPI

Review
Nutritional Therapy in Liver Transplantation

Ahmed Hammad [1,2], Toshimi Kaido [1,*], Vusal Aliyev [1], Claudia Mandato [3] and Shinji Uemoto [1]

1   Division of Hepato-Biliary-Pancreatic and Transplant Surgery, Department of Surgery,
    Graduate School of Medicine, Kyoto University, Kyoto 606-8501, Japan;
    ahmedhammad2005@yahoo.com (A.H.); dr.vusal@outlook.com (V.A.); uemoto@kuhp.kyoto-u.ac.jp (S.U.)
2   Department of General Surgery, Mansoura University, Mansoura 35516, Egypt
3   L'AORN Children's Hospital Santobono and Pausilipon, Napoli 80122, Italy; cla.mandato@gmail.com
*   Correspondence: kaido@kuhp.kyoto-u.ac.jp; Tel.: +81-75-751-4323; Fax: +81-75-751-4348

Received: 23 August 2017; Accepted: 12 October 2017; Published: 16 October 2017

Abstract: Protein-energy malnourishment is commonly encountered in patients with end-stage liver disease who undergo liver transplantation. Malnutrition may further increase morbidity, mortality and costs in the post-transplantation setting. The importance of carefully assessing the nutritional status during the work-up of patients who are candidates for liver replacement is widely recognized. The metabolic abnormalities induced by liver failure render the conventional assessment of nutritional status to be challenging. Preoperative loss of skeletal muscle mass, namely, sarcopenia, has a significant detrimental impact on post-transplant outcomes. It is essential to provide sufficient nutritional support during all phases of liver transplantation. Oral nutrition is preferred, but tube enteral nutrition may be required to provide the needed energy intake. Herein, the latest currently employed perioperative nutritional interventions in liver transplant recipients are thoroughly illustrated including synbiotics, micronutrients, branched-chain amino acid supplementation, immunonutrition formulas, fluid and electrolyte balance, the offering of nocturnal meals, dietary counselling, exercise and rehabilitation.

Keywords: liver transplantation; immunonutrition; synbiotics; nutritional intervention; sarcopenia; branched-chain amino acids; nutraceuticals

1. Introduction

The liver is the largest and most crucial metabolic organ, playing a pivotal role in integrating several biochemical pathways of carbohydrate, fat, protein, and vitamin metabolism as well as the transport of lipids and the secretion and excretion of bile, all of which are processes involved in muscle and protein metabolism and central for well-nourished status [1–3].

Advances in post-transplant care and management of graft rejection have greatly improved outcomes for patients after orthotopic liver transplantation (LT). However, malnutrition is a relevant factor when determining the progress of hepatic disease, as it contributes to hypoalbuminemia and intensifies the hydroelectrolytic imbalance determined by renal alterations [3–7].

Protein energy malnutrition (PEM) is a common problem in patients with end-stage liver disease (ESLD) awaiting LT [5]. This applies to nearly every etiology of ESLD with the exception of fulminant hepatic failure. The diagnosis of PEM in ESLD is established by marked muscle wasting and subcutaneous fat loss [5,6]. PEM is more prevalent in those with decompensated liver disease i.e., those with ascites, portosystemic hepatic encephalopathy (HE), portal hypertensive bleeding and patients hospitalized for alcoholic liver disease than in patients with nonalcoholic liver disease [7].

Clinical features of deteriorated liver function tend to normalize following successful LT. However, PEM can significantly increase the operative risk at the time of surgery and is a risk factor for morbidity, short- and long-term mortality in patients undergoing LT [7,8] and decreased graft survival after LT [9].

Moreover, PEM predisposes a patient to complications such as compromised respiratory function, wound-healing problems, longer dependency on mechanical ventilation, increased rates of septic complications, use of antibiotics, blood products usage, length of hospital stay, intensive care unit admissions, delayed physical rehabilitation, with substantially higher cost of the transplant [8,9]. Prolonged waiting times worsen outcomes when patients are already malnourished [10].

A patient's nutritional status can worsen rapidly in the immediate postoperative period due to perioperative malnutrition, surgical stress, immunosuppressive therapy, post-interventional complications, postoperative protein catabolism, and fasting periods [5,6]. This suggests the need for preemptive nutritional support with liver-adapted formulas containing additional carbohydrates, fat and proteins especially branched-chain amino acids (BCAAs) [7,8].

Body cell mass (BCM) is defined as the sum of intracellular water and fat-free mass, including skeletal muscle and viscera, without bone mineral mass. BCM comprises the metabolically active and protein-rich compartments in the body responsible for basal energy expenditure (BEE) and is known to be depleted in patients with PEM [9]. Loss of skeletal muscle mass (SMM) or sarcopenia, reflecting preoperative malnutrition is a common complication of liver cirrhosis (LC). Sarcopenia could interfere with early postoperative mobilization and has been found to be closely associated with post-LT mortality in patients undergoing living donor LT (LDLT) [9]. Sarcopenia confers a vulnerability to preoperative infection, including spontaneous bacterial peritonitis, pneumonia, post-LT bacteremia, sepsis and wound dehiscence and pulmonary complications, including aspiration pneumonia and atelectasis secondary to deteriorated immune functions [10,11]. Although less apparent, muscle wasting may be present in obese patients, which is identified as "sarcopenic obesity" [10,11] and underscores the importance of considering muscle depletion in such patients. This observation is relevant because the number of obese patients, with ESLD due to Non-alcoholic steato-hepatitis, is increasing among those awaiting LT [11,12].

An aggressive approach to ensure adequate nutritional repletion, as well as correcting vitamin and micronutrient deficiencies is central to maintain remaining hepatic function, improve the patient's metabolic reserves, and the outcomes after LT [1]. Hence, timely nutrition assessment and patient tailored intervention for anticipated recipients or those on the waiting list may improve outcomes surrounding LT [1–3].

1.1. Etiology of Malnutrition

1.1.1. Decreased Energy Intake

Patients with liver disease have decreased energy intake due to anorexia caused by zinc deficiency, hyperglycemia and increased pro-inflammatory cytokine levels; tumor necrosis factor-alpha (TNF-α), interleukin (IL)-6 and leptin [12–15]. Other causes of loss of appetite in those patients are the unpalatable specialized diets; low-salt and low-protein diets for ascites and HE, respectively, and altered gustatory sensation due to hypomagnesemia and autonomic neuropathy in LC, which also causes gastroparesis and delayed bowel transit time, together with conditional bacterial overgrowth on top of tense ascites, early satiety due to less gastrointestinal peristalsis and gastric restrictive expansion due to large volume ascites, maldigestion, impaired hepato-intestinal extraction, malabsorption and intestinal mucosal atrophy associated with portal hypertensive gastroenteropathy [12–16]. Increased protein losses due to gastrointestinal bleeding and frequent large volume paracentesis also contribute to malnutrition, which may further be worsened by protein-losing enteropathy, exacerbating hypoalbuminemia. In liver cirrhosis, up to 45% of patients may have a coexisting infection with *Helicobacter pylori* may cause dyspepsia and a decreased desire for food [13]. Moreover, limited intake due to diagnostic procedural events can lead to prolonged nil per os may further contribute to PEM [14–17].

1.1.2. Hypercatobolic Status

A number of cirrhotic patients may also have increased BEE that may be related to increased sympathetic nervous system activity and inflammation. Fever, spontaneous peritonitis and bacterial translocation are undoubtedly considered as the most common inducing factors contributing to accelerating catabolism [18]. Although hyperinsulinemia is present, glucose intolerance ensues due to insulin resistance, decreased glycogen stores and impaired glycogenolysis. This subsequently leads to gluconeogenesis from lipid peroxidation and mobilization of amino acids from the skeletal muscles and visceral proteins demonstrating muscle depletion and decrease in subcutaneous fat [17–19].

Patients with protein malnutrition have increased protein requirements in order to maintain a positive nitrogen balance [19,20]. Low plasma levels of insulin growth factor (IGF-1), which mediates most of the growth-promoting effects of growth hormone, also explain the severe growth hormone resistance seen in patients with ESLD [20].

Moreover, patients with ESLD may have impaired synthesis of polyunsaturated fatty acids from their essential fatty acid precursors with increases in levels of *n*-6 and *n*-9 fatty acids and decreases in *n*-3 moieties in plasma and adipose tissue [21]. Enhanced gluconeogenesis, especially after fasting, with preference for fat metabolism, lipid peroxidation and lipolysis, also increases upon impaired glycogen storage and utilization [22].

1.1.3. Decreased Nutrient Absorption

Other contributing factors include drug-induced diarrhea (like neomycin, lactulose, diuretics, antimetabolites, cholestryamine) [12,23]. Fat malabsorption in alcoholic and cholestatic liver diseases, especially sclerosing cholangitis with inflammatory bowel disease or concomitant pancreatic insufficiency can result in specific fat-soluble vitamin deficiencies [23]. Also, metabolic stresses from surgery, gastrointestinal reperfusion injury, immunosuppressive therapy and corticosteriods use lead to delayed bowl function recovery and disorder of nutrients absorption (Figure 1).

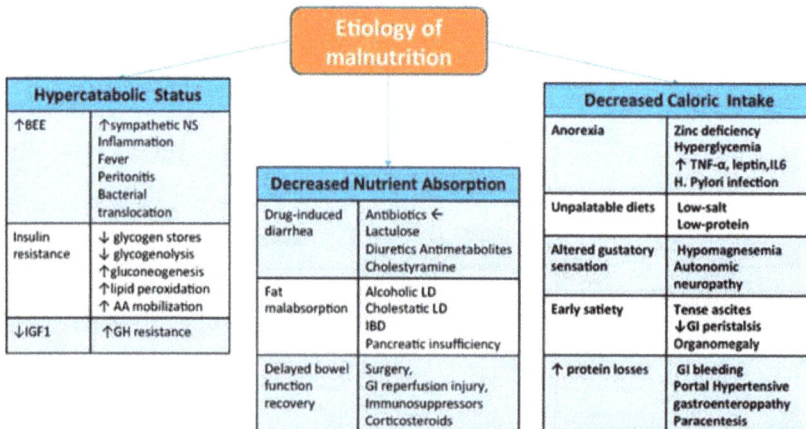

Figure 1. Etiology of Malnutrition in End Stage Liver Disease. BEE: basal energy expenditure; IBD: inflammatory bowel disease; IGF1: insulin growth factor 1; IL6: interleukin-6; GI: gastrointestinal tract; GH: growth hormone; LD: liver disease; NS: nervous system; TNF-α: tumour necrosis factor alpha.

1.2. Assessment of Nutritional Status

All patients being prepared for LT should undergo a thorough nutritional evaluation. Traditional assessment tools as BMI and anthropometry are not accurate in patients with liver disease due to fluid retention and organomegaly found in a significant number of patients. No gold-standard evaluation exists to determine the extent of malnutrition in patients with ESLD [6,24].

1.2.1. Subjective Global Assessment

The initial assessment should begin with a careful history to document weight loss, nausea, anorexia, and specialized diets and supplements. A complete physical examination should search for changes in oral mucosa, skin and hair, loss of subcutaneous fat, muscle-wasting and stigmata of chronic liver disease. Subjective global assessment (SGA) combines a thorough history-taking and physical examination and rates patients either "well-nourished", "moderately malnourished", or "severely malnourished" [6]. This test has shown high specificity with very low sensitivity for diagnosing malnutrition in patients with alcoholic liver disease. However, it has not been found to be a reliable tool for evaluating nutritional status in LT patients [6,24]. First, SGA depends on personal information that can be difficult to obtain from patients with cognitive impairment or somnolence. Second, the only anthropometric measure utilized is the body weight, which is often changed by ascites and edema [6,24].

1.2.2. Biochemical Parameters and Immune-Competence

Biochemical tests used as nutritional indicators include serum transferrin and retinol binding protein levels [25,26]. A reduced level of serum transferrin is additionally indicative of decreased energy protein intake related to LT patients [25]. However, such parameters have not been shown to be accurate indices of nutritional status given the fact that their levels correlate with severity of liver damage and inflammatory states rather than malnutrition due to the catabolic nature of liver disease and associated protein turnover.

Serum albumin frequently serves as an important indicator of liver function. However, it has a long half-life (17–21 days) and because exogenous albumin supplements are frequently administered in clinical practice, serum albumin levels cannot sensitively or dynamically reflect early liver damage. The shorter half-life (2–3 days) of prealbumin (transthyretin) renders it a more sensitive indicator of damaged synthesis functioning in the liver and fluctuations in nutritional status than albumin [27]. Creatinine-height index, 24-h urine nitrogen and 3-methylhistidine excretion were suggested as indirect measure of body muscle mass, as 1 g of excreted creatinine equals 18.5 kg of muscle mass [26].

Immune competence, which is considered a functional test of nutritional status, may be affected by hypersplenism, abnormal immunologic reactivity and alcohol abuse [26]. Low total lymphocyte, CD8 cell counts, and abnormal response to skin anergy tests; delayed cutaneous hypersensitivity response ($\geq$5 mm induration to two or more skin tests) were suggested parameters for malnutrition [27]. The measurement of lean cell mass with total body potassium has been postulated for nutritional assessment of children but it is not a part of routine nutritional assessment of children [28].

1.2.3. Anthropometry

Anthropometric measurements, such as body mass index, mid-arm muscle circumference, triceps skin fold thickness, biceps or subscapular skin fold thickness are simple, quick, cheap and noninvasive assessment methods in patients with liver disease [25–27,29]. However, these measures have been questioned regarding their reliability in patients with ascites and peripheral edema but correction by subtracting estimated amounts of ascites and other fluid collections may compensate for this disadvantage to some extent [25–27,29]. Triceps skinfold thickness remained inadequate in 70% of malnourished patients at the end of the first year [30]. In a prospective cohort study, cirrhotic patients who were severely malnourished while on the waiting list showed further deterioration at 3 months after transplantation; however, they improved at 6 and 12 months. Once again, primary changes were observed for fat mass (median triceps skinfold: basal 10.8 mm vs. 15.2 mm, 12 mm $p = 0.03$) [30].

1.2.4. Hand Grip Dynamometry

Functional assessment such as handgrip strength dynamometry and the six-minute walk test have been advocated as potential good parameters not only to assess but also to follow up nutritional interventions [27]. Hand grip strength is good reflector of upper limb strength and can used serially in conjunction with bioelectrical impedance analysis (BIA) to follow up adopted nutritional therapy regimen [29–32].

1.2.5. Indirect Calorimetry

The BEE can be predicted with several formulas such as the Harris-Benedict or Schofield equations [33]. The REE is an estimated value of BEE accounting for the effects of food, temperature, stress and activity factors [19,30]. The non-protein respiratory quotient (npRQ), a unitless number measured by 24 h urinary urea nitrogen, body carbon dioxide production and oxygen consumption was used to evaluate the nutritional status of patients with LC [34]. Moreover, npRQ provides useful information regarding substrate utilization in the post-operative period which can be very helpful in the development of a nutrition support strategy [34].

1.2.6. Bioelectrical Impedance

In nutritional assessment for patients undergoing LDLT, Kaido et al. [10–12] used direct segmental multi-frequency BIA with the InBody720 (Biospace, Tokyo, Japan) device, by which body mass index, intra- and extracellular water, and body fat percentage could be automatically and measured within 2 min. SMM was measured and shown as a percent against standard SMM calculated by sex and height of each patient. BCM was automatically calculated by the InBody 720 and displayed as a normal range (e.g., 23.0–28.1 kg).

The BIA measures the body's resistance to flow (impedance) of alternating electrical current at a designated frequency between points of contact on the body. Water in body tissue is conductive; therefore, BIA can indirectly provide information on the body's tissue content including total body water, fat-free mass, and SMM [7,9]. BIA is increasingly being used because it is easy to perform, portable, non-invasive, and quick despite some limitations in patients with ascites. It has been highly correlated with hydrostatic weighing, dual energy X-ray absorptiometry, in vivo-neutron activation analysis, and deuterium isotope dilution, without the radiation exposure hazards [35–38]. BIA might be considered comparable to measuring the psoas muscle cross sectional area at the L_3 vertebral level by computed tomography (CT) scan or magnetic resonance imaging (MRI) as it might be appropriate to evaluate not only the psoas muscle mass, but also the whole body SMM [39–41].

Considering feasibility, the current guidelines of the European Society for Clinical Nutrition and Metabolism (ESPEN) recommend only SGA and/or anthropometry parameters to identify patients at risk for poor nutritional status, and BIA to quantify undernutrition in spite of the limitations of all techniques in patients with ascitic decompensation [40–42]. According to the ESPEN, other composite nutrition scores provide no additional prognostic information [42–44] (Figure 2).

EXPLORED AREA	CLINICAL & LAB TOOLS
Subjective global assessment (SGA)	SGA scale • well-nourished • moderately malnourished • severely malnourished
Biochemical parameters of nutritional status	Serum transferrin Retinol binding protein Serum albumin Prealbumin (transthyretin) Creatinine-height index 24-hour urine nitrogen 3-methylhistidine excretion Total body potassium
Immune competence	Hypersplenism ↓ total lymphocyte and CD8 cell counts Skin anergy tests
Anthropometry	Body mass index (BMI) Midarm muscle circumference Skin folds thickness (ascites)
Hand grip dynamometry	Handgrip strength dynamometry Six minute walk test
Indirect Calorimetry	Non-protein respiratory quotient (npRQ)
Bioelectrical impedance	Direct segmental multi-frequency bioelectrical analysis
Others	Dual energy X-ray absorptiometry In vivo-neutron activation analysis Deuterium isotope dilution Psoas muscle cross sectional area

Figure 2. Assessment of nutritional status in End Stage Liver Disease Patients.

2. Nutritional Therapy before Liver Transplantation

The main goals of pre-LT nutritional therapy are to prevent further nutrient and muscle depletion and to correct any vitamin and mineral deficiencies present in order to minimize the risk of infections and debility [23].

Because in deceased donor transplantation (DDLT), no one can predict when a patient will receive a transplant [2], an aggressive early post-operative nutritional support (by enteral route if possible) should be allocated to those patients with highest MELD scores, especially when they are undernourished and, if it is anticipated that patients will be unable to eat within for more than two days. Also, this approach should be considered when patients cannot maintain oral intake above 60% of the recommended intake for more than 10 days [18]. On the other hand, an early, planned, preoperative nutritional intervention can be performed in most cases of LDLT, since the date of LT is known in advance, unlike in DDLT. Nutritional therapy, as well as rehabilitation at the time of referral of a potential recipient, starts approximately a few months before LT to most effectively increase SMM and BCM [7].

2.1. Route of Nutritional Support

Enteral nutrition (EN) with a gastric or jejunal small-bore feeding tube is the preferable route of delivery of nutrition for all patients who are not able to maintain adequate oral intake to still benefit from topical nutritional factors in the gut, and maintain the integrity of the gastric mucosa and gut barrier. It is also less costly, with fewer complications and decreased hospital length of stay compared with parenteral nutrition (PN) which carries risk of infection, fluid overload and electrolyte imbalance [45]. ESPEN guidelines (2006) on enteral nutrition in organ transplantation recommended use of nutritional support in patients with severe nutritional risk for 10–14 days prior to major surgery even if surgery has to be delayed [41,42].

EN provides antigenic stimulation to the gut-associated lymphoid tissue and is a stimulus for biliary secretion of immunoglobulin A [10,46]. These factors maintain the barrier against translocation of luminal bacteria to the portal circulation, thus decreasing infectious complications indicated by the differential urinary excretion of carbohydrates of varying molecular weights [10,47].

With EN, excessive feeding will lead to intolerance with diarrhea, bloating, and vomiting. Because the gut provides a "gate-keeper" role, major complications related to excessive tube feed administration are generally kept to a minimum. With PN however, there are no means of regulation and the patient is forced to assimilate the entire substrate load [10,45].

Feeding tubes do not increase the risk for esophageal variceal hemorrhage, but may be associated with an increased risk of epistaxis, sinusitis, impaired gastric emptying and tube feeding-associated diarrhea on long-term use as well as tube retraction, clogging and small intestinal obstruction. However, complications related to mal-positioned feeding tubes are usually preventable if placement is correctly achieved and regularly monitored [10,47].

Feeding tubes are preoperatively placed endoscopically by transillumination across the abdominal wall. The presence of ascites may increase the difficulty in finding a safe window for tube placement. Fluid in the peritoneal cavity can prevent proper apposition of the gastric body to the abdominal wall to ensure the healing of a proper tube tract. Ascites that accumulates can also drain through the tract and increase the risk of infection. Particularly in the setting of hypocomplementemia in cirrhosis, the decreased opsonization and the open communication from the skin to subcutaneous tissue and ascitic fluid could further increase the risk of bacterial peritonitis. The concern is for puncture of a variceal vessel during the procedure. In addition, portal hypertension can lead to many small collateral vessels subcutaneously that also elevate bleeding risk [18,43].

The indications for PN use in liver disease have recently been reviewed and published by ESPEN for patients with fulminant hepatic failure and coma, and for patients who are moderately or severely malnourished and cannot achieve adequate energy intake, either orally or through EN due to gastrointestinal dysfunction such as esophageal bleeding, ileus or intestinal obstruction or those who should be [41,48]. Given the low glycogen stores in patients with liver disease, it is important to provide a glucose infusion in patients who require fasting and are not able to take oral nutrients or EN for more than 12 h [41,42]. Use of "standardized" formulas should be restricted to stable patients with no fluid overload who need maintenance fluid administration only [48]. As for stable patients, the option exists to use fluid maintenance containing water, electrolytes, water- and fat-soluble vitamins or the liver-adapted solutions containing higher BCAA and lower content of aromatic amino acids [49].

2.2. Considerations for Carbohydrate Supplementation

Carbohydrate intake should exclusively be provided by glucose and cover 50–60% of non-protein energy requirements. Glucose infusion should supply 2–3 g/kg body weight per day of glucose. Administration of glucose in excess will result in severe hyperglycemia, lipogenesis and increased carbon dioxide production [47,48]. Patients with liver failure can have alterations in glucose homeostasis; therefore, careful monitoring of serum glucose is needed to avoid complications associated with hyperglycemia [48]. In the early postoperative phase, a dysfunction of glucose metabolism associated with insulin resistance is often prevalent. Increased ischemia-related damage of neurons and glia cells, dysfunctional leukocyte function or oxidative stress have been found to be associated with hyperglycaemia. Thus, hyperglycaemia should be treated by reducing the glucose intake to 2.0 g/kg/day, and up to 4 IU/h insulin, if needed, to maintain euglycaemia because higher insulin doses do not improve glucose oxidation. When tacrolimus is used for immunosuppression, its diabetogenic potential can be lowered by reducing the dose and aiming for trough levels of 3–8 ng/mL without undue risk of rejection [49].

2.3. Considerations for Lipid Supplementation

Patients with advanced LC have decreased plasma levels of essential fatty acids and their polyunsaturated derivatives such as arachidonate levels that have been associated with lower survival. Both are cell membrane components and precursors of a wide array of biologically active compounds. Lipid should be provided by using emulsions with a reduced content of polyunsaturated fatty acids, as compared to pure soy bean oil emulsions, and cover 40–50% of non-protein energy requirements [22,50].

Because fat is important in nutrient repletion of the malnourished patient, dietary fat should not be restricted unless true fat malabsorption has been diagnosed using a fecal fat test. Incorporating medium chain triglycerides; an alternative form of fat not requiring bile salts for absorption, can provide a concentrated source of calories to patients with fat malabsorption and are available in both EN and PN formulations [22,50].

Many EN formulas provide a wide range of lipid dosages from a variety of sources for fatty acids. When prescribing total parenteral nutrition (TPN) many hospitals compound "three-in-one" TPN solutions containing amino acids, dextrose, and lipids. The minimum lipid dose in such combinations should be 20 g/L or 2% final concentration. More dilute lipid formulas are unstable in the presence of hypertonic dextrose and amino acids, resulting in separation of the lipid emulsion into oil and water [50]. However, Clinical essential fatty acid deficiency takes approximately 5 to 6 weeks to develop without linoleic acid or linolenic acid intake, so it is not likely to become an issue for most patients with liver failure except in those severely malnourished. Therefore, a short course of "fat-free" TPN might be used [22,51].

Other hospitals favor separate "piggyback" lipid infusion which may be preferred due to increased infection risk that comes from TPN solutions hanging for up to 24 h and the use of multi-dose lipid vials for compounding TPN [40,52]. A large dose of PN lipid can result in reticuloendothelial system blocking which aggravates infection risk and is exacerbated by rapid "piggyback" infusion techniques, and ameliorated by slower continuous infusion. Lipid administration should not exceed 1 g/kg/day using pre-hospital dry weight and should be given over 24 h if possible [49,52].

The use of an omega-3 fatty acid-predominant lipid emulsion can prevent the occurrence of dietary-induced and parenteral nutrition-induced steatosis and improves the resolution of cholestasis. Omega-3 can decrease de novo lipogenesis, interfere with the arachidonic acid pathway of inflammation thereby reducing the availability for eicosanoid-synthesizing enzymes and inflammation. It is thought that appropriate intake of omega-3 fatty acids would improve immunological resistance and offer some protection against inflammatory tissue damage and capillary permeability [52,53].

2.4. Considerations for Protein Supplementation

The dilemma of sarcopenic chronically malnourished hepatopathic patients with ESLD and cirrhosis, having a subtle border between the need for hypercaloric diets rich in proteins and the risk of hyperammoniemia and HE is still to be solved. In these patients, the need for severe protein restriction, however, may be alleviated by measures, such as lactulose and neomycin or probiotics to decrease intestinal ammoniogenesis and BCAAs [54].

Hyperammonemia results from the production of ammonia in the gut and kidneys and the decreased breakdown by liver and skeletal muscle, caused by sarcopenia in malnourished patients with liver disease. It is well known that ammonia has a direct toxicity on brain astrocytes. This effect definitely contributes to HE. In addition, inflammation, infection, and oxidative stress also play a role [54].

Protein intake should not be limited as this may aggravate protein deficiency, and improvement in nitrogen balance may be achieved without aggravating HE [55]. Supplementation with vegetable, rather than animal, source protein may be advantageous [56].

In practice, whole-protein formulas are generally recommended, and BCAA-enriched formulas should be used in patients who develop HE during re-feeding. Protein intake should be at least 1 g/kg/day initially, and then 24-h urinary urea nitrogen can be measured to assess the catabolic rate in patients with normal renal function. Further increases in protein intake can be adjusted accordingly. Progressive increments in protein supplementation should be implemented, up to 1.8–2.0 g/kg/day as tolerated [52,56].

2.5. Branched-Chain Amino Acid Supplementation

BCAAs (leucine, isoleucine and valine) do not require the liver for metabolism, and thus are preferentially used in liver failure. On the other hand, aromatic amino acids (AAAs) (phenylalanine, tryptophan and tyrosine) are not metabolized effectively in liver failure and thus accumulate [52–57]. The expected ratio, the so-called Fisher's ratio, or the BCAAs/tyrosine ratio (BTR) should be 3.5:1; however, this ratio falls to 1:1 in patients with ESLD, allowing preferential transport of the AAAs to occur across the blood-brain barrier [58]. These are metabolized to octopamine, phenylethylamine, and phenylethanolamine, which are weak false neurotransmitters that compete with endogenous neurotransmitters, inhibit excitatory stimulation of the brain, competing with endogenous neurotransmitters, thus aggravating HE [57,58]. In addition, tryptophan is metabolized to 5-hydroxytryptophan (serotonin), which can produce further lethargy [55,56] (Figure 3).

Aromatic amino acids—serum levels increased

—Tyrosine
—Phenylalanine*
—Free Tryptophan*

Branched-chain amino acids BCAAs—serum levels decreased

—Valine*
—Leucine*
—Isoleucine*

Other amino acids—serum levels increased

Methionine*, Asparagine

Figure 3. Amino Acids Altered in Liver Disease. The expected BCAAs/tyrosine ratio (Fisher's ratio), should be 3.5:1; it falls to 1:1 in patients with end stage liver disease. * Essential amino acids.

There is a debate on the use of BCAA-enriched versus standard amino acid formulas [59–61] based on the hypothesis that decreased BTR contributes to HE [62]. However, ESPEN guidelines do not recommend using specialized formulas [41,42].

BCAAs induce secretion of hepatocyte growth factor and glutamine production [63–66]. Leucine activates the mammalian target of rapamycin signaling pathway, thus inhibiting protein degradation and activating glycogen synthase [7,11].

Shirabe et al. [67] reported preoperative oral BCAA supplementation reduced the incidence of post-transplant bacteremia and sepsis in LDLT patients. Nakamura et al. [68] reported that the phagocytic functions of neutrophils and killer lymphocytes obtained from LC patients were restored by oral BCAAs supplementation.

Recently, a pre-LT BCAA-enriched formula has been demonstrated to lower ammonia, and improve albumin, prealbumin, total lymphocyte count, BTR, glucose intolerance, liver regeneration, immune system function, maturation of dendritic cells and the ability of peripheral blood mononuclear cells to proliferate in response to mitogens, thus preventing postoperative sepsis [7,65,67].

Initiation of oral BCAAs in patients in the early stage of liver disease may contribute to solving current LT problems, such as the donor shortage, the availability of only small liver grafts for patients awaiting LDLT. The use of oral BCAAs might also play a role in improving post-LT mortality by preserving the hepatic reserve of scheduled LT recipients [68,69].

BCAA supplementation post-exercise attenuated the decline in myofibrillar protein synthesis, which is vital in preserving lean mass during weight loss. Thus, the addition of BCAA supplements may have allowed for the maintenance of lean muscle mass because of its potential to enhance lean muscle protein synthesis [65,70]. Oral ingestion of a BCAA supplement before or after exercise improved the recovery of damaged muscles by suppressing the endogenous muscle-protein breakdown [64,66,70].

2.6. Micronutrient Supplementation

Patients with ESLD are susceptible to severe deficiencies in folate and pyridoxal-5'-phosphate, the biologically active vitamin B6. Thiamine liver stores are depleted in alcoholic and hepatitis C-related LC [71–73]. This depletion is associated with increased brain ammonia concentrations due to decreased activity of a-ketoglutarate dehydrogenase, a rate-limiting tricarboxylic acid cycle enzyme [71,72]. Deficiencies in antioxidant micronutrients (selenium, vitamin E, vitamin C) are related to oxidative stress common in such patients [73].

A typical feature of alcoholic or cholestatic liver diseases is an increasingly severe reduction in hepatic vitamin A stores, which sometimes leads to infertility and night blindness [73–75]. In vitamin A-deficient cirrhotic patients, the supplementation of vitamin A, even at relatively moderate doses, may further aggravate liver injury since high-dose vitamin A preparations may be hepatotoxic due to polar retinoid metabolites that cause hepatocellular apoptosis and may promote fibrogenesis [74,75]. Decreased levels of folate, B12, calcium, phosphorus and vitamin K with subsequent coagulopathy are also common [75–78].

Magnesium and zinc deficiency are common in patients with decompensated LC due to decreased absorption and diuretic-induced increased urinary excretion [31,32]. Clinically, zinc deficiency presents with alterations of smell and taste, alterations in protein metabolism, and HE. Zinc supplementation improves glucose intolerance and decreases ammonia levels [31,32,76].

Bitetto et al. [79] observed that vitamin D may act as an immune modulator in LT, favoring immune tolerance of liver allograft. Additionally, Bitetto et al. found that early vitamin D supplementation, in addition to preventing osteoporosis, was independently associated with a lack of acute rejection, which is important because low vitamin D levels are prevalent among LT candidates.

On the other hand, an excess of micronutrients can also be dangerous. Serum ferritin is associated with increased body iron or can be a consequence of systemic necro-inflammatory states. The level of serum ferritin acts as a predictor of mortality in LC patients [77].

2.7. Correction of Liver Osteodystrophy

Osteopenia and osteoporosis are highly prevalent in patients with ESLD, and represent a major cause of morbidity before and after LT [80]. They can be caused by hormonal changes in parathormone and calcitonin, increased circulating levels of bilirubin and cytokines, corticosteroids, and immunosuppressive therapy in cholestatic diseases [81–83]. Ingestion of alcohol can directly and indirectly promote bone loss. However, poor diet, physical inactivity, and degree of liver insufficiency further contribute to deterioration of bone [81,82].

LT candidates should be encouraged to consume foods high in calcium and vitamin D. If consumption is low, calcium and vitamin D supplementation (1200–1500 mg/day) is highly recommended for patients with osteopenia and in combination with bisphosphonates for patients with established osteoporosis and/or history of fractures. If steatorrhea is diagnosed, as in cholestatic diseases water-miscible forms of fat-soluble vitamins including vitamin D should be prescribed [81].

Protein metabolism generates a large amount of acid, which must be buffered by the skeleton and kidneys. The skeleton responds to high serum acidity by releasing a buffering agent calcium into the bloodstream, activating bone resorption. With more calcium entering the bloodstream, the kidneys respond by increasing urinary excretion, resulting in a net loss of calcium. There is also a link between high-fat diets and bone loss, as fat is suggested to inhibit osteoblast formation [80–83].

2.8. Over-Supplementation and Physical Rehabilitation Program

Patients with liver disease commonly suffer from obesity because of continued oral intake along with limitations in physical activity that are often recommended due to fear that exertion would hasten the progress of ESLD progression or worsen complications. However, exercise is documented not to adversely affect liver function tests or worsen symptoms. In fact, the adverse effects of inactivity and bed rest may not only worsen the complications of reduced physical functioning, muscle wasting and osteopenia, but may also be linked to decreased post-LT success [83,84].

Obesity is also considered a predictor of hepatic steatosis in deceased [85] and living donors [12]. A donor's fatty liver is strongly associated with decreased allograft function and decreased patient survival [86], and the presence of fatty liver is the main reason for the discarding of potential donor livers [85]. Pre-LT obese patients may be more likely to have primary graft dysfunction or delayed graft function after LT [87,88]. Weight loss is used to reduce the amount of liver fat among obese patients [87].

Dietitians need to resist the temptation to reach the impractical goal of producing anabolism. Attempts to replete the malnourished metabolically stressed pre-LT patient in excess of the patient's energy expenditure lead to hyperglycemia and increased incidence of infection [48]. The goal of nutritional support for the patient with liver failure is to provide adequate protein and energy equivalent to, or slightly less than, the patient's energy expenditure. Therefore, energy restriction to 25–30 kcal/kg/day is routinely used to encourage the mobilization of native fat stores [89].

Recently, a rehabilitation program has been introduced to encourage early postoperative mobilization and avert pulmonary dysfunction. Because LDLT is an elective procedure that differs from DDLT, a pre-LT rehabilitation program can be implemented until the day of LT [7].

2.9. Immunonutrition

Use an immuno-modulating diet (IMD) as a part of EN or PN is based on its down-regulatory effects on inflammatory cytokine production, its modulation of eicosanoid synthesis, and its amelioration of the necrotized liver injury and post-LT immunosuppression, rather than its effects on nutrition per se [90,91].

Glutamine dipeptide, arginine, nucleotides and omega-3 fatty acids (fish oil emulsion) intake has been suggested to minimize ischemia or reperfusion damage of the donor organ [10,63,92]. Arginine stimulates the release of growth hormone, insulin release, improves nitrogen balance, promotes wound healing, strengthens immune function and enhances nitric oxide biosynthesis [89].

An IMD enriched with hydrolyzed whey peptide (HWP), which is a protein complex derived from milk, has been proved to decrease post-LT bacteremia, infections and mortality compared with a conventional elemental diet [93]. These benefits are attributed to the antioxidant, antihypertensive, antiviral, anti-inflammatory, and antibacterial properties of HWP because it is rich in lactoferrin, β-lactoglobulin, α-lactalbumin, glycomacropeptide, and immunoglobulins [10,94]. Lactoferrin protects against the development of hepatitis caused by the sensitization of Kupffer cells by lipopolysaccharide and inhibits the production of inflammatory cytokines such as TNF-α, IL-1β, and IL-6 in monocytes [4,7,73].

The considerable amount of steroids administered to patients after LT, as well as surgical diabetes and insulin resistance, can cause intra- and postoperative hyperglycemia, which has been associated with surgical site infections [92]. IMD enriched with HWP contains isomaltulose disaccharide (glucose plus fructose with a glycosidic bond). Isomaltulose is often used instead of sugar in diets for patients with diabetes mellitus since it prevents postprandial hyperglycemia due to slow resolution. An IMD enriched with HWP has been found to significantly decrease the incidence of post-LT hyperglycemia [93,95].

2.10. Use of Synbiotics

Bacterial translocation usually occurring in LC is related to bacterial overgrowth, increased intestinal permeability and immune alterations, and leads to intestinal edema, decreased peristalsis, and infection. It also contributes to pathogenesis of a hyperdynamic circulatory state and multiple organ dysfunction via pro-inflammatory cytokine responses [11,96,97].

Probiotics are living bacteria found in fermented beverages, yogurt and sauerkraut that foster a hostile colonic environment against bad bacteria. Prebiotics are non-digestible dietary fiber that pass unchanged through the gastrointestinal tract and nourish probiotics. Synbiotics are a combination of both [97,98].

Sugawara et al. [99] reported that preoperative oral administration of synbiotics can enhance the immune response, attenuate the systemic postoperative inflammatory response, and decrease the occurrence of post-LT infection and the duration of antibiotic therapy. These benefits of synbiotics are attributed to the ability of *Lactobacillus* to initiate immunoglobulin production, restore macrophage function, stimulate apoptosis, and modulate lymphocyte function. In addition, *Lactobacillus* is reported to attenuate cytokine release, increase mucin production, eliminate toxins, and stimulate mucosal growth [100].

Probiotics such as Enterococcus faecalis, Clostridium butyricum, Echerichia coli strain Nissle 1917, Lactobacillus casei strain Shirota, Bacillus mesentericus, Lactobacillus, and Bifidobacterium with fructooligosaccharides can all alter gut microbiota, prevent bacterial translocation, decrease endotoxin levels and restore neutrophil phagocytic capacity [97], since neutrophil function is impaired by endotoxemia upon bacterial translocation in LC [101].

Lower ammonia levels, significant rates of minimal HE reversal and good adherence by patients, with greater improvement in all neuropsychological tests, have been all observed upon use of probiotics compared with use of conventional lactulose [102]. Furthermore, lactulose treatment was associated with occasional abdominal pain, cramping, diarrhea and flatulence. Synbiotic supplements were free of such adverse effects [102–105].

2.11. Nocturnal Meals

Periods of fasting should be avoided in cirrhotic patients. Frequent meals should be implemented to combat catabolic state during the overnight fasting period. Because of this, nocturnal supplementation of a small bedtime snack and nocturnal glucose supplementation increase carbohydrate along with decreased lipid and protein oxidation rates in the next morning without significant BEE changes, thus improving nitrogen balance, total body protein gain and preventing catabolic states and undernutrition [106,107]. It has been reported that nocturnal BCAAs administration as a late evening snack (LES) improves the serum albumin level and glucose tolerance in LC patients [31,106,107].

Some reports found that carbohydrate-predominant LES promote improved nutritional status [108,109]. Others reported that LES with BCAA were useful in improving protein metabolism and lipolysis in cirrhotic patients and that energy efficiency of BCAA is higher than that of glucose or carbohydrates [31,106,107].

For adult recipients preparing for LDLT, Kaido et al. [10,11] illustrated a detailed preoperative nutritional therapy regimen. It starts approximately 2 weeks before LDLT after BIA assessment. The therapy consists of the following three components: a nutrient mixture enriched with BCAAs or BCAAs nutrients as late evening nutrients; synbiotics using a supplementation product enriched with glutamine, dietary fiber and oligosaccharide three times daily, and a lacto-fermented beverage containing 5×10^8/mL of *Lactobacillus casei Shirota* strain once a day via feeding tube or orally until discharge. Additionally, patients with low serum zinc level receive 1.0 g/day of polaprezinc.

Dietitians should adjust the type and amount of food for each patient to maintain a total energy intake at least 1.3 times the BEE (e.g., a protein intake of 1.2 to 1.5 g/kg including BCAAs nutrients (scaled according to degree of hepatic decompensation) adherent to ESPEN guidelines ESPEN [41,42]. Of the total non-protein energy requirements, 60–70% should be administered as high-complex and simple carbohydrates, whereas lipids should make up the other 40–50%. In malnourished patients, a daily intake of 50 kcal/kg is required for energy repletion [23]. Excess calories should be avoided, as this promotes hepatic lipogenesis, liver dysfunction and increased carbon dioxide production, leading to increased work of breathing [23,42,43].

3. Nutritional Support after LT

Liver disease, nutrition abnormalities are expected to correct when a new functioning liver is in place. However, unlike other complications, a reverse of malnutrition and more specifically of sarcopenia is not a rule after LT. Therefore, despite the regain of liver function after LT and the improvement in body weight after surgery, the alterations in body composition may persist. In particular, muscle depletion seems to persist for at least 12 months or more [38,39]. Moreover, other features of malnutrition, such as overweight and obesity, may occur in liver recipients during long-term follow-up.

During the stay of surgical intensive care unit (SICU), nutritional support should be emphasized on the destination of graft function recovery and overall convalescence which is faced with stress from critical illness and multiple treatments (mechanical ventilation, hemodiafiltration, use of corticosteroid and immunosuppressive agents and so on) [28,44].

3.1. Factors That May Influence Nutritional Modifications after LT

3.1.1. Liver Gut Brain Axis

The normal hepatic innervations and more specifically, vagus innervation, are lost during transplantation. It has been suggested that the isolation of the liver from the autonomic regulatory control may influence not only nutrient absorption and metabolism, glucose and lipids homeostasis but also appetite signaling and eating behavior [104]. All of these modifications may contribute to the body composition and weight changes observed in liver transplanted patients [105,106].

3.1.2. Diet

The majority of the published studies reported a significant increase in dietary intake when the patients were followed after liver transplantation. These changes are particularly evident in those patients following severe dietary restrictions or in those suffering from relevant gastrointestinal symptoms or anorexia before LT [107,108]. Calories reportedly improved from a median of 27 kcal/kg/day to 32 kcal/kg/day and proteins from a median of 0.8 g/kg/day to 1.3 g/kg/day (comparing dietary intake before LT and 12 months post-transplant [73]. Moreover, overweight or obesity in LT long-term recipients was correlated with the increase in energy intake (from 1542 ± 124 kcal/day to 2227 ± 141 kcal/day), a higher consumption of both proteins and carbohydrates and an approximately doubled intake of fat (from 62 g/day to 102 g/day) compared to pre-transplant [107].

3.1.3. Immunosuppressive Therapy

Corticosteroids need attention as they increase appetite and fat deposition and decrease fat oxidation; moreover, they are responsible for increased proteolysis and impaired protein synthesis [89]. Calcineurin inhibitors, such as cyclosporine and tacrolimus, may affect energy metabolism and muscle mass [95]. Cyclosporine was found to be an independent predictor of post-transplant weight gain [89], whereas tacrolimus has been reported to increase energy expenditure [95]. Both cyclosporine and tacrolimus may contribute to the impairment of muscle growth and muscle regeneration by inhibiting calcineurin, which exerts its effects on skeletal muscle differentiation, hypertrophy, protein accretion and fiber-type determination [89,95]. Other immunosuppressive agents, such as sirolimus and everolimus, negatively influence muscle mass by inhibiting the mammalian target of rapamycin complex, which is a key regulator of protein synthesis [95].

After liver transplant, patients will have to take immunosuppressant medication to the end of their lives. Although modern drugs with less side effects are available, increased survival rates and decreased overall complications have led to many nutrition status implications associated with the use of cyclosporine, tacrolimus and corticosteroids. New onset diabetes or glucose impairment is common initially after the operation as the consequence of immunosuppressant regiment [105,106].

Diabetic dietary advice is usual required, and if necessary, the use of oral hypoglycemic or insulin regimens should be tethered according to the progression of diet. If hyperglycemia persists, it should be managed by reducing excess glucose intake, since higher insulin might hamper increased glucose oxidation in this period. Also, the diabetogenic potential of the immunosuppressant tacrolimus may be lowered by reducing its dose, without undue risk of rejection [109].

Many patients may concomitantly present with high potassium levels shortly after the operation. This usually results from the nephrotoxicity of the prescribed immunosuppressant medication. Thus, in the early post-transplant periods, it might be important to control potassium food sources as well as, it the recommendation of the use of dietary techniques which are able to reduce its content in nutrients [106]. In the long term, this is not indicated, as this condition mostly disappears. Hypomagnesemia also rises as a consequence of immunosuppression and, patients generally receive magnesium supplementation, however, some progress with diarrhea. The intake of magnesium rich food sources should be encouraged, such as dark cocoa, whole grains, nuts, legumes, fruits and green vegetables. Important to point that the consumption of this kind of food should not be restricted, even considering the immunocompromised host as a result of anti-graft rejection drugs. Patients should receive food safety advice to prevent food borne infections, which can be achieved with the correct handling of fruits and vegetables [95]. "As a result of immunosuppressive medications, the transplant recipient, in addition to other at-risk people such as those suffering from diabetes, kidney disease; infants; and the elderly—are 15–20% more susceptible to foodborne illness than the general population as shigella, yersinia, norovirus, rotaviruses, cryptosporidium, Toxoplasma gondii, Trichinella and Giardia lamblia. The commonly assumed mode of food contamination traditionally involved undercooked meats fish, poultry, eggs, fermented foods, and unwashed raw fruits, and vegetables, fresh salad dressings containing aged cheese raw, non-heat treated honey or unpasteurized dairy products [110]. Pasteurization and sufficient cooking kill Listeria; however, contamination with hepatitis A, *E. coli*, Listeria, Salmonella, may occur after cooking and before packaging by fecal contamination if handled by food handlers. Flies, may act as carriers of contamination either directly by laying eggs on the meat by transporting contaminants from one source to another. the transplant recipient may experience a more rapid onset of symptoms compared with the general population, in the form of severe dehydration and organ failure/hemolytic uremic syndrome (*E. coli*), sepsis, or death (Listeria and Clostridia botulinum). Prevention of foodborne illness involve thorough cleaning, hand washing, avoiding raw meat or canned food, maintaining appropriate storage temperature [7,110]. Grapefruit, turmeric, pomelo, ginger, pomegranates, Seville oranges, black pepper, cranberry juice, black tea, beer, cruciferous vegetables, kava, licorice root, wine, and olive oil, contain compounds that modulate P450 activity juice should be avoided as elevate blood immunosuppressant's levels. Other interactions to be avoided include K-rich foods (e.g., broccoli, spinach) and Coumadin. Foods containing the substance tyramine, including chocolate, beer, wine, avocados, some aged cheeses, and some processed meats, and monoamine oxidase (MAO) inhibitors, a type of antidepressant result in a dangerous rise in blood pressure. Natural licorice, which contains the compound glycyrrhizin, can reduce the effectiveness of blood pressure medications and diuretics such as Aldactone (spironolactone). It can also increase the risk of Lanoxin (digoxin) toxicity. Resveratrol, an antioxidant compound found in red wine and peanuts, inhibits platelet aggregation, and high intakes could increase the risk of bleeding when consumed with anticoagulant drugs such as Coumadin [111].

3.1.4. Energy Metabolism

Hypermetabolism after transplantation was significantly associated with hypermetabolism before LT and a higher cumulative dose of prednisone. Energy expenditure normalized only when insulin sensitivity was restored. However, those patients with a reduced energy expenditure showed the higher increase in fat mass [107–109].

After the LT operation, energy and protein requirements are still increased for weeks. Metabolism in liver recipients only improves at 4 weeks after LT, especially considering the non-protein respiratory quotient, serum non esterified fatty acids and nitrogen balance [109]. In the immediate phase after the operation, protein catabolism is markedly increased and patients should receive about 1.5–2.0 g/kg of protein. Non-protein energy requirements, in this period, vary according to the metabolic and inflammatory status, with unstable patients demanding lower intakes while the others more. When indirect calorimetry is not available, estimates between 25 and 30 kcal/kg/day maybe used [108,109].

Total body water decreases and body fat increases, whereas BCM remains unchanged after LT [107]. Deficiencies in vitamin A and zinc immediately normalize after LT [108,109]. Increased REE may persist for a long period after LT [108,112]; however, overweight status and hypercholesterolemia have been observed after LT [110,111], accompanied by an increase in the saturated fatty acid content of fat tissue [109,113].

Nutritional status after LT depends on the allograft function; if the allograft fails or is rejected, many of the nutritional derangements present before LT will persist. Even in a well-functioning graft, some nutritional disturbances do not completely normalize in the long term after LT. Increased protein breakdown is often present during the first 2 weeks post-LT; thus, optimizing the nutrient intake over this period is needed for wound healing and hepatocyte recovery [109,114].

3.2. Nutritional Support during the Immediate Post-LT Phase and Short-Term after LT

The goal of nutrition therapy in the acute post-LT phase is to ensure adequate protein and energy provisions to avoid protein breakdown [115]. Hypermetabolism has been found predictive of transplant-free survival independently of MELD and Child-Pugh scores and tends to persist for at least a year post-LT [116].

Resuming EN within 12 h of LT has been shown to reduce postoperative viral infections and to produce better nitrogen retention. Patients should be advanced from nutritional support to an oral diet using smaller and more frequent feedings as soon as tolerated after LT. EN should not be discontinued until patients are able to maintain an adequate oral intake consistent with their nutritional requirements [10,11,94].

Intra-operative placement of the tip of the feeding tube in the proximal jejunum allows early EN after LT. For adult LDLT recipients, Kaido et al. [10,11,94] described in detail an early postoperative EN regimen using a 9F Witzel enteral tube jejunostomy placed in the proximal jejunum at surgery, through which an EN is started within 24 h after surgery. The starting total daily energy intake until postoperative day (POD) 3 is 10–15 kcal/kg and gradually increased to 25–35 kcal/kg using an IMD enriched with HWP. The initial infusion rate is 20 mL/h. If well tolerated, it is increased to 40 mL/h by POD 5. In case of severe edema of the small intestine or severe diarrhea, the speed of IMD is decreased to 20 mL/h (=20 kcal/h) or an oral rehydration solution is used. After confirmation of improvement in edema or diarrhea, the regimen can be resumed. Oral nutrition is started after swallowing ability is confirmed, usually around POD 5. Dietitians calculate the daily amounts of protein and carbohydrates required for each recipient and adjust the speed of the EN according to the oral intake. EN is stopped when the patient can tolerate adequate oral intake containing solid food. All patients resume preoperative synbiotic supplementation three times daily and a lactic fermented beverage once a day via the feeding tube or orally until discharge. This technique allows long-term feeding without discomfort or risk of pneumonia carried by trans-nasal feeding and avoids the need for concomitant TPN with risk of infection.

Metabolic alkalosis and depletion of serum potassium, phosphorus, and magnesium levels in the acute post-LT period due to routine chronic diuretic use in cirrhotic patients, amount of fluid from abdominal drains, gastrointestinal losses or fluid overload should be monitored. Also, refeeding syndrome should be taken as a risk factor for these disorders. In cases of metabolic alkalosis, 90% are chloride-sensitive and easily correctable. Chloride can be delivered using TPN as a vehicle [9–11,117].

Glucose utilization by the transplanted liver is reduced in the first hours of engraftment, due to impaired mitochondrial respiration and inactivity of the tricarboxylic acid cycle [118,119]. During this time, energy is generated mostly from fatty acid oxidation and after approximately 6 h, a shift from fat to glucose utilization occurs in normally-functioning liver grafts, while a failing liver continues to utilize mainly fat [119,120]. Glucose administration immediately after LT has been recommended in small quantities and without insulin in order not to suppress peripheral fat mobilization, judged clinically by blood glucose, lactate, triglyceride levels and arterial ketone bodies [119–122].

Diabetic patients with liver failure receiving EN should be covered with long-acting isophane insulin suspension on a sliding scale for episodes of hyperglycemia [123].

Patients with fulminant hepatic failure are generally well nourished and do not have a pre-hospital history of weight loss. Patients without PEM will tolerate 5–7 days of NPO before needing nutritional support, however, an adequate nutritional supplementation is required as early as comatose patients are put on liver dialysis and on through to support regenerating hepatocytes. Patients with malnutrition should start nutritional support sooner. Withholding nutritional support and inducing a cumulative energy deficit of over 10,000 kcal has been associated with decreased survival [89].

3.3. Long-Term Nutritional Support after LT

In the long-term after liver transplantation, weight gain is mostly observed. It is important to recover the nutritional status, since the patients lose an average of 9.1 kg during the course of liver disease [117]. Greatest relative weight gain occurs in the first six months after the operation [47] and, recovery of all weight loss happens in the first post-transplant year [124]. However, unfortunately, patients do not stop gaining weight in the subsequent years [125], resulting in the alarming prevalence of overweight and obesity [47]. During the first 12 months, the fat mass progressively increases in those patients who had previously depleted overall body mass, but muscle mass recovery is subtle and non-significant by the end of the first year [126]. Therefore, despite the weight gain, the high prevalence of sarcopenia does not change after transplantation [7,47].

Metabolic syndrome, hyperlipidemia and obesity are common in patients after the first 6 months post-LT, especially with immobility, and is associated with an increased risk of major vascular events, diabetes mellitus, hypertension, cancer and fibrosis progression. These conditions contribute to long-term morbidity and mortality [7,47,117,124].

Weight gain is mostly between 2 and 16 months after LT, attributed to stimulated appetite by corticosteroids. Immediately after LT, patients are often instructed to ingest a high-protein, high-energy diet to counteract weight loss associated with pre-LT cachexia and increased energy requirements for surgical recovery but can induce unwanted weight gain. Depressive moods have been implicated in over- and under-eating and should be considered a factor in LT recipients; therefore, patients should be instructed on a diet that promotes a healthy body composition which is low in fat, with adequate amounts of lean protein foods to promote muscle gain. Calories should be sufficient to spare protein from being used as energy, yet not in excess of energy requirements. Regular follow-up with a dietitian will ensure patient compliance. Dietitians should re-assess nutritional status to optimize the patient's diet during the transition from the acute to chronic post-LT phase [41,49,125–127].

Tacrolimus is thought to be associated with a less adverse cardiovascular risk profile than cyclosporin, with significantly reduced prevalence of hypertension, hypercholesterolemia and obesity, together with significantly lower triglyceride levels. Corticosteroids also contribute to post-LT disturbances of these parameters. In patients with stable graft function, withdrawal of prednisolone over time reduces prevalence of such disorders [117,128]. Long-term administration of glucocorticoids results in lipid accumulation, weight gain, osteoporosis and muscle-wasting by impairing REE and substrate oxidation rates. Insulin resistance, postoperative cytokine response, and postmenopausal status in women are other suggested mechanisms that inhibit gain of muscle mass after LT [129].

Standard recommendations after LT include a "no added salt" diet (3 g sodium/day) to prevent water retention associated with steroid therapy. However, health professionals often encourage the addition of flavoring agents, including sodium, to foods to improve taste in order to promote appetite. Therefore, sodium intake may be higher than suspected [89].

Several risk factors for bone loss after LT include steroid use, malnutrition, muscle-wasting, immobilization, pre-LT osteopenia or osteoporosis, previous fractures, and immunosuppressive agents. Bone loss occurs mostly within the first 3–6 months after LT and increases the risk of fractures within the first year. However, osteopenia related to cholestasis tends to become stable at 1 year after LT following improved allograft function. Bisphosphonates may prevent bone loss after LT [78,130–135] (Figure 4).

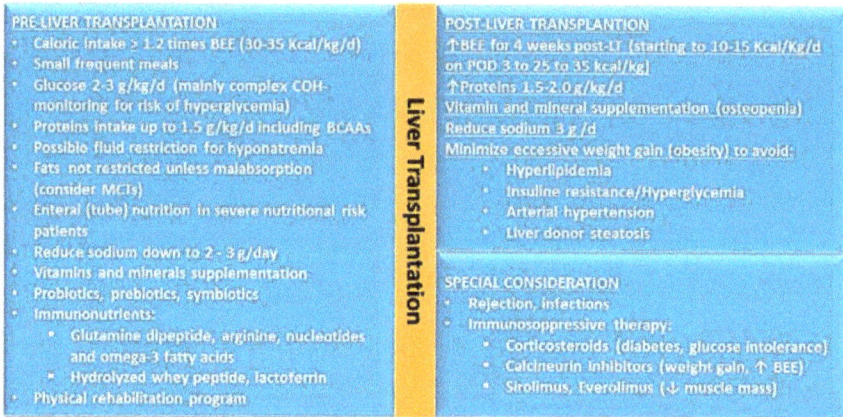

PRE-LIVER TRANSPLANTATION	POST-LIVER TRANSPLANTION
• Caloric intake > 1.2 times BEE (30-35 Kcal/kg/d)	↑BEE for 4 weeks post-LT (starting to 10-15 Kcal/Kg/d
• Small frequent meals	on POD 3 to 25 to 35 kcal/kg)
• Glucose 2-3 g/kg/d (mainly complex COH-monitoring for risk of hyperglycemia)	↑Proteins 1.5-2.0 g/kg/d
• Proteins intake up to 1.5 g/kg/d including BCAAs	Vitamin and mineral supplementation (osteopenia)
• Possible fluid restriction for hyponatremia	Reduce sodium 3 g /d
• Fats not restricted unless malabsorption (consider MCTs)	Minimize eccessive weight gain (obesity) to avoid:
• Enteral (tube) nutrition in severe nutritional risk patients	• Hyperlipidemia
	• Insuline resistance/Hyperglycemia
	• Arterial hypertension
• Reduce sodium down to 2 - 3 g/day	• Liver donor steatosis
• Vitamins and minerals supplementation	
• Probiotics, prebiotics, symbiotics	SPECIAL CONSIDERATION
• Immunonutrients:	• Rejection, infections
▪ Glutamine dipeptide, arginine, nucleotides and omega-3 fatty acids	• Immunosoppressive therapy:
	• Corticosteroids (diabetes, glucose intolerance)
▪ Hydrolyzed whey peptide, lactoferrin	• Calcineurin inhibitors (weight gain, ↑ BEE)
• Physical rehabilitation program	• Sirolimus, Everolimus (↓ muscle mass)

Liver Transplantation

Figure 4. Nutritional interventions before and after liver transplantation. BEE: basal energy expenditure; BCAA: branched chain amino acids; COH: carbohydrates; MCTs: mean chain triglycerides; LT: liver transplantation; POD: post operative day.

4. Special Considerations in Pediatric LT

In children, malnutrition and growth retardation are usually present in all cases before LT, specifically linked to the most common indication; biliary atresia. Partial substitution of usual fats with medium chain triglycerides, and carefully monitored supplementation of fat soluble vitamin are needed. Anthropometry derangement starts to recover as soon as 6 months after LT. Height recovery occurs late [128]. Marked catch-up growth is observed in those children with the most severe growth retardation before LT. However, transplanted children do not have complete catch up growth and achieve a final height below their genetic potential and even some children experience failure to thrive after LT [110].

Although individually rare, when considered together, liver-based metabolic diseases represent approximately 10% of pediatric liver transplants [136]. Strict galactose- or fructose-free preoperative diets are needed in galactosemia and hereditary fructose intolerance, respectively. Frequent feedings are needed in glycogen storage diseases, which often includes continuous nighttime nasogastric feedings in infants. Uncooked cornstarch ingested every few hours in older patients has been shown to release glucose slowly and steadily and allows avoidance of hypoglycemia [137]. In tyrosinemia, tyrosine free-diet and Nitisinone (NTBC), which blocks the second step in tyrosine degradation are fundamental [138].

Medical treatment during the acute presentation of urea cycle disorders is based initially on reducing blood ammonia levels by (a) discontinuing protein intake and supplying sufficient glucose intravenously to limit catabolism (b) providing biochemical alternatives for nitrogen excretion as intravenous or oral sodium benzoate and phenylacetate [138,139]. Long-term dietary protein restriction is paramount. Enzyme defects block synthesis of arginine and overall protein-restricted diet will lead to arginine deficiency. Arginine supplementation is therefore essential in argininosuccinic aciduria or argininemia to increase nitrogen excretion. However, in carbamyl phosphate synthetase or ornithine transcarbamylase deficiency, citrulline supplementation is preferred [137–139].

In maple syrup disease, dietary restriction of BCAA and aggressive management of episodic metabolic decompensation are required. The B12 supplements are added for methylmalonic aciduria. Tin-protoporphyrin or zinc-mesoporphyrin may decrease the hours of phototherapy required per day or the need for exchange transfusions in crigler najjar cases. Hydrophilic bile acids are used for erythropoietic protoporphyria. Copper-free diet and zinc salts supplements when used in a timely manner can augment chelation therapy to prevent progression of Wilson disease. Likewise, iron-free diet in haemochromatosis. Mannose or Fucose supplementations are essential in some congenital disorders of glycosylation. Dextrose 10% infusion suppresses heme synthesis in porphyria [137–139]. A further comprehensive and detailed discussion of age-specific nutritional treatment in pediatric LT is warranted.

5. Conclusions

Nutritional therapy should be considered an essential adjunct to clinical therapies, especially when the patient is a candidate for LT. Accurate assessment of nutritional status and adequate intervention are prerequisites for perioperative nutritional treatment in patients who undergo LT. However, the metabolic abnormalities induced by liver failure cause the traditional assessment of nutritional status to be difficult. Preoperative malnutrition and sarcopenia estimated by recently-developed body BIA have a significant negative impact on post LT outcome. It is essential to provide adequate nutritional support during all phases of liver transplantation, including preoperative administration of BCAA-enriched nutrient mixture and postoperative use of an IMD enriched with HWP. Perioperative nutritional therapy is now indispensable to improve outcomes after LT. Further studies are warranted to refine patient-tailored nutritional regimens and optimize nutritional recovery and rehabilitation long-term after LT.

Acknowledgments: There is no funding to disclose by all authors.

Author Contributions: A.H. and T.K. conceived and designed the article; A.H. and V.A. performed the literature review; A.H., T.M. and C.M. organized drafting and analysis; T.M. and C.M. contributed figures and revised the article; S.Y. revised the paper; A.H. wrote the paper.

Conflicts of Interest: The authors declare no conflict of interest.

References

1. Dudrick, S.J.; Kavic, S.M. Hepatobiliary nutrition: History and future. *J. Hepatobiliary Pancreat. Surg.* **2002**, *9*, 459–468. [CrossRef] [PubMed]
2. Cabre, E.; Gassull, M.A. Nutrition in liver disease. *Curr. Opin. Clin. Nutr. Metab. Care* **2005**, *8*, 545–551. [CrossRef] [PubMed]
3. O'Brien, A.; Williams, R. Nutrition in end-stage liver disease, principles and practice. *Gastroenterology* **2008**, *134*, 1729–1740. [CrossRef] [PubMed]
4. Mendenhall, C.L.; Moritz, T.E.; Roselle, G.A.; Morgan, T.R.; Nemchausky, B.A.; Tamburro, C.H.; Schiff, E.R.; McClain, C.J.; Marsano, L.S.; Allen, J.I.; et al. A study of oral nutritional support with oxandrolone in malnourished patients with alcoholic hepatitis, results of a Department of Veterans Affairs cooperative Study. *Hepatology* **1993**, *17*, 564–576. [CrossRef] [PubMed]
5. Merli, M.; Giusto, M.; Gentili, F.; Novelli, G.; Ferretti, G.; Riggio, O.; Corradini, S.G.; Siciliano, M.; Farcomeni, A.; Attili, A.F.; et al. Nutritional status, its influence on the outcome of patients undergoing liver transplantation. *Liver Int.* **2010**, *30*, 208–214. [CrossRef] [PubMed]
6. Stephenson, G.R.; Moretti, E.W.; El-Moalem, H.; Clavien, P.A.; Tuttle-Newhall, J.E. Malnutrition in liver transplant patients, preoperative subjective global assessment is predictive of outcome after liver transplantation. *Transplantation* **2001**, *72*, 666–670. [CrossRef] [PubMed]

7. Kaido, T.; Mori, A.; Ogura, Y.; Ogawa, K.; Hata, K.; Yoshizawa, A.; Yagi, S.; Uemoto, S. Pre and perioperative factors affecting infection after living donor liver transplantation. *Nutrition* **2012**, *28*, 1104–1108. [CrossRef] [PubMed]
8. Iida, T.; Kaido, T.; Yagi, S.; Yoshizawa, A.; Hata, K.; Mizumoto, M.; Mori, A.; Ogura, Y.; Oike, F.; Uemoto, S. Posttransplant bacteremia in adult living donor liver transplant recipients. *Liver Transpl.* **2010**, *16*, 1379–1385. [CrossRef] [PubMed]
9. Durczynski, A.; Strzelczyk, J.; Wojciechowska-Durczynska, K.; Borkowska, A.; Hogendorf, P.; Szymanski, D.; Justyna, C.; Leszek, C. Major liver resection results in early exacerbation of insulin resistance, and may be a risk factor of developing overt diabetes in the future. *Surg. Today* **2013**, *43*, 534–538. [CrossRef] [PubMed]
10. Kaido, T.; Ogawa, K.; Fujimoto, Y.; Ogura, Y.; Hata, K.; Ito, T.; Tomiyama, K.; Yagi, S.; Mori, A.; Uemoto, S. Impact of sarcopenia on survival in patients undergoing living donor liver transplantation. *Am. J. Transplant.* **2013**, *13*, 1549–1556. [CrossRef] [PubMed]
11. Kaido, T.; Mori, A.; Ogura, Y.; Hata, K.; Yoshizawa, A.; Lida, A.; Yagi, S.; Uemoto, S. Impact of enteral nutrition using a new immuno-modulating diet after liver transplantation. *Hepatogastroenterology* **2010**, *57*, 1522–1525. [PubMed]
12. Kaido, T.; Mori, A.; Oike, F.; Mizumoto, M.; Ogura, Y.; Hata, K.; Yoshizawa, A.; Iida, T.; Uemoto, S. Impact of pretransplant nutritional status in patients undergoing liver transplantation. *Hepatogastroenterology* **2010**, *57*, 1489–1492. [PubMed]
13. Aranda-Michel, J. Nutrition in hepatic failure and liver transplantation. *Curr. Gastroenterol. Rep.* **2001**, *3*, 362–370. [CrossRef] [PubMed]
14. Kamalaporn, P.; Sobhonslidsuk, A.; Jatchavala, J.; Atisook, K.; Rattanasiri, S.; Parmoolsinsap, C. Factors predisposing to peptic ulcer disease in asymptomatic cirrhotic patients. *Aliment. Pharmacol. Ther.* **2005**, *21*, 1459–1465. [CrossRef] [PubMed]
15. Madden, A.M.; Bradbury, W.; Morgam, M.Y. Taste perception in cirrhosis, its relationship to circulating micronutrients and food preferences. *Hepatology* **1997**, *26*, 40–48. [CrossRef] [PubMed]
16. Thuluvath, P.J.; Triger, D.R. Autonomic neuropathy and chronic liver disease. *Q. J. Med.* **1989**, *72*, 737–747. [PubMed]
17. Maheshwari, A.; Thuluvath, P.J. Autonomic neuropathy may be associated with delayed orocaecal transit time in patients with cirrhosis. *Auton. Neurosci.* **2005**, *118*, 135–139. [CrossRef] [PubMed]
18. Aqel, B.A.; Scolapio, J.S.; Dickson, R.C.; Bruton, D.D.; Bouras, E.P. Contribution of ascites to impaired gastric function and nutritional intake in patients with cirrhosis and ascites. *Clin. Gastroenterol. Hepatol.* **2005**, *3*, 1095–1100. [CrossRef]
19. Muller, M.J.; Lautz, H.U.; Plogmann, B.; Bürger, M.; Körber, J.; Schmidt, F.W. Energy expenditure and substrate oxidation in patients with cirrhosis, the impact of cause, clinical staging and nutritional state. *Hepatology* **1992**, *15*, 782–794. [CrossRef] [PubMed]
20. Petrides, A.S.; DeFronzo, R.A. Glucose metabolism in cirrhosis, a review with some perspective for the future. *Diabetes Metab. Rev.* **1989**, *5*, 691–709. [CrossRef] [PubMed]
21. Stanley, A.J.; Gilmour, H.M.; Ghosh, S.; Ferguson, A.; McGilchrist, A.J. Transjugular intrahepatic portosystemic shunt as a treatment for protein-losing enteropathy caused by portal hypertension. *Gastroenterology* **1996**, *111*, 1679–1682. [CrossRef]
22. Thomas, E.L.; Taylor-Robinson, S.D.; Barnard, M.L.; Frost, G.; Sargentoni, J.; Davidson, B.R.; Cunnane, S.C.; Bell, J.D. Changes in adipose tissue composition in malnourished patients before and after liver transplantation, a carbon-13 magnetic resonance spectroscopy and gas liquid chromatography study. *Hepatology* **1997**, *25*, 178–183. [CrossRef] [PubMed]
23. Cabre, E.; Abad-Lacruz, A.; Nunez, M.C.; Gonzalez-Huix, F.; Fernandez-Banares, F.; Gil, A.; Esteve-Comas, M.; Moreno, J.; Planas, R.; Guilera, M. The relationship of plasma polyunsaturated fatty acid deficiency with survival in advanced liver cirrhosis, multivariate analysis. *Am. J. Gastroenterol.* **1993**, *88*, 718–722. [PubMed]
24. Campos, A.C.; Matias, J.E.; Coelho, J.C. Nutritional aspects of liver transplantation. *Curr. Opin. Clin. Nutr. Metab. Care* **2002**, *5*, 297–307. [CrossRef] [PubMed]
25. Detsky, A.S.; McLaughlin, J.R.; Baker, J.P.; Johnston, N.; Whittaker, S.; Mendelson, R.A. What is subjective global assessment of nutritional status? *J. Parenter. Enter. Nutr.* **1987**, *11*, 8–13. [CrossRef] [PubMed]
26. Driscoll, D.F.; Palombo, J.D.; Bistrian, B.R. Nutritional and metabolic considerations of the adult liver transplant candidate and donor organ. *Nutrition* **1995**, *11*, 255–263. [PubMed]

27. Mullen, J.L.; Buzby, G.P.; Waldman, M.T.; Gertner, M.H.; Hobbs, C.L.; Rosato, E.F. Prediction of operative morbidity and mortality by preoperative nutritional assessment. *Surg. Forum* **1979**, *30*, 8–11.

28. Stephen, M.R.; Roger, W. Nutrition and liver transplantation. *Hepatology* **1999**, *31*, 955–962.

29. Shenkin, A. Serum prealbumin, Is it a marker of nutritional status or of risk of malnutrition? *Clin. Chem.* **2006**, *52*, 2177–2179. [CrossRef] [PubMed]

30. Giusto, M.; Lattanzi, B.; Di Gregorio, V.; Giannelli, V.; Lucidi, C.; Merli, M. Changes in nutritional status after liver transplantation. *World J. Gastroenterol.* **2014**, *20*, 10682–10690. [CrossRef] [PubMed]

31. Sugihara, K.; Yamanaka-Okumura, H.; Teramoto, A.; Urano, E.; Katayama, T.; Morine, Y.; Imura, S.; Utsunomiya, T.; Shimada, M.; Takeda, E. Recovery of nutritional metabolism after liver transplantation. *Nutrition* **2015**, *31*, 105–110. [CrossRef] [PubMed]

32. Tsuchiya, M.; Sakaida, I.; Okamoto, M.; Okita, K. The effect of a late evening snack in patients with liver cirrhosis. *Hepatol. Res.* **2005**, *31*, 95–103. [CrossRef] [PubMed]

33. Stickel, F.; Inderbitzin, D.; Candinas, D. Role of nutrition in liver transplantation for end-stage chronic liver disease. *Nutr. Rev.* **2008**, *66*, 47–54. [CrossRef] [PubMed]

34. Sanchez, A.J.; Aranda-Michel, J. Nutrition for the liver transplant patient. *Liver Transpl.* **2006**, *12*, 1310–1316. [CrossRef] [PubMed]

35. Kawaguchi, T.; Taniguchi, E.; Itou, M.; Ibi, R.; Okada, T.; Mutou, M.; Shiraishi, S.; Uchida, Y.; Otsuka, M.; Umeki, Y.; et al. Body cell mass is a useful parameter for assessing malnutrition and severity of disease in non-ascitic cirrhotic patients with hepatocellular carcinoma or esophageal varices. *Int. J. Mol. Med.* **2008**, *22*, 589–594. [CrossRef] [PubMed]

36. Anderson, L.J.; Erceg, D.N.; Schroeder, E.T. Unity of multifrequency bioelectrical impedance compared with dual-energy x-ray absorptiometry for assessment of total and regional body composition varies between men and women. *Nutr. Res.* **2012**, *32*, 479–485. [CrossRef] [PubMed]

37. Hoyle, G.E.; Chua, M.; Soiza, R.L. Volaemic assessment of the elderly hyponatraemic patient, reliability of clinical assessment and validation of bioelectrical impedance analysis. *QJM* **2011**, *104*, 35–39. [CrossRef] [PubMed]

38. Jensky-Squires, N.E.; Dieli-Conwright, C.M.; Rossuello, A.; Erceg, D.N.; McCauley, S.; Schroeder, E.T. Validity and Reliability of Body Composition Analyzers in Children and Adults. *Br. J. Nutr.* **2008**, *100*, 859–865. [CrossRef] [PubMed]

39. Delmonico, M.J.; Harris, T.B.; Lee, J.S.; Visser, M.; Nevitt, M.; Kritchevsky, S.B.; Tylavsky, F.A.; Newman, A.B. Health, Aging and Body Composition Study. Alternative definitions of sarcopenia, lower extremity performance, and functional impairment with aging in older men and women. *J. Am. Geriatr. Soc.* **2007**, *55*, 769–774. [CrossRef] [PubMed]

40. Englesbe, M.J.; Patel, S.P.; He, K.; Lynch, R.J.; Schaubel, D.E.; Harbaugh, C.; Holcombe, S.A.; Wang, S.C.; Segev, D.L.; Sonnenday, C.J. Sarcopenia and mortality after liver transplantation. *J. Am. Coll. Surg.* **2010**, *211*, 271–278. [CrossRef] [PubMed]

41. Tandon, P.; Ney, M.; Irwin, I.; Ma, M.M.; Gramlich, L.; Bain, V.G.; Esfandiari, N.; Baracos, V.; Montano-Loza, A.J.; Myers, R.P. Severe muscle depletion in patients on the liver transplant wait list, Its prevalence and independent prognostic value. *Liver Transpl.* **2012**, *18*, 1209–1216. [CrossRef] [PubMed]

42. Plauth, M.; Cabre, E.; Riggio, O.; Assis-Camilo, M.; Pirlich, M.; Kondrup, J. ESPEN guidelines on enteral nutrition, liver disease. *Clin. Nutr.* **2006**, *25*, 285–294. [CrossRef] [PubMed]

43. Plauth, M.; Cabre, E.; Campillo, B.; Kondrup, J.; Marchesini, G.; Schütz, T. ESPEN guidelines on parenteral nutrition, hepatology. *Clin. Nutr.* **2009**, *28*, 436–444. [CrossRef] [PubMed]

44. Figueiredo, F.; Dickson, E.R.; Pasha, T.; Kasparova, P.; Therneau, T.; Malinchoc, M.; DiCecco, S.; Francisco-Ziller, N.; Charlton, M. Impact of nutritional status on outcomes after liver transplantation. *Transplantation* **2000**, *70*, 1347–1352. [CrossRef] [PubMed]

45. Nompleggi, D.J.; Bonkovsky, H.L. Nutritional supplementation in chronic liver disease, an analytical review. *Hepatology* **1994**, *19*, 518–523. [CrossRef] [PubMed]

46. Metheny, N.A.; Meert, K.L.; Clouse, R.E. Complications related to feeding tube placement. *Curr. Opin. Gastroenterol.* **2007**, *23*, 178–182. [CrossRef] [PubMed]

47. Burns, D.; Schaeffer, D.; Bosco, J. Nutritional assessment of endoscopically placed nasojejunal feeding tubes. *Gastrointest. Endosc.* **1995**, *41*, 263–269. [CrossRef]

48. Baskin, W.N. Acute complications associated with bedside placement of feeding tubes. *Nutr. Clin. Pract.* **2006**, *21*, 40–55. [CrossRef] [PubMed]

49. Plauth, M.; Schuetz, T. Hepatology—Guidelines on Parenteral Nutrition, Chapter 16. *Ger. Med. Sci.* **2009**, *7*, 12–17.

50. Martindale, R.G.; McClave, S.A.; Vanek, V.W.; McCarthy, M.; Roberts, P.; Taylor, B.; Ochoa, J.B.; Napolitano, L.; Cresci, G.; Gervasio, J.M.; et al. Guidelines for the provision and assessment of nutrition support therapy in the adult critically ill patient, Society of Critical Care Medicine and American Society for Parenteral and Enteral Nutrition. *Crit. Care Med.* **2009**, *37*, 1–30. [CrossRef] [PubMed]

51. Yamamoto, T. Metabolic response to glucose overload in surgical stress, Energy disposal in brown adipose tissue. *Surg Today* **1996**, *26*, 151–157. [CrossRef] [PubMed]

52. Cabré, E.; Periago, J.L.; Abad Lacruz, A.; González Huix, F.; González, J.; Esteve Comas, M. Plasma fatty acid profile in advanced cirrhosis, unsaturation deficit of lipid fractions. *Am. J. Gastroenterol.* **1990**, *85*, 1597–1604. [CrossRef]

53. Abrams, S.A. Impact of new-generation parenteral lipid emulsions in pediatric nutrition. *Adv. Nutr.* **2013**, *4*, 518–520. [CrossRef] [PubMed]

54. Driscoll, D.F.; Newton, D.W.; Bistrian, B.R. Precipitation of calcium phosphate from parenteral nutrient fluids. *Am. J. Hosp. Pharm.* **1994**, *51*, 2834–2836. [PubMed]

55. Moro, M.L.; Maffei, C.; Manso, E.; Morace, G.; Polonelli, L.; Biavasco, F. Nosocomial outbreak of systemic candidosis associated with parenteral nutrition. *Infect. Control Hosp. Epidemiol.* **1990**, *11*, 1127–1135. [CrossRef]

56. Seyan, A.S.; Hughes, R.D.; Shawcross, D.L. Changing face of hepatic encephalopathy, role of inflammation and oxidative stress. *World J. Gastroenterol.* **2010**, *16*, 3347–3357. [CrossRef] [PubMed]

57. Shawcross, D.; Jalan, R. The pathophysiologic basis of hepatic encephalopathy, central role for ammonia and inflammation. *Cell. Mol. Life Sci.* **2005**, *62*, 2295–2304. [CrossRef] [PubMed]

58. Bianchi, G.R.; Marchesini, G.; Fabbri, A.; Rondelli, A.; Buglanesi, E.; Zoli, M.; Pisi, E. Vegetable versus animal protein diet in cirrhotic patients with chronic encephalopathy. A randomised cross-over comparison. *J. Intern. Med.* **1993**, *233*, 385–392. [CrossRef] [PubMed]

59. Swart, G.R.; Van den Berg, J.W.; Wattimena, J.L.; Rietveld, T.; Van Vuure, J.K.; Frenkel, M. Elevated protein requirements in cirrhosis of the liver investigated by whole body protein turnover studies. *Clin. Sci.* **1988**, *75*, 101–107. [CrossRef] [PubMed]

60. Hiyama, D.T.; Fischer, J.E. Nutritional support in hepatic failure, the current role of disease-specific therapy. *Total Parenter. Nutr.* **1991**, *2*, 263–278.

61. Als-Nielsen, B.; Koretz, R.L.; Gluud, L.L.; Gluud, C. Branched-chain amino acids for hepatic encephalopathy. *Cochrane Database Syst. Rev.* **2003**, *2*, 1935–1939.

62. Le Cornu, K.A.; McKiernan, F.J.; Kapadia, S.A.; Neuberger, J.M. A prospective randomized study of preoperative nutritional supplementation in patients awaiting elective orthotopic liver transplantation. *Transplantation* **2000**, *69*, 1364–1369. [CrossRef] [PubMed]

63. Reilly, J.; Mehta, R.; Teperman, L.; Cemaj, S.; Tzakis, A.; Yanaga, K.; Ritter, P.; Rezak, A.; Makowka, L. Nutritional support after liver transplantation, a randomized prospective study. *J. Parenter. Enter. Nutr.* **1990**, *14*, 386–391. [CrossRef] [PubMed]

64. Fischer, J.E.; Baldessarini, R.J. False neurotransmitters and hepatic failure. *Lancet* **1971**, *2*, 75–80. [CrossRef]

65. Khanna, S.; Gopalan, S. Role of branched-chain amino acids in liver disease, the evidence for and against. *Curr. Opin. Clin. Nutr. Metab. Care* **2007**, *10*, 297–303. [CrossRef] [PubMed]

66. Holecek, M. Three targets of branched-chain amino acid supplementation in the treatment of liver disease. *Nutrition* **2010**, *26*, 482–490. [CrossRef] [PubMed]

67. Shirabe, K.; Yoshimatsu, M.; Motomura, T.; Takeishi, K.; Toshima, T.; Muto, J.; Matono, R.; Taketomi, A.; Uchiyama, H.; Maehara, Y. Beneficial effects of supplementation with branched-chain amino acids on postoperative bacteremia in living donor liver transplant recipients. *Liver Transpl.* **2011**, *17*, 1073–1080. [PubMed]

68. Nakamura, I.; Ochiai, K.; Imawari, M. Phagocytic function of neutrophils of patients with decompensated liver cirrhosis is restored by oral supplementation of branched-chain amino acids. *Hepatol. Res.* **2004**, *29*, 207–211. [CrossRef] [PubMed]

69. Bassit, R.A.; Sawada, L.A.; Bacurau, R.F.; Navarro, F.; Martins, E.J.; Santos, R.V.; Caperuto, E.C.; Rogeri, P.; Costa Rosa, L.F. Branched-chain amino acid supplementation and the immune response of long-distance athletes. *Nutrition* **2002**, *18*, 376–379. [CrossRef]

70. Kawamura, E.; Habu, D.; Morikawa, H.; Enomoto, M.; Kawabe, J.; Tamori, A.; Sakaguchi, H.; Saeki, S.; Kawada, N.; Shiomi, S. A randomized pilot trial of oral branched-chain amino acids in early cirrhosis, validation using prognostic markers for preliver transplant status. *Liver Transpl.* **2009**, *15*, 790–797. [CrossRef] [PubMed]

71. Takeshita, S.; Ichikawa, T.; Nakao, K.; Miyaaki, H.; Shibata, H.; Matsuzaki, T.; Muraoka, T.; Honda, T.; Otani, M.; Akiyama, M.; et al. A snack enriched with oral branched chain amino acids prevents a fall in albumin in patients with liver cirrhosis undergoing chemoembolization for hepatocellular carcinoma. *Nutr. Res.* **2009**, *29*, 89–93. [CrossRef] [PubMed]

72. Butterworth, R.F. Thiamine deficiency-related brain dysfunction in chronic liver failure. *Metab. Brain Dis.* **2009**, *24*, 189–196. [CrossRef] [PubMed]

73. Merli, M.; Giusto, M.; Riggio, O.; Gentili, F.; Molinaro, A.; Attili, A.F.; Ginanni Corradini, S.; Rossi, M. Improvement of nutritional status in malnourished cirrhotic patients one year after liver transplantation. *Eur. e-J. Clin. Nutr. Metab.* **2011**, *6*, 142–147. [CrossRef]

74. Levy, S.; Herve, C.; Delacoux, E.; Erlinger, S. Thiamine deficiency in hepatitis C virus and alcohol-related liver diseases. *Dig. Dis. Sci.* **2002**, *47*, 543–548. [CrossRef] [PubMed]

75. Moscarella, S.; Duchini, A.; Buzzelli, G. Lipoperoxidation, trace elements and vitamin E in patients with liver cirrhosis. *Eur. J. Gastroenterol. Hepatol.* **1994**, *6*, 633–636. [CrossRef]

76. Gloria, L.; Cravo, M.; Camilo, M.E.; Resende, M.; Cardoso, J.N.; Oliveira, A.G.; Leitão, C.N.; Mira, F.C. Nutritional deficiencies in chronic alcoholics, relation to dietary intake and alcohol consumption. *Am. J. Gastroenterol.* **1997**, *92*, 485–489. [PubMed]

77. Leo, M.A.; Lieber, C.S. Alcohol, vitamin A, and beta-carotene, adverse interactions including hepatotoxicity and carcinogenensis. *Am. J. Clin. Nutr.* **1999**, *69*, 1071–1085. [PubMed]

78. Marchesini, G.; Fabbri, A.; Bianchi, G.; Brizi, M.; Zoli, M. Zn supplementation and amino acid-nitrogen metabolism in patients with advanced cirrhosis. *Hepatology* **1996**, *23*, 1084–1092. [CrossRef] [PubMed]

79. Bitetto, D.; Fabris, C.; Falleti, E.; Fornasiere, E.; Fumolo, E.; Fontanini, E.; Cussigh, A.; Occhino, G.; Baccarani, U.; Pirisi, M.; et al. Vitamin D and the risk of acute allograft rejection following human liver transplantation. *Liver Int.* **2010**, *30*, 417–444. [CrossRef] [PubMed]

80. Walker, N.M.; Stuart, K.A.; Ryan, R.J.; Desai, S.; Saab, S.; Nicol, J.A.; Fletcher, L.M.; Crawford, D.H. Serum ferritin concentration predicts mortality in patients awaiting liver transplantation. *Hepatology* **2010**, *51*, 1683–1691. [CrossRef] [PubMed]

81. Barzel, U.S.; Massey, L.K. Excess dietary protein can adversely affect bone. *J. Nutr.* **1998**, *128*, 1051–1053. [PubMed]

82. Parhami, F.; Jackson, S.; Tintut, Y.; Le, V.; Balucan, J.P.; Territo, M.; Demer, L.L. Atherogenic diet and minimally oxidized low density lipoprotein inhibit osteogenic and promote adipogenic differentiation of marrow stromal cells. *J. Bone Miner. Res.* **1999**, *14*, 2067–2078. [CrossRef] [PubMed]

83. Hay, J.E.; Guichelaar, M.M. Evaluation and management of osteoporosis in liver disease. *Clin. Liver Dis.* **2005**, *9*, 747–766. [CrossRef] [PubMed]

84. Beyer, N.; Aadahl, M.; Strange, B.; Mohr, T.; Kjaer, M. Exercise capacity of patients after liver transplantation. *Med. Sci. Sports Exerc.* **1995**, *6*, 80–84.

85. Ritland, S.; Foss, N.; Skrede, S. The effect of standardized work load on "liver tests" in patients with chronic active hepatitis. *J. Gastroenterol.* **1982**, *17*, 1013–1016.

86. Escartin, A.; Castro, E.; Dopazo, C.; Bueno, J.; Bilbao, I.; Margarit, C. Analysis of discarded livers for transplantation. *Transplant. Proc.* **2005**, *37*, 3859–3860. [CrossRef] [PubMed]

87. Marsman, W.A.; Wiesner, R.H.; Rodriguez, L.; Batts, K.P.; Porayko, M.K.; Hay, J.E.; Gores, G.J.; Krom, R.A. Use of fatty donor liver is associated with diminished early patient and graft survival. *Transplantation* **1996**, *62*, 1246–1251. [CrossRef] [PubMed]

88. Perkins, J.D. Saying 'Yes' to obese living liver donors, short-term intensive treatment for donors with hepatic steatosis in living-donor liver transplantation. *Liver Transpl.* **2006**, *12*, 1012–1013. [CrossRef] [PubMed]

89. Malik, S.M.; deVera, M.E.; Fontes, P.; Shaikh, O.; Ahmad, J. Outcome after liver transplantation for NASH cirrhosis. *Am. J. Transplant.* **2009**, *9*, 782–793. [CrossRef] [PubMed]

90. Driscoll, D.F.; Blackburn, G.L. A review of its current status in hospitalized patients, and the need for patient-specific feeding. *Drugs* **1990**, *40*, 346–363. [CrossRef] [PubMed]

91. Plank, L.D.; McCall, J.L.; Gane, E.J.; Rafique, M.; Gillanders, L.K.; McIlroy, K.; Munn, S.R. Pre- and postoperative immunonutrition in patients undergoing liver transplantation, a pilot study of safety and efficacy. *Clin. Nutr.* **2005**, *24*, 288–296. [CrossRef] [PubMed]

92. Senkal, M.; Zumtobel, V.; Bauer, K.H.; Marpe, B.; Wolfram, G.; Frei, A.; Eickhoff, U.; Kemen, M. Outcome and cost-effectiveness of perioperative enteral immunonutrition in patients undergoing elective upper gastrointestinal tract surgery, a prospective randomized study. *Arch. Surg.* **1999**, *134*, 1309–1316. [CrossRef] [PubMed]

93. Jiang, H.; Li, B.; Yan, L.N.; Lu, S.C.; Wen, T.F.; Zhao, J.C.; Wan, W.T.; Jiang, Z.M. Effect of Intravenous glutamine-dipeptide fortified enteral nutrition on clinical outcomes in patients after liver transplantation, A prospective randomized controlled study. *Chin. J. Clin. Nutr.* **2007**, *15*, 21–25.

94. Kaido, T.; Ogura, Y.; Ogawa, K.; Hata, K.; Yoshizawa, A.; Yagi, S.; Uemoto, S. Effects of post-transplant enteral nutrition with an immunomodulating diet containing hydrolyzed whey peptide after liver transplantation. *World J. Surg.* **2012**, *36*, 1666–1671. [CrossRef] [PubMed]

95. Kume, H.; Okazaki, K.; Sasaki, H. Hepatoprotective effects of whey protein on D-galactosamine-induced hepatitis and liver fibrosis in rats. *Biosci. Biotechnol. Biochem.* **2006**, *70*, 1281–1285. [CrossRef] [PubMed]

96. Park, C.; Hsu, C.; Neelakanta, G.; Nourmand, H.; Braunfeld, M.; Wray, C.; Steadman, R.H.; Hu, K.Q.; Cheng, R.T.; Xia, V.W. Severe intraoperative hyperglycemia is independently associated with surgical site infection after liver transplantation. *Transplantation* **2009**, *87*, 1031–1036. [CrossRef] [PubMed]

97. Bellot, P.; Frances, R.; Such, J. Bacterial translocation in cirrhosis. *Gastroenterol. Hepatol.* **2008**, *31*, 508–514. [CrossRef] [PubMed]

98. Riordan, S.M.; Williams, R. The intestinal flora and bacterial infection in cirrhosis. *J. Hepatol.* **2006**, *45*, 744–757. [CrossRef] [PubMed]

99. Sugawara, G.; Nagino, M.; Nishio, H.; Ebata, T.; Takagi, K.; Asahara, T. Perioperative synbiotic treatment to prevent postoperative infectious complications in biliary cancer surgery, a randomized controlled trial. *Ann. Surg.* **2006**, *244*, 706–714. [CrossRef] [PubMed]

100. Rayes, N.; Seehofer, D.; Hansen, S.; Boucsein, K.; Müller, A.R.; Serke, S. Early enteral supply of lactobacillus and fiber versus selective bowel decontamination, a controlled trial in liver transplant recipients. *Transplantation* **2002**, *74*, 123–127. [CrossRef] [PubMed]

101. Rayes, N.; Seehofer, D.; Theruvath, T.; Schiller, R.A.; Langrehr, J.M.; Jonas, S. Supply of pre- and probiotics reduces bacterial infection rates after liver transplantation—A randomized, double-blind trial. *Am. J. Transplant.* **2005**, *5*, 125–130. [CrossRef] [PubMed]

102. Bajaj, J.S.; Saeian, K.; Christensen, K.M.; Hafeezullah, M.; Varma, R.R.; Franco, J. Probiotic yogurt for the treatment of minimal hepatic encephalopathy. *Am. J. Gastroenterol.* **2008**, *103*, 1707–1715. [CrossRef] [PubMed]

103. Malaguarnera, M.; Gargante, M.P.; Malaguarnera, G.; Salmeri, M.; Mastrojeni, S.; Rampello, L. Bifidobacterium combined with fructo-oligosaccharide versus lactulose in the treatment of patients with hepatic encephalopathy. *Eur. J. Gastroenterol. Hepatol.* **2010**, *22*, 199–206. [CrossRef] [PubMed]

104. Lata, J.; Novotný, I.; Príbramská, V.; Juránková, J.; Fric, P.; Kroupa, R.; Stibůrek, O. The effect of probiotics on gut flora, level of endotoxin and Child-Pugh score in cirrhotic patients, results of a double blind randomized study. *Eur. J. Gastroenterol. Hepatol.* **2007**, *19*, 1111–1113. [CrossRef] [PubMed]

105. Swart, G.R.; Zillikens, M.C.; van Vuure, J.K.; Van den Berg, J.W. Effect of a late evening meal on nitrogen balance in patients with cirrhosis of the liver. *Br. Med. J.* **1989**, *299*, 1202–1203. [CrossRef]

106. Plank, L.D.; Gane, E.J.; Peng, S.; Muthu, C.; Mathur, S.; Gillanders, L. Nocturnal nutritional supplementation improves total body protein status of patients with liver cirrhosis, a randomized 12-month trial. *Hepatology* **2008**, *48*, 557–566. [CrossRef] [PubMed]

107. Richardson, R.A.; Garden, O.J.; Davidson, H.I. Reduction in energy expenditure after liver transplantation. *Nutrition* **2001**, *17*, 585–589. [CrossRef]

108. Hou, W.; Li, J.; Lu, J.; Wang, J.H.; Zhang, F.Y.; Yu, H.W.; Zhang, J.; Yao, Q.W.; Wu, J.; Shi, S.Y.; et al. Effect of a carbohydrate-containing late-evening snack on energy metabolism and fasting substrate utilization in adults with acute-on-chronic liver failure due to Hepatitis B. *Eur. J. Clin. Nutr.* **2013**, *67*, 1251–1256. [CrossRef] [PubMed]

109. Ymanaka-Okumura, H.; Nakamura, T.; Takeuchi, H.; Miyake, H.; Katayama, T.; Arai, H.; Taketani, Y.; Fujii, M.; Shimada, M.; Takeda, E. Effect of late evening snack with rice ball on energy metabolism in liver cirrhosis. *Eur. J. Clin. Nutr.* **2006**, *60*, 1067–1072. [CrossRef] [PubMed]
110. Fagiuoli, S.; Colli, A.; Bruno, R.; Craxì, A.; Battista, G.; PaoloGrossi, G. Management of infections pre- and post-liver transplantation: Report of an AISF consensus conference. *Hepatology* **2014**, *60*, 1075–1089. [CrossRef] [PubMed]
111. Egashira, K.; Sasaki, H.; Higuchi, S.; Ieiri, I. Food-drug interaction of tacrolimus with pomelo, ginger, and turmeric juice. *Drug Metab. Pharmacokinet.* **2012**, *27*, 242–247. [CrossRef] [PubMed]
112. Bianchi, G.; Marzocchi, R.; Agostini, F.; Marchesini, G. Update on nutritional supplementation with branched-chain amino acids. *Curr. Opin. Clin. Nutr. Metab. Care* **2005**, *8*, 83–87. [CrossRef] [PubMed]
113. Janczewska, I.; Ericzon, B.G.; Eriksson, L.S. Influence of orthotopic liver transplantation on serum vitamin A levels in patients with chronic liver disease. *Scand. J. Gastroenterol.* **1995**, *30*, 68–71. [CrossRef] [PubMed]
114. Pescovitz, M.D.; Mehta, P.L.; Jindal, R.M.; Milgrom, M.L.; Leapman, S.B.; Filo, R.S. Zinc deficiency and its repletion following liver transplantation in humans. *Clin. Transplant.* **1996**, *10*, 256–260. [PubMed]
115. Palmer, M.; Schaffner, F.; Thung, S.N. Excessive weight gain after liver transplantation. *Transplantation* **1991**, *51*, 797–800. [CrossRef] [PubMed]
116. Chin, S.E.; Shepherd, R.W.; Cleghorn, G.J.; Patrick, M.K.; Javorsky, G.; Frangoulis, E. Survival, growth and quality of life in children after orthotopic liver transplantation: A 5 year experience. *J. Pediatr. Child Health* **1991**, *27*, 38–85. [CrossRef]
117. Holt, R.I.; Broide, E.; Buchanan, C.R.; Miell, J.P.; Baker, A.J.; Mowat, A.P.; Mieli Vergani, G. Orthotopic liver transplantation reverses the adverse nutritional changes of end stage liver disease in children. *Am. J. Clin. Nutr.* **1997**, *65*, 534–542. [PubMed]
118. Porayko, M.K.; DiCecco, S.; O'Keefe, S.J. Impact of malnutrition and its therapy in liver transplantation. *Semin. Liver Dis.* **1991**, *11*, 305–314. [CrossRef] [PubMed]
119. Muller, M.J.; Loyal, S.; Schwarze, M.; Lobers, J.; Selberg, O.; Ringe, B.; Pichlmayr, R. Resting energy expenditure and nutritional state in patients with liver cirrhosis before and after liver transplantation. *Clin. Nutr.* **1994**, *13*, 145–152. [CrossRef]
120. Canzanello, V.J.; Schwartz, L.; Taler, S.J.; Textor, S.C.; Wiesner, R.H.; Porayko, M.K.; Krom, R.A. Evolution of cardiovascular risk after liver transplantation, a comparison of cyclosporine A and tacrolimus (FK506). *Liver Transpl. Surg.* **1997**, *3*, 1–9. [CrossRef]
121. Kaido, T.; Egawa, H.; Tsuji, H.; Ashihara, E.; Maekawa, T.; Uemoto, S. In-hospital mortality in adult recipients of living donor liver transplantation, experience of 576 consecutive cases at a single center. *Liver Transpl.* **2009**, *15*, 1420–1425. [CrossRef] [PubMed]
122. Osaki, N.; Ringe, B.; Gubernatis, G.; Takada, Y.; Yamaguchi, T.; Yamaoka, Y.; Oellerich, M.; Ozawa, K.; Pichlmayr, R. Changes in energy substrates in relation to arterial ketone body ratio after human orthotopic liver transplantation. *Surgery* **1993**, *113*, 403–409.
123. Takada, Y.; Ozawa, K.; Yamaoka, Y.; Uemoto, S.; Tanaka, A.; Morimoto, T.; Honda, K.; Shimahara, Y.; Mori, K.; Inamoto, T.; et al. Arterial ketone body ratio and glucose administration as an energy substrate in relation to changes in ketone body concentration after live-related liver transplantation in children. *Transplantation* **1993**, *55*, 1314–1319. [CrossRef] [PubMed]
124. Hasse, J. Liver transplantation, the benefits of nutrition therapy in the liver transplant patient. *Liver Transpl.* **1996**, *2*, 81–100.
125. Shanbhogue, R.L.; Bistrian, B.R.; Jenkins, R.L.; Randall, S.; Blackburn, G.L. Increased protein catabolism without hypermetabolism after human orthotopic liver transplantation. *Surgery* **1987**, *101*, 146–149. [PubMed]
126. Pomposelli, J.J.; Baxter, J.K., III; Babineau, T.J.; Pomfret, E.A.; Driscoll, D.F.; Forse, R.A. Early postoperative glucose control predicts nosocomial infection rate in diabetic patients. *J. Parenter. Enter. Nutr.* **1998**, *22*, 77–81. [CrossRef] [PubMed]
127. Stegall, M.D.; Everson, G.; Schroter, G.; Bilir, B.; Karrer, F.; Kam, I. Metabolic complications after liver transplantation. Diabetes, hypercholesterolemia, hypertension, and obesity. *Transplantation* **1995**, *60*, 1057–1060. [PubMed]
128. Muñoz, S.J.; Deems, R.O.; Moritz, M.J.; Martin, P.; Jarrell, B.E.; Maddrey, W.C. Hyperlipidemia and obesity after orthotopic liver transplantation. *Transplant. Proc.* **1991**, *23*, 1480–1483. [PubMed]

129. Richards, J.; Gunson, B.; Johnson, J.; Neuberger, J. Weight gain and obesity after liver transplantation. *Transpl. Int.* **2005**, *18*, 461–466. [CrossRef] [PubMed]
130. Anastácio, L.R.; Ferreira, L.G.; Ribeiro, H.S.; Liboredo, J.C.; Lima, A.S.; Correia, M.I. Metabolic syndrome after liver transplantation, prevalence and predictive factors. *Nutrition* **2011**, *27*, 931–937. [CrossRef] [PubMed]
131. Weseman, R.A.; McCashland, T.M. Nutritional care of the chronic post-transplant patient. *Top. Clin. Nutr.* **1998**, *13*, 27–34. [CrossRef]
132. Green, G.A.; Moore, G.E. Exercise and organ transplantation. *J. Back Musculoskelet. Rehabil.* **1998**, *10*, 3–11. [CrossRef]
133. Van Den Ham, E.C.; Kooman, J.P.; Christiaans, M.H.; van Hooff, J.P. Relation between steroid dose, body composition and physical activity in renal transplant patients. *Transplantation* **2000**, *69*, 1591–1598. [CrossRef] [PubMed]
134. Giannini, S.; Nobile, M.; Ciuffreda, M.; Iemmolo, R.M.; Dalle Carbonare, L.; Minicuci, N. Long-term persistence of low bone density in orthotopic liver transplantation. *Osteoporosis* **2000**, *11*, 417–424. [CrossRef] [PubMed]
135. Peris, P.; Navasa, M.; Guañabens, N.; Monegal, A.; Moya, F.; Brancós, M.A. Sacral stress fracture after liver transplantation. *Br. J. Rheumatol.* **1993**, *32*, 702–704. [CrossRef] [PubMed]
136. Millonig, G.; Graziadci, I.W.; Eichler, D.; Pfeiffer, K.P.; Finkenstedt, G.; Muchllechner, P.; Koenigsrainer, A.; Margreiter, R.; Vogel, W. Alendronate in combination with calcium and vitamin D prevents bone loss after orthotopic liver transplantation, a prospective single-center study. *Liver Transpl.* **2005**, *11*, 960–966. [CrossRef] [PubMed]
137. Schilsky, M.L. Transplantation for Inherited Metabolic Disorders of the Liver. *Transplant. Proc.* **2013**, *45*, 455–462. [CrossRef] [PubMed]
138. Moini, M.; Mistry, P.; Schilsky, M.L. Liver transplantation for inherited metabolic disorders of the liver. *Curr. Opin. Organ Transplant.* **2010**, *15*, 269–276. [CrossRef] [PubMed]
139. Scorza, M.; Elce, A.; Zarrilli, F.; Liguori, R.; Amato, F.; Castaldo, G. Genetic diseases that predispose to early liver cirrhosis. *Int. J. Hepatol.* **2014**, *4*, 616–627. [CrossRef] [PubMed]

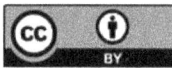

nutrients

MDPI

Article

Protective Effects of Ethanolic Extracts from Artichoke, an Edible Herbal Medicine, against Acute Alcohol-Induced Liver Injury in Mice

Xuchong Tang [1,*], Ruofan Wei [1], Aihua Deng [2] and Tingping Lei [3]

1   College of Chemical Engineering, Huaqiao University, Xiamen 361021, China; rovanwei@yahoo.com
2   College of Life and Environmental Science, Hunan University of Arts and Science, Changde 415000, China; dengaihua@yahoo.com
3   College of Mechanical Engineering and Automation, Huaqiao University, Xiamen 361021, China; tplei@hqu.edu.cn
*   Correspondence: xctang@hqu.edu.cn; Tel.: +86-0592-6162302

Received: 7 August 2017; Accepted: 6 September 2017; Published: 11 September 2017

Abstract: Oxidative stress and inflammation are well-documented pathological factors in alcoholic liver disease (ALD). Artichoke (*Cynara scolymus* L.) is a healthy food and folk medicine with anti-oxidative and anti-inflammatory properties. This study aimed to evaluate the preventive effects of ethanolic extract from artichoke against acute alcohol-induced liver injury in mice. Male Institute of Cancer Research mice were treated with an ethanolic extract of artichoke (0.4, 0.8, and 1.6 g/kg body weight) by gavage once daily. Up to 40% alcohol (12 mL/kg body weight) was administered orally 1 h after artichoke treatment. All mice were fed for 10 consecutive days. Results showed that artichoke extract significantly prevented elevated levels of aspartate aminotransferase, alanine aminotransferase, triglyceride, total cholesterol, and malondialdehyde. Meanwhile, the decreased levels of superoxide dismutase and glutathione were elevated by artichoke administration. Histopathological examination showed that artichoke attenuated degeneration, inflammatory infiltration and necrosis of hepatocytes. Immunohistochemical analysis revealed that expression levels of toll-like receptor (TLR) 4 and nuclear factor-kappa B (NF-κB) in liver tissues were significantly suppressed by artichoke treatment. Results obtained demonstrated that artichoke extract exhibited significant preventive protective effect against acute alcohol-induced liver injury. This finding is mainly attributed to its ability to attenuate oxidative stress and suppress the TLR4/NF-κB inflammatory pathway. To the best of our knowledge, the underlying mechanisms of artichoke on acute ALD have been rarely reported.

Keywords: artichoke; acute alcohol liver disease; oxidative stress; inflammation; TLR4/NF-κB pathway

1. Introduction

Drinking alcohol has always been deemed essential in many areas, such as in social gatherings, status functions, personal interactions, and conformance. However, long-term excessive alcohol intake can result in alcoholic liver disease (ALD). ALD is the leading cause of cirrhosis and liver-related death worldwide for decades and is responsible for 4% of global mortality [1–3]. ALD encompasses a histological spectrum of liver injury that ranges from steatosis (fatty liver) to alcoholic steatohepatitis (ASH), and in severe cases, fibrosis, cirrhosis, and ultimately hepatocellular carcinoma [4,5]. Thus, the control of ALD at an early stage, for example, at a stage prior to the occurrence of ASH, could be of great significance in preventing development of ALD.

Potential mechanisms of acute alcohol-induced liver injury are associated with oxidative stress, steaotosis, endotoxin, dysregulated immunity, and inflammation. However, in recent decades, studies have focused on the inflammatory pathway in ALD, and increasing evidence demonstrates that ASH is caused by the lipopolysaccharide (LPS) binding to toll-like receptor (TLR)-induced nuclear factor-kappa B (NF-κB) activation pathway [6–8]. TLRs are pattern-recognition receptors that enable the innate immune system to react immediately to infections by recognizing both bacterial and viral constituents. Among the TLRs, TLR4 can initiate activation of NF-κB and cascade response further causing the accumulation of pro-inflammation cytokines, ultimately resulting in the aggravation of inflammatory progress [9–12].

Although various treatments, such as nutritional therapy, pharmacological therapy, psychotherapy, and surgery, are currently available for the spectrums of ALD, no satisfactory therapy is available except for abstinence [13–15]. Medications that act as anti-inflammatories and anti-oxidants, are frequently used as therapeutic drugs in ALD. For example, there is silymarin, which alleviates liver injury mainly by reducing free radical activity and lipid peroxidation, protecting the liver cell membrane, and promoting hepatocytes regeneration, and bifendate, which alleviates liver injury mainly by reducing serum level of alanine aminotransferase (ALT), inflammatory cell infiltration and liver histological changes. However, clinical applications are limited because of side effects among other reasons. For example, silymarin has poor oral-bioavailability, and bifendate may cause liver hypertrophy [16–18]. Thus, finding convincingly effective treatment drugs with fewer side effects without compromising therapeutic effect continues to be an important goal.

Artichoke (*Cynara scolymus* L.), an edible herbal medicine of the family Compositae, is a perennial herb widely studied because of its possible antioxidative and hepatoprotective effects [19–22]. The extracts and derivatives from artichoke contain a variety of dicaffeoylquinic acids and many kinds of flavonoid functional compounds, such as cynarin (1,5-dicaffeoylquinic acids), chlorogenic acid (3-caffe-oylquinic acid), luteolin glucoside, and apigenin glucoside [23,24], which exhibit anti-microbial, anti-allergic, anti-inflammatory, and anticancer effects. One study indicated that artichoke extract had potential in reducing hypercholesterolemia through preventing lipid peroxidation and ameliorating hepatic antioxidant status [25]. Another report demonstrated that artichoke aqueous leaf extract reduced serum total cholesterol (TC), triglycerides (TG), very low density lipoprotein, glucose levels, and plasma malondialdehyde (MDA) levels in streptozotocin-treated diabetic rats [26]. Reports also demonstrated that artichoke showed marked anti-inflammatory effects on tissue plasminogen activator-induced inflammation and antitumor activity in an in vivo two-stage carcinogenesis test in mice [27]. Besides, it was reported that artichoke extract was very safe to the human body as no obvious side effects were observed after continuous medication for several months [28]. Therefore, artichoke has a broad application prospects in ALD treatment due to its anti-oxidant and anti-inflammatory effects.

The purpose of this study was to investigate the prophylactic protective effects of ethanolic extract from artichoke on acute alcohol-induced injury in an acute ALD mice model. To date, the indicators of aspartate aminotransferase (AST), ALT, TG, TC, MDA, glutathione (GSH), and superoxide dismutase (SOD) were assessed. The possible mechanism for acute alcohol-induced liver injury was discussed using the signals of TLR4 and NF-κB.

2. Materials and Methods

2.1. Materials

Artichokes in freeze-dried powder (8.89% caffeic acid derivatives, 0.98% chlorogenic acid, 0.56% cynarin) were supplied by Huimei Agricultural Science and Technology Co., Ltd. (Hunan, China), and the artichokes were diluted into 0.04 g/mL, 0.08 g/mL, and 0.16 g/mL suspensions with distilled water, respectively. Edible alcohol was obtained from Beijing Red Star Co., Ltd. (Beijing, China), and edible alcohol was diluted with distilled water to a concentration of 40% (w/v). Regular chow diet (40–43% corn, 26% bran, 29% bean cake, 1% salt, 1% bone meal, 1% lysine) for mice was purchased from Huayueyang Biotechnology CO., Ltd. (Beijing, China). Bifendate was provided by Beijing Union Pharmaceutical Factory (Beijing, China), and bifendate was diluted as a 0.036 g/mL suspension with distilled water. Diagnostic kits for AST, ALT, TG, TC, SOD, MDA, and GSH were received from the Nanjing Jiancheng Institute of Biotechnology (Nanjing, China). Antibodies for TLR4 and NF-κB p50 were purchased from OriGene Technologies, Inc. (Rockville, MD, USA) and Novus Biologicals, Inc. (Littleton, CO, USA), respectively. All other chemicals used were of analytical reagent and obtained from Sinopharm Chemical Reagent Co., Ltd. (Shanghai, China).

2.2. Experimental Animals

Seven-week-old male Institute of Cancer Research (ICR) mice (25 ± 2 g) were supplied by the Shanghai Laboratory Animal Center (Shanghai, China) and acclimated for one week prior to use. These mice were kept under environmentally controlled conditions (12-h normal light/dark cycles, 22 ± 2 °C and 50 ± 10% relative humidity) with chow diet and water ad libitum. All animal experiments were approved by the Animal Care and Use Committee of the Huaqiao University (Approval No. SCXK (HU) 2012-0002) and followed the National Institutes of Health Guidelines for animal care (Approval No. HQ-ECLA-20160517).

The ICR mice were randomly divided into 6 groups of 10 mice per group:

(1) Control group: mice were gavaged with same volume of 0.9% saline twice per day (interval time, one hour).
(2) EtOH group (model group): mice were gavaged with same volume of 0.9% saline and with 12 mL/kg body weight (BW) alcohol one hour after saline administration per day.
(3) Positive control group (EtOH + bifendate): mice were gavaged with 0.36 g/kg BW of bifendate and with 12 mL/kg BW alcohol one hour after bifendate pretreatment each day.
(4) Low-dose artichoke group (EtOH + artichoke 0.4): mice were gavaged with 0.4 g/kg BW of artichoke and with 12 mL/kg BW alcohol one hour after artichoke pretreatment each day.
(5) Middle-dose artichoke group (EtOH + artichoke 0.8): mice were gavaged with 0.8 g/kg BW of artichoke and with 12 mL/kg BW alcohol one hour after artichoke pretreatment each day.
(6) High-dose artichoke group (EtOH + artichoke 1.6): mice were gaveged with 1.6 g/kg BW of artichoke and with 12 mL/kg BW alcohol one hour after artichoke pretreatment each day.

All groups were fed for 10 consecutive days. Then, all groups were fasted for 12 h and subsequently anesthetized by pentobarbital solution (60 mg/kg BW) before the experiment.

2.3. Serum Biochemical Assays

Blood samples were collected from the retrobulbar vessels of the mice. The samples were centrifuged at 1500 rpm for 10 min at 4 °C (GTR16-2, Beijing Era Beili Centrifuge Co., Ltd, Beijing, China) to separate the serum after standing for 1 h at room temperature. Serum ALT, AST, TG, and TC activities were subsequently subjected to diagnostic kit testing (Nanjing Jiancheng Institute of Biotechnology) according to the instructions provided using spectrophotometer determination (UV2550, Shimadzu Crop., Kyoto, Japan). Briefly, for assessment of ALT and AST, the samples were mixed with substrates or buffer solution. After incubation at room temperature for 5 min, the absorbance at 505 nm was measured. The final data of ALT and AST were represented as U/L. For assessment of TG and TC, the samples were transferred into a 96-well plate containing substrates or buffer solution. After incubation at 37 °C for 10 min, the plate was incubated for an additional time after adding color developing agent and the absorbance at 510 nm was measured. The final data are represented as μmol/L.

2.4. Hepatic Antioxidant and Oxidative Stress Marker Assays

The livers were weighed accurately. A total of 0.5 g liver tissue was cut and washed with distilled water, then excess water was dried up. Then the liver tissue was cut into slices and homogenated with nine volumes of phosphate buffer (4.5 mL) in an ice bath (pH 7.2–7.4). The resulting suspension was centrifuged at 12,000 rpm for 10 min at 4 °C (GTR16-2, Beijing Era Beili Centrifuge Co., Ltd, Beijing, China), and the supernatant was measured by diagnostic kits of SOD, MDA, and GSH (Nanjing Jiancheng Institute of Biotechnology) according to the manufacturer's instructions. In brief, the concentrations of SOD, MDA and GSH were assayed by hydroxylamine method, thiobarbituric acid-reactive method and microplate method, respectively.

2.5. Histological Examination of Liver Tissue

Liver tissues were fixed in 10% neutral formalin buffer for 24 h, and 5-μm sections were cut and stained with hematoxylin and eosin (H&E), and then observed using a Nikon DS-Fi2 fluorescent microscope (Nikon, Tokyo, Japan). The magnification was 200×. At least 10 areas of each tissue slice were observed. Representative images were presented. Analyses of pathological changes were based on proportion of inflammation, necrosis (0 point, 0 foci; 1 point, <2 foci; 2 points, 2–4 foci; 3 points, >4 foci, per 200× field) and steatosis (0 point, <5%; 1 point, 6–33%; 2 points, 34–66%; 3 points, >66%), which were assessed by three examiners independently [29].

2.6. Immunohistochemical Analysis of TLR4 and NF-κB

Liver tissues were fixed in 10% neutral formalin buffer and embedded in paraffin. Five-millimeter-thick paraffin sections were cut and were then heated in unmasking solution at 95 °C for 15 min after deparaffinization. Nonspecific binding sites were blocked with goat serum. Sections were then incubated overnight at 4 °C in a humidified chamber with the following primary antibodies: rabbit anti-TLR4 (1:50) and rabbit anti-NF-κB p50 (1:250). The examiners, blinded to the experimental groups, counted the cells labeled with TLR4 and NF-κB p50 throughout five random lesion regions in the stained areas under a 200× light microscope. Then, the expression levels of TLR4 and NF-κB p50 were analyzed by mean integrated optical density (IOD).

2.7. Statistical Analysis

All quantifications for assays were repeated for three times and a mean value was used by taking mean of the triplicate plus/minus standard deviation (mean ± SD) for each group. Statistically significant differences ($p < 0.05$) were evaluated by one-way analysis of variance using SPSS 18.0 (SPSS Inc., Chicago, IL, USA).

3. Results and Discussion

3.1. Liver Index of ICR Mice

The liver index was calculated as a ratio (%) of the liver weight (g) to body weight (g) [30,31]. At the first stage of ALD formation, excessive drinking implies a large number of calories, resulting in a dramatic increase in liver weight, body weight and liver index. Thus, the liver index is an informative ratio for predicting ALD. Table 1 shows the liver indices of mice of six groups. No significant difference was observed in the final body weight in bifendate or artichoke treatment mice compared with the EtOH group. However, the weight gain of mice treated with alcohol decreased significantly ($p < 0.05$) when compared to control group, which could be explained as a symptom of anorexia caused by liver damage, indicating the successful establishment of an acute alcohol-induced mice model. Liver index was significantly increased by 8.79% ($p < 0.05$) in the EtOH group in comparison to the control group, whereas no significant decrease was shown in the bifendate group or artichoke treatment groups compared with the EtOH group. However, the medication groups under bifendate and artichoke treatment all showed a protective effect on the liver as evidenced by comparatively low liver indexes when compared with EtOH group, suggesting that artichoke is helpful for attenuating ethanol-induced liver injury.

Table 1. Effect of artichoke on liver index of acute alcoholic liver disease (ALD) mice [a].

Treatment Group	Dosage (g/kg)	Liver Weight (g)	Initial Body Weight (g)	Final Body Weight (g)	Liver Index (%)
Control	–	1.75 ± 0.22	26.46 ± 0.64	36.96 ± 4.26 [#]	4.78 ± 0.64 [#]
EtOH	–	1.53 ± 0.17	26.24 ± 0.70	29.94 ± 2.98 *	5.20 ± 0.22 *
EtOH + Bifendate	0.36	1.53 ± 0.18	26.17 ± 0.95	30.18 ± 2.13 *	5.05 ± 0.38
Low-dose artichoke	0.4	1.47 ± 0.23	26.35 ± 0.72	28.79 ± 3.00 *	5.12 ± 0.64
Middle-dose artichoke	0.8	1.57 ± 0.20	26.39 ± 0.52	29.06 ± 2.03 *	5.04 ± 0.44
High-dose artichoke	1.6	1.54 ± 0.12	25.94 ± 0.85	29.84 ± 1.27 *	5.14 ± 0.31

[a] Data are expressed as means ± standard deviation (SD) ($n = 10$); * $p < 0.05$, vs. the control group; [#] $p < 0.05$, vs. the EtOH group.

3.2. Serum Biochemical Markers

The levels of serum ALT, AST, TG and TC are early biochemical and pathological markers of hepatocyte damage. ALT is a cytosolic enzyme which is mainly presented in the cell cytoplasm, while AST is a mitochondrial enzyme which is released from the liver and other organs in the body. ALT and AST are released into the blood, resulting in an increase of serum transaminase when damage (e.g., inflammation and necrosis) occurs in liver cells. Meanwhile, TG and TC are characterized as indicators of fat accumulation in the liver and responses to alcohol consumption [11,32].

As shown in Figure 1, serum levels of ALT, AST, TG, and TC in the EtOH group greatly increased by 44.63% ($p < 0.05$), 23.69% ($p < 0.05$), 43.98% ($p < 0.05$), and 57.83% ($p < 0.05$), respectively, compared with the control group. In AST and TG levels, significant decreases were observed between low-dose (0.4 g/kg BW) and high-dose (1.6 g/kg BW) artichoke groups. Notably, the ALT, AST, TG, and TC levels in the artichoke pretreatment groups were abated in a dose-dependent manner compared with the EtOH group. Pretreatment with high-dose artichoke (1.6 g/kg BW) markedly recovered serum ALT, AST, TG, and TC levels to near those of control group mice. The results demonstrated that artichoke pretreatment was also effective in reversing the acute alcohol-induced liver dysfunction.

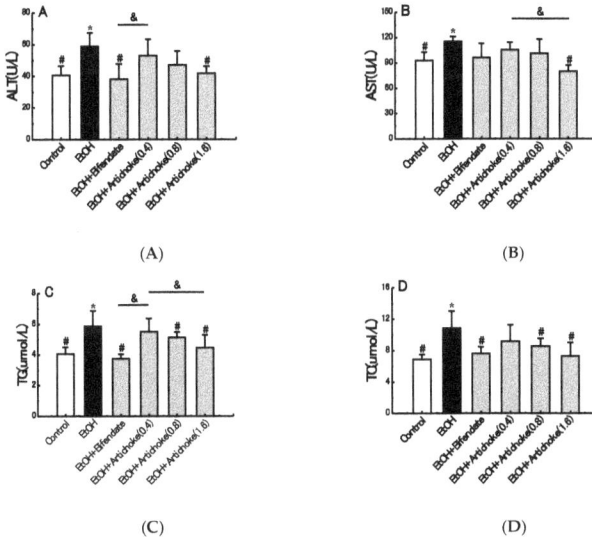

(A)

(B)

(C)

(D)

Figure 1. Effects of artichoke on levels of ALT (**A**), AST (**B**), TG (**C**), and TC (**D**). Values represent means ± standard deviation (SD) ($n = 10$); * $p < 0.05$ vs. the control group; [#] $p < 0.05$ vs. the EtOH group; [&] $p < 0.05$. ALT: alanine aminotransferase; AST: aspartate aminotransferase; TG: triglycerides; TC: total cholesterol.

3.3. Histopathological Analysis

The effect of artichoke on the histopathology of the acute ALD mice is presented in Figure 2. Staining with H&E revealed normal hepatic architecture within the complete structure, similar size, tight arrangement, regular hepatic cords with central vein, and clear hepatic sinusoid in control group (Figure 2A). Nevertheless, the EtOH group demonstrated evident pathological changes, including loose arrangement, disarrangement of cell cords, leukocytes infiltration, necrosis, and hepatocytes steatosis, which confirmed the establishment of liver injury with inflammation (Figure 2B). Slight leukocyte infiltration and hepatocyte steatosis was still observed in the low-dose artichoke (0.4 g/kg) group (Figure 2D). However, pretreatment with bifendate and artichokes exerted a regenerative effect of hepatocytes and a decrease of necrotic and inflamed areas. This indicated that artichoke pretreatment promoted structure restoration of the liver to a certain extent.

As shown in score results (Figure 2G–I), the pathological scores of steatosis, inflammation and necrosis increased significantly ($p < 0.001$) in the EtOH group when compared to control group. However, compared with EtOH group, the degree of hepatic change had made an improvement in the artichoke and bifendate pretreatment group, suggesting that artichoke had preventive effect of alleviating alcohol-induced liver steatosis, inflammation and necrosis. Significant differences were observed between artichoke low-dose (0.4 g/kg BW) and high-dose (0.8 g/kg BW) groups in all score results. Interestingly, the decrease effect of artichoke was in a dose-dependent manner.

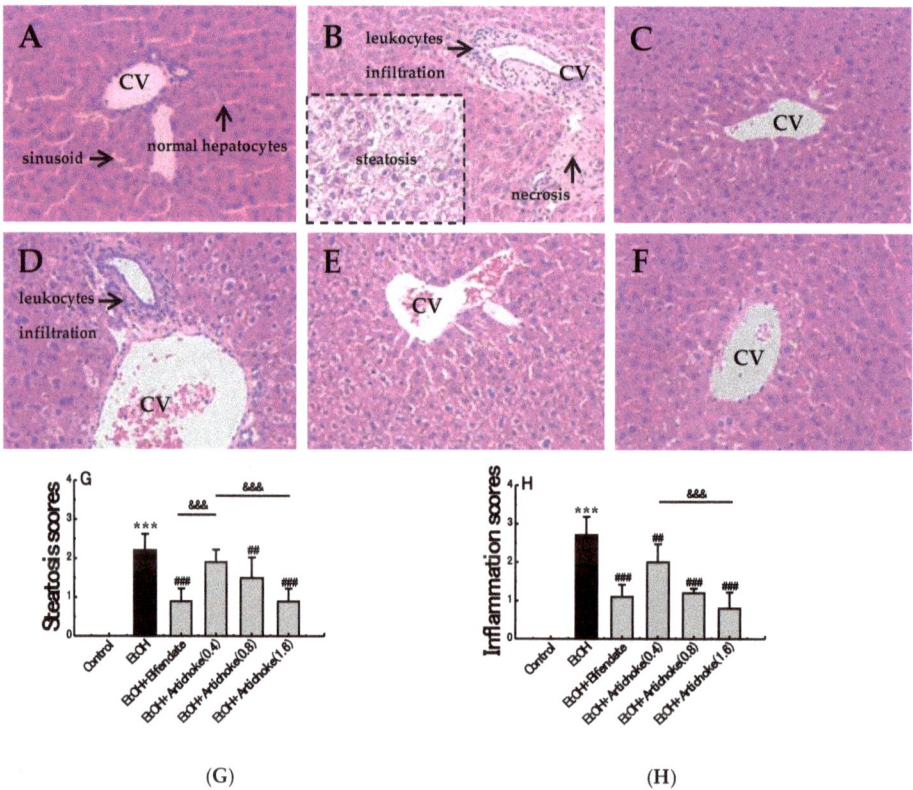

(G)   (H)

Figure 2. *Cont.*

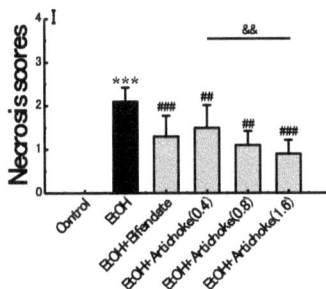

(I)

Figure 2. Effect of artichoke on alcohol-induced histopathological changes in liver tissues. (**A**) Control group, (**B**) EtOH group, (**C**) positive control group, (**D**) low-dose group, (**E**) middle-dose group, (**F**) high-dose group, (**G**) steatosis scores, (**H**) inflammation scores, (**I**) necrosis scores, and central vein (CV). Hematoxylin and eosin staining. Original magnification, 200×. Values represent means ± SD ($n = 10$); *** $p < 0.001$ vs. the control group; ## $p < 0.01$, ### $p < 0.001$ vs. the EtOH group; && $p < 0.01$, &&& $p < 0.001$.

3.4. Hepatic Antioxidant and Oxidative Stress Markers

Oxidative stress plays a central role in alcohol-induced liver injury and ALD pathogenesis [33]. To counterbalance oxidative stress, a number of enzymatic (e.g., SOD) and non-enzymatic (e.g., GSH) mechanisms have evolved to protect against reactive oxygen species (ROS) caused by oxidative stress in alcoholic liver injury. SOD reduces the generation of free radical and lipid peroxide and even accelerates its clearance, thus reducing the damage of liver cells [34,35]. GSH serves as a reservoir for cysteine to counteract ROS [36]. SOD and GSH activities reflect the body's ability of clearing oxygen free radicals indirectly. Meanwhile, MDA is the main product of lipid peroxidation induced by ROS; in addition, MDA content can reflex the severity of free radical attacks on the body cells indirectly [37,38]. Regarding oxidative stress, excessive ROS and MDA will consume a large quantity of antioxidation factors, such as SOD and GSH. The in vivo SOD and GSH would be unable to fight against the excessively increasing ROS and MDA once the balance is lost. Maintaining suitable levels of SOD, GSH, and MDA plays an important role in liver protection from attacks of free radicals.

As shown in Figure 3, the SOD and GSH in the EtOH group decreased by 20.24% ($p < 0.05$) and 39.08% ($p < 0.05$) respectively compared with the control group. By contrast, hepatic MDA activity increased significantly by 255.14% ($p < 0.001$) in the EtOH group compared with the control group. Results showed that the activities of SOD and GSH in the blood increased significantly, whereas MDA decreased significantly when artichoke was subjected to an alcohol diet. Notably, a dose-dependent mechanism was found for all SOD, GSH and MDA activities. High-dose artichoke (1.6 g/kg BW) administrations significantly protected against the acute alcohol-induced elevation of MDA activity ($p < 0.001$) and reduction of SOD ($p < 0.05$) and GSH ($p < 0.05$). This suggested that pretreatment of artichoke could protect the liver from acute alcohol-induced hepatic oxidative stress.

(A)

(B)

(C)

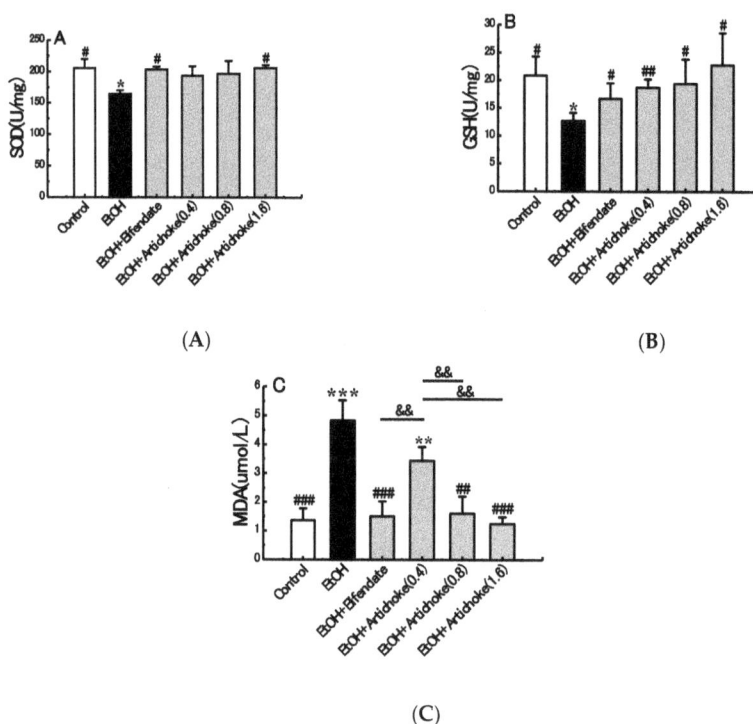

Figure 3. Effects of artichoke on levels of SOD (**A**), GSH (**B**), and MDA (**C**). Values represent means ± SD ($n = 10$); * $p < 0.05$, ** $p < 0.01$, *** $p < 0.001$ vs. the control group; # $p < 0.05$, ## $p < 0.01$, ### $p < 0.001$ vs. the EtOH group; && $p < 0.01$. SOD: superoxide dismutase; GSH: glutathione; MDA: malondialdehyde.

3.5. TLR4 and NF-κB Expression Levels

TLRs are a family of pattern-recognition receptors that enable the innate immune system to react immediately to infections by recognizing both the bacterial and viral constituents [39]. Among these, TLR4 is responsible for LPS-induced inflammatory reaction. Acute excessive alcohol exposure increases gut permeability, which allows gut-derived endotoxins (LPS) to bind with TLR4. The interaction of TLR4 and LPS result in the activation of NF-κB, which is composed of the p50 and p65 subunits. Generally, NF-κB is sequestered as an inactive complex in cytoplasm by inhibitory subunit-inhibitory κB (IκB). Once activated, IκB is phosphorylated and degraded, which allows NF-κB p50 to translocate to the nucleus and induce the expression of its target genes, hence resulting in release of pro-inflammatory cytokines, such as tumor necrosis factor α (TNF-α), the interleukin (IL)-1 receptor (IL-1β), IL-6, and IL-8. All of these pro-inflammatory mediators can aggravate inflammatory progress, ultimately leading to hepatic fibrosis, cirrhosis, and hepatocellular carcinoma [8,40,41]. Thus, the expression levels of upstream index TLR4 and downstream index NF-κB in an inflammatory pathway are two pivotal indicators implicated in inflammation.

As shown in Figure 4, the positive cells of TLR4 were stained as brown or yellow, which were distributed mainly in the cytoplasm and cell membrane, whereas the positive cells of NF-κB p50 were stained as brown in the nucleus. The mean IOD result showed that expression levels of TLR4 and NF-κB p50 in the EtOH group were elevated significantly, by 147.88% ($p < 0.001$) and 103.58% ($p < 0.001$), respectively, compared with the control group. However, these increases were attenuated by artichoke pretreatment in a dose-dependent manner compared with the EtOH group. In the mean IOD of TLR4 expression, a significant difference ($p < 0.05$) was observed between low-dose (0.4 g/kg BW) and high-dose (1.6 g/kg BW) artichoke pretreatment groups. Based on the results, the preventive effect of artichoke against acute alcohol-induced liver injury was associated with TLR4 downregulation. The activation of NF-κB was therefore inhibited. Thus, the release of pro-inflammatory cytokines was limited. The inflammatory effect was then ultimately suppressed.

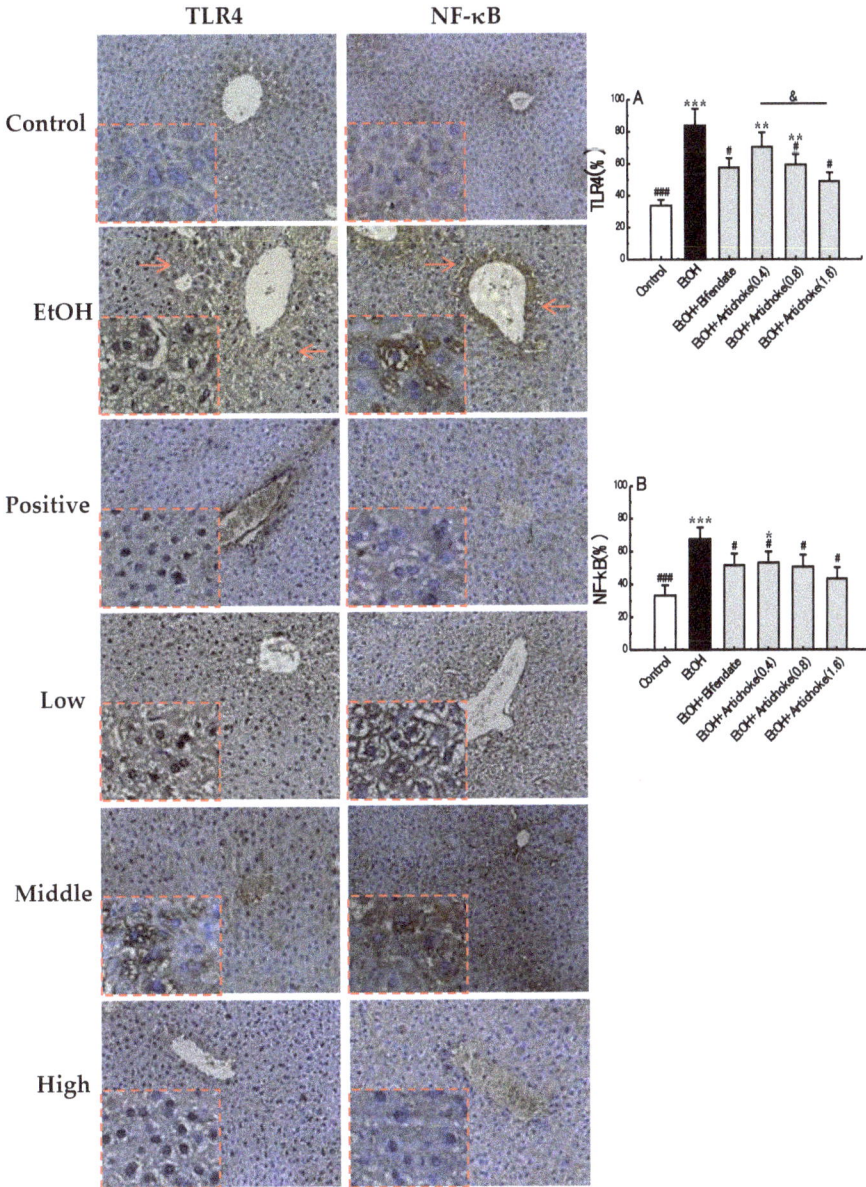

Figure 4. Immunohistochemical analysed results of mice liver in TLR4 and NF-κB. (**A**) mean IOD of TLR4, (**B**) mean IOD of NF-κB, and (**Red Arrows**) positive cells. Original magnification, 200×. * $p < 0.05$, ** $p < 0.01$, *** $p < 0.001$ vs. the control group; # $p < 0.05$, ### $p < 0.001$ vs. the EtOH group; & $p < 0.05$. TLR: toll-like receptor; NF-κB: nuclear factor-kappa B; IOD: integrated optical density.

4. Conclusions

Data presented clearly showed that artichoke reduced levels of AST, ALT, TG, TC, and MDA, while increasing the levels of SOD and GSH in an acute ALD mice model. Degeneration and necrosis of hepatic cells were also significantly attenuated by artichoke. Besides, TLR4 and NF-κB expression levels in liver tissue were effectively downregulated by artichoke. Our study demonstrated that 1.6 g/kg BW artichoke exhibited significant preventative potentiality for acute alcohol-induced liver injury, whereas the effect of 0.4 g/kg BW artichoke was not significant. The preventative effect of artichoke was mainly due to its ability to attenuate oxidative stress and inhibit the inflammatory pathway by suppressing the expression levels of TLR4 and NF-κB. Overall, 1.6 g/kg BW artichoke could be an effective adjuvant in the prevention of acute ALD. Moreover, interventions in the pathogenesis of the TLR4/NF-κB pathway showed its potential as a therapeutic target in acute alcohol-induced liver injury.

Acknowledgments: This work was supported by the Xiamen Science and Technology Program (No. 3502Z20173501), the Education Department of Hunan Province (No. 17A154), the Joint Funds of Hunan Provincial Natural Science Foundation of China (No. 2017JJ4043), and the Fujian Province Young and Middle-aged Teacher Education Research Project (No. JAT170049).

Author Contributions: Tang conceived and designed the experiments; Tang and Wei performed the experiments; Tang and Wei analyzed the data; Wei wrote the paper; Deng contributed reagents/materials tools; Lei revised the manuscript.

Conflicts of Interest: The authors declare that they have no conflict of interets.

References

1. Szabo, G. Gut–liver axis in alcoholic liver disease. *Gastroenterology* **2015**, *148*, 30–36. [CrossRef] [PubMed]
2. Yang, Y.; Han, Z.; Wang, Y.; Wang, L.; Pan, S.; Liang, S.; Wang, S. Plasma metabonomic analysis reveals the effects of salvianic acid on alleviating acute alcoholic liver damage. *RSC Adv.* **2015**, *5*, 36732–36741. [CrossRef]
3. Kawaratani, H.; Tsujimoto, T.; Douhara, A.; Takaya, H.; Moriya, K.; Namisaki, T.; Noguchi, R.; Yoshiji, H.; Fujimoto, M.; Fukui, H. The effect of inflammatory cytokines in alcoholic liver disease. *Mediat. Inflamm.* **2013**, *2013*, 495156. [CrossRef] [PubMed]
4. Cao, Y.-W.; Jiang, Y.; Zhang, D.-Y.; Zhang, X.-J.; Hu, Y.-J.; Li, P.; Su, H.; Wan, J.-B. The hepatoprotective effect of aqueous extracts of penthorum chinense pursh against acute alcohol-induced liver injury is associated with ameliorating hepatic steatosis and reducing oxidative stress. *Food Funct.* **2015**, *6*, 1510–1517. [CrossRef] [PubMed]
5. Gao, B.; Bataller, R. Alcoholic liver disease: Pathogenesis and new therapeutic targets. *Gastroenterology* **2011**, *141*, 1572–1585. [CrossRef] [PubMed]
6. Tilg, H.; Moschen, A.R.; Kaneider, N.C. Pathways of liver injury in alcoholic liver disease. *J. Hepatol.* **2011**, *55*, 1159–1161. [CrossRef] [PubMed]
7. Akira, S.; Uematsu, S.; Takeuchi, O. Pathogen recognition and innate immunity. *Cell* **2006**, *124*, 783–801. [CrossRef] [PubMed]
8. Gilmore, T.D. Introduction to nf-kappab: Players, pathways, perspectives. *Oncogene* **2006**, *25*, 6680–6684. [CrossRef] [PubMed]
9. Wada, S.; Yamazaki, T.; Kawano, Y.; Miura, S.; Ezaki, O. Fish oil fed prior to ethanol administration prevents acute ethanol-induced fatty liver in mice. *J. Hepatol.* **2008**, *49*, 441–450. [CrossRef] [PubMed]
10. Hritz, I.; Mandrekar, P.; Velayudham, A.; Catalano, D.; Dolganiuc, A.; Kodys, K.; Kurt-Jones, E.; Szabo, G. The critical role of toll-like receptor (TLR) 4 in alcoholic liver disease is independent of the common TLR adapter MyD88. *Hepatology* **2008**, *48*, 1224–1231. [CrossRef] [PubMed]
11. Purohit, V.; Gao, B.; Song, B.J. Molecular mechanisms of alcoholic fatty liver. *Alcohol. Clin. Exp. Res.* **2009**, *33*, 191–205. [CrossRef] [PubMed]
12. He, W.; Zhang, Y.; Zhang, J.; Yu, Q.; Wang, P.; Wang, Z.; Smith, A.J. Cytidine-phosphate-guanosine oligonucleotides induce interleukin-8 production through activation of TLR9, MyD88, NF-κB, and ERK pathways in odontoblast cells. *J. Endod.* **2012**, *38*, 780–785. [CrossRef] [PubMed]

13. Suk, K.T.; Kim, M.Y.; Baik, S.K. Alcoholic liver disease: Treatment. *World J. Gastroenterol.* **2014**, *20*, 12934–12944. [CrossRef] [PubMed]
14. O'Shea, R.S.; Dasarathy, S.; McCullough, A.J.; Practice Guideline Committee of the American Association for the Study of Liver Diseases; Practice Parameters Committee of the American College of Gastroenterology. Alcoholic liver disease. *Hepatology* **2010**, *51*, 307–328.
15. Massey, V.L.; Arteel, G.E. Acute alcohol-induced liver injury. *Front. Physiol.* **2012**, *3*, 193. [CrossRef] [PubMed]
16. Leggio, L.; Kenna, G.A.; Ferrulli, A.; Zywiak, W.H.; Caputo, F.; Swift, R.M.; Addolorato, G. Preliminary findings on the use of metadoxine for the treatment of alcohol dependence and alcoholic liver disease. *Hum. Psychopharmacol.* **2011**, *26*, 554–559. [CrossRef] [PubMed]
17. Pan, S.Y.; Yang, R.; Dong, H.; Yu, Z.L.; Ko, K.M. Bifendate treatment attenuates hepatic steatosis in cholesterol/bile salt- and high-fat diet-induced hypercholesterolemia in mice. *Eur. J. Pharmacol.* **2006**, *552*, 170–175. [CrossRef] [PubMed]
18. Kumar, N.; Rai, A.; Reddy, N.D.; Raj, P.V.; Jain, P.; Deshpande, P.; Mathew, G.; Kutty, N.G.; Udupa, N.; Rao, C.M. Silymarin liposomes improves oral bioavailability of silybin besides targeting hepatocytes, and immune cells. *Pharmacol. Rep.* **2014**, *66*, 788–798. [CrossRef] [PubMed]
19. Pistón, M.; Machado, I.; Branco, C.S.; Cesio, V.; Heinzen, H.; Ribeiro, D.; Fernandes, E.; Chisté, R.C.; Freitas, M. Infusion, decoction and hydroalcoholic extracts of leaves from artichoke (*cynara cardunculus* L. Subsp. *Cardunculus*) are effective scavengers of physiologically relevant ros and rns. *Food Res. Int.* **2014**, *64*, 150–156.
20. Bianco, V.V. *Present Situation and Future Potential of Artichoke in the Mediterranean Basin*; International Society for Horticultural Science (ISHS): Leuven, Belgium, 2005; pp. 39–58.
21. Wittemer, S.M.; Ploch, M.; Windeck, T.; Muller, S.C.; Drewelow, B.; Derendorf, H.; Veit, M. Bioavailability and pharmacokinetics of caffeoylquinic acids and flavonoids after oral administration of artichoke leaf extracts in humans. *Phytomedicine* **2005**, *12*, 28–38. [CrossRef] [PubMed]
22. Wegener, T.; Fintelmann, V. Pharmacological properties and therapeutic profile of artichoke (*cynara scolymus* L.). *Wien. Med. Wochenschr.* **1999**, *149*, 241–247. [PubMed]
23. Joy, J.F.; Haber, S.L. Clinical uses of artichoke leaf extract. *Am. J. Health Syst. Pharm.* **2007**, *64*, 1904, 1906–1909. [CrossRef] [PubMed]
24. Moglia, A.; Lanteri, S.; Comino, C.; Acquadro, A.; de Vos, R.; Beekwilder, J. Stress-induced biosynthesis of dicaffeoylquinic acids in globe artichoke. *J. Agric. Food Chem.* **2008**, *56*, 8641–8649. [CrossRef] [PubMed]
25. Wider, B.; Pittler, M.H.; Thompson-Coon, J.; Ernst, E. Artichoke leaf extract for treating hypercholesterolaemia. *Cochrane Database Syst. Rev.* **2013**, *7*, CD003335.
26. Heidarian, E.; Soofiniya, Y. Hypolipidemic and hypoglycemic effects of aerial part of cynara scolymus in streptozotocin-induced diabetic rats. *J. Med. Plants Res.* **2011**, *5*, 2717–2723.
27. Yasukawa, K.; Matsubara, H.; Sano, Y. Inhibitory effect of the flowers of artichoke (*cynara cardunculus*) on TPA-induced inflammation and tumor promotion in two-stage carcinogenesis in mouse skin. *J. Nat. Med.* **2010**, *64*, 388–391. [CrossRef] [PubMed]
28. Gebhardt, R. Inhibition of cholesterol biosynthesis in HepG2 cells by artichoke extracts is reinforced by glucosidase pretreatment. *Phytother. Res.* **2002**, *16*, 368–372. [CrossRef] [PubMed]
29. Zhang, W.; Wang, L.W.; Wang, L.K.; Li, X.; Zhang, H.; Luo, L.P.; Song, J.C.; Gong, Z.J. Betaine protects against high-fat-diet-induced liver injury by inhibition of high-mobility group box 1 and toll-like receptor 4 expression in rats. *Dig. Dis. Sci.* **2013**, *58*, 3198–3206. [CrossRef] [PubMed]
30. Chen, Y.X.; Lai, L.N.; Zhang, H.Y.; Bi, Y.H.; Meng, L.; Li, X.J.; Tian, X.X.; Wang, L.M.; Fan, Y.M.; Zhao, Z.F.; et al. Effect of artesunate supplementation on bacterial translocation and dysbiosis of gut microbiota in rats with liver cirrhosis. *World J. Gastroenterol.* **2016**, *22*, 2949–2959. [CrossRef] [PubMed]
31. Liu, N.; Yang, M.; Huang, W.; Wang, Y.; Yang, M.; Wang, Y.; Zhao, Z. Composition, antioxidant activities and hepatoprotective effects of the water extract of ziziphus jujuba cv. Jinsixiaozao. *RSC Adv.* **2017**, *7*, 6511–6522. [CrossRef]
32. Ozer, J.; Ratner, M.; Shaw, M.; Bailey, W.; Schomaker, S. The current state of serum biomarkers of hepatotoxicity. *Toxicology* **2008**, *245*, 194–205. [CrossRef] [PubMed]
33. Koch, O.R.; Pani, G.; Borrello, S.; Colavitti, R.; Cravero, A.; Farre, S.; Galeotti, T. Oxidative stress and antioxidant defenses in ethanol-induced cell injury. *Mol. Asp. Med.* **2004**, *25*, 191–198. [CrossRef] [PubMed]

34. Afonso, V.; Champy, R.; Mitrovic, D.; Collin, P.; Lomri, A. Reactive oxygen species and superoxide dismutases: Role in joint diseases. *Jt. Bone Spine* **2007**, *74*, 324–329. [CrossRef] [PubMed]

35. Ding, R.B.; Tian, K.; Cao, Y.W.; Bao, J.L.; Wang, M.; He, C.; Hu, Y.; Su, H.; Wan, J.B. Protective effect of panax notoginseng saponins on acute ethanol-induced liver injury is associated with ameliorating hepatic lipid accumulation and reducing ethanol-mediated oxidative stress. *J. Agric. Food Chem.* **2015**, *63*, 2413–2422. [CrossRef] [PubMed]

36. De Matos, D.G.; Furnus, C.C. The importance of having high glutathione (GSH) level after bovine in vitro maturation on embryo development: Effect of β-mercaptoethanol, cysteine and cystine. *Theriogenology* **2000**, *53*, 761–771. [CrossRef]

37. Li, G.; Ye, Y.; Kang, J.; Yao, X.; Zhang, Y.; Jiang, W.; Gao, M.; Dai, Y.; Xin, Y.; Wang, Q.; et al. L-theanine prevents alcoholic liver injury through enhancing the antioxidant capability of hepatocytes. *Food Chem. Toxicol.* **2012**, *50*, 363–372. [CrossRef] [PubMed]

38. Tuma, D.J. Role of malondialdehyde-acetaldehyde adducts in liver injury. *Free Radic. Biol. Med.* **2002**, *32*, 303–308. [CrossRef]

39. Akira, S.; Takeda, K.; Kaisho, T. Toll-like receptors: Critical proteins linking innate and acquired immunity. *Nat. Immunol.* **2001**, *2*, 675–680. [CrossRef] [PubMed]

40. Kawai, T.; Akira, S. Signaling to nf-kappab by toll-like receptors. *Trends Mol. Med.* **2007**, *13*, 460–469. [CrossRef] [PubMed]

41. Palsson-McDermott, E.M.; O'Neill, L.A. Signal transduction by the lipopolysaccharide receptor, toll-like receptor-4. *Immunology* **2004**, *113*, 153–162. [CrossRef] [PubMed]

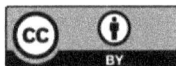

nutrients

MDPI

Review

Parenteral Nutrition-Associated Liver Disease: The Role of the Gut Microbiota

Monika Cahova [1],*, Miriam Bratova [1] and Petr Wohl [2]

[1] Centre for Experimental Medicine, Institute for Clinical and Experimental Medicine, Department of Metabolism and Diabetes, Videnska 1958/9, 14021 Prague 4, Czech Republic; miriam.bratova@ikem.cz

[2] Centre of Diabetology, Institute for Clinical and Experimental Medicine, Department of Metabolism and Diabetes, Videnska 1958/9, 14021 Prague 4, Czech Republic; petr.wohl@ikem.cz

*   Correspondence: monika.cahova@ikem.cz; Tel.: +420-261-365-366; Fax: +420-261-363-027

Received: 20 June 2017; Accepted: 30 August 2017; Published: 7 September 2017

Abstract: Parenteral nutrition (PN) provides life-saving nutritional support in situations where caloric supply via the enteral route cannot cover the necessary needs of the organism. However, it does have serious adverse effects, including parenteral nutrition-associated liver disease (PNALD). The development of liver injury associated with PN is multifactorial, including non-specific intestine inflammation, compromised intestinal permeability, and barrier function associated with increased bacterial translocation, primary and secondary cholangitis, cholelithiasis, short bowel syndrome, disturbance of hepatobiliary circulation, lack of enteral nutrition, shortage of some nutrients (proteins, essential fatty acids, choline, glycine, taurine, carnitine, etc.), and toxicity of components within the nutrition mixture itself (glucose, phytosterols, manganese, aluminium, etc.). Recently, an increasing number of studies have provided evidence that some of these factors are directly or indirectly associated with microbial dysbiosis in the intestine. In this review, we focus on PN-induced changes in the taxonomic and functional composition of the microbiome. We also discuss immune cell and microbial crosstalk during parenteral nutrition, and the implications for the onset and progression of PNALD. Finally, we provide an overview of recent advances in the therapeutic utilisation of pro- and prebiotics for the mitigation of PN-associated liver complications.

Keywords: Parenteral nutrition; microbiota; PNALD; intestinal permeability; gut-associated immune system; bile acids; FXR signalling; pre/probiotics

1. Introduction

Parenteral nutrition (PN) provides life-saving nutritional support in situations where caloric supply via the enteral route is either not possible or cannot cover the necessary needs of the organism, e.g., preterm neonates with immature gut, perioperatively in patients requiring massive intestinal surgery, or in patients with short bowel syndrome (SBS). PN preserves lean body mass, supports immune functions, and reduces metabolic complications in patients who are otherwise unable to feed [1]. Nevertheless, PN does have serious adverse effects, one of which is the deterioration of liver function. PN-induced cholestasis generally refers to the onset of liver disease in the context of the administration of intravenous nutrition in patients with temporary or permanent intestinal failure. Other terms commonly used to describe the condition are parenteral nutrition-associated cholestasis (PNAC) and intestinal failure-associated liver disease (IFALD), but the most frequently used is parenteral nutrition-associated liver disease (PNALD) [2]. PNALD clinical manifestations—which range from steatosis, cholestasis, gallbladder sludge/stones, fibrosis, and cirrhosis—can occur separately or in combination [3,4]. Steatosis (defined as fat accumulation in hepatocytes) can present as mild to moderate elevations in liver function tests and is usually benign. Cholestasis results from impaired secretion or obstruction of bile, and is associated with elevations in alkaline phosphatase, gamma-glutamyl transferase, and conjugated bilirubin [5].

There are some differences between child and adult patients totally dependent on parenteral nutrition (TPN) with regard to the pathogenesis of PNALD. Cholestasis occurs in 40–60% of infants, steatosis in 40–55% of adults, while biliary sludge and cholelithiasis occur in both adults and children. Child TPN patients (premature infants) typically exhibit prematurity (impaired transsulfuration, lack of cystathionase, etc.) and bowel lengths <25 cm, while necrotising enterocolitis is frequently the cause of intestinal failure. In addition, the high-energy requirements (80–100 kcal/kg per day) for growth are associated with the rapid onset of PNALD within months. All of these factors make children patients significantly more susceptible to PNALD/IFALD. In adults, a history of PNALD is characterised by elevated liver enzymes and associated steatosis, which can last for years. Ensuing complications include steatohepatitis, cholestatic hepatitis, as well as fibrosis and cirrhosis. In contrast, histology findings in child-type PNALD are defined by cholestasis, portal fibrosis, peri-cellular fibrosis, bile duct proliferation, pigmented Kupffer cells and non-progressive cirrhosis. Risk factors in children include lack of taurine, excess of calories, excess of lipids (>3.5 g/kg/day, mainly omega-6 fatty acids), phytosterols, bowel inflammation, catheter infections, and an absence of the ileo-caecal valve. In adults, risk factors include lack of choline, excess of calories, excess of lipids >1 g/kg/day, phytosterols, bowel inflammation, small bowel bacterial overgrowth, and absence of the ileo-caecal valve. In both groups, sepsis is a significant complication. The detailed differences of the pathomechanisms that underlie liver damage in both PN-dependent paediatric and adult patients are beyond the scope of this paper. More information is available in some excellent recent reviews [6,7].

Although the pathogenesis of PNALD is undoubtedly a multifactorial phenomenon, the privileged role may be attributed to the impaired function of the intestine. It harbours most of the immune cells in the body and represents the largest area for contact with antigens from the environment. The gut microbiome plays an essential role in intestinal development and homeostasis maintenance [8]. In humans, the gut microbiome is composed of approximate 1000 species and it is estimated that their genomes exceed the human genome by more than one hundred-fold. This represents a major stimulus to the immune system and facilitates the performance of many physiological functions [9]. The gut microbiota is the most abundant cohort of antigen-presenting cells. Based on the above facts, it is conceivable that the radical alteration of gut microbiome composition and function as a result of switching to total parenteral nutrition could lead to detrimental effects on the intestine and significantly contribute to PNALD development.

2. PN and the Gut Microbiota

Data on the gut microbiota in the context of PN have been obtained under three different group settings: animal models (mouse, rat, piglet), neonate babies (most of them premature), and adult patients who have lost a substantial portion of functional gut tissue and cannot feed themselves via the enteral route. Although PN is present in all cases, each of these groups has specific features that strongly influence microbiome composition (Table 1).

Table 1. The effect of parenteral nutrition on gut microbiome composition.

Model	Bowel Resection	TPN Duration	Enteral Feeding		References
Rat-adult	No	14 days	No	*Firmicutes/Bacteroidetes* ratio; shift in favour of Bacteroidetes	[10]
Mouse-adult	No	5 days	No	Shift from *Firmicutes* to *Proteobactoria* and *Bacteroidetes*, i.e., *Salmonella, Proteus, Escherichia, Bacteroides*	[11]
Mouse-adult	No	5 days	No	Shift from *Firmicutes* to *Bacteroidetes* and *Proteobacteria*	[12]
Piglet-newborn	Yes	6 weeks	No	Changes in the composition of the *Firmicutes* phylum (decrease of *Anaerotruncus, Clostridium, Ruminococcus, Peptostreptococcus;* increase in *Acidaminococcus* and *Mitsuokella*)	[13]
Piglet-newborn	No	7 days	No	Lower total bacterial counts and reduced bacterial diversity, enriched in *Clostridium difficile*	[14]
Piglet-newborn	No	7 days	No	Enriched in *C. perfringens* and sulphated monosaccharide-degrading bacteria	[15]
Piglet-newborn	No	14 days	No	PN + ω-3: increased *Parabacteroides* PN + ω-6: increased *Enterobacteriaceae*	[16]
Human-pre-term newborn	Yes	Long-term	Yes	Higher diversity, higher abundance of Gram-negative bacteria, lower odds of death and late-onset sepsis cases	[17]
			No	Less diversity, lower abundance of Gram-negative bacteria, increased odds of death and late-onset sepsis cases	
Human-paediatric/adult	Yes	Long-term	Yes	Increased *Staphylococcus, Pseudomonas, Campylobacter, Propionibacterium, Chryseomonas*	[18]
			No	Increased *Enterobacter, Shigella, Klebsiella, Fusobacterium*	
Human-adult	Yes	Long-term	Yes	Enrichment in *Lactobacillus/Leuconostoc*; depletion of anaerobes, especially *Clostridiaceae*	[19,20]
Human-adult	Yes	Long-term	Yes	High abundance of *Proteobacteria*, especially *Enterobacteriaceae* and *Fusobacteria*; changes in the *Firmicutes* spectrum, depletion of *Lachnospiraceae* and *Ruminococcaceae*	[21]

2.1. Adult Animal Models

In rats, Hodin et al. demonstrated that after 14 days of PN, total bacterial numbers per gram of luminal content did not differ between PN-fed and control rats; however, the composition of the bacterial population significantly changed. *Firmicutes* abundance dropped while the abundance of *Bacteroidetes* did not differ between groups. Consequently, the proportional representation of these two phyla in PN rats significantly shifted in favour of *Bacteroidetes* [10]. In a mouse model (5 days of PN), Miyasaka demonstrated that at the phylum level, the vast majority of mucosa-associated bacteria in the small bowels of control mice were *Firmicutes*. However, in the PN group, the dominant phyla were *Proteobacteria* and *Bacteroidetes*. At the genus level, PN mice had more bacteria in the genera *Salmonella, Escherichia, Proteus,* and *Bacteroides*. These genera are often associated with clinical infections, potentially indicating the development of a pathological state within the intestinal microbial community. Furthermore, enteral nutrient deprivation resulted in a loss of diversity in the large and small intestines [11]. Similar results indicating a shift from *Firmicutes* to *Bacteroides* have also been reported by an independent group [12]. A common feature of all these models is the overall deprivation of enteral nutrition for the entire duration of the experiments.

2.2. Neonates: Humans

In preterm neonates, the immature gut is much more prone to insults resulting from reduced intestinal motility, inappropriate immune responses, decreased protective gastrointestinal secretions, reduced digestive and absorptive function, and increased intestinal epithelial permeability [22]. In a prospective two-centre study, Parm et al. compared the effect of enteral-versus-parenteral feeding on the pattern of gut colonisation in preterm neonates at risk of late-onset sepsis and necrotising enterocolitis. PN was associated with the reduced acquisition of both Gram-positive and Gram-negative colonising microorganisms. *Candida albicans* colonisation was more frequent in neonates receiving PN. Despite greater mucosal colonisation by potentially pathogenic microorganisms (e.g., *Enterobacteriaceae* and *Enterococcus*), an enteral feeding regimen was associated with lower odds of late-onset sepsis and mortality in premature neonates than a PN regimen [17]. *Enterococcus faecalis* is the main immune modulator among human intestinal lactic acid bacteria, and is able to downregulate the expression of the host immune genes that participate in inflammation [23]. Thus, in the context of the naïve gut, colonisation with some *Enterococci* may be beneficial due to the suppression of specific toll-like receptors (TLR)-signalling pathways. Nevertheless, the conclusions drawn by Parm et al. are limited in that their study only included individuals under third-level neonatal intensive care, with all participants receiving at least one but usually more antibiotics, all of which may have significantly influenced gut microflora composition.

2.3. Neonates: Animal Models

In controlled animal model experiments that investigate the effect of PN on gut colonisation in neonates, enterally fed piglets exhibited a higher bacterial diversity, higher concentrations of bacteria (CFU/g), and increased colonisation of all segments of the intestinal tract compared to PN pigs. Translocation of bacteria from the intestinal tract to tissues or blood was similar in both groups. PN-treated piglets were at higher risk of colonisation by toxin-expressing strains of *C. difficile* [14]. Using the same model but a different method of bacterial taxa identification (16S rRNA NGS sequencing versus DGGE analysis), Deplancke found that the bacterial community structure was equally complex in the ilea of enterally and parenterally fed piglets; however, profiles clustered according to the mode of nutrition. The opportunistic pathogen *C. perfringens*, as well as mucus-associated bacteria, were specifically enriched in the guts of animals dependent on PN [15]. Bacteria capable of using sulphated monosaccharides were also more abundant in PN samples.

A recently published study by Lavallee et al. demonstrated that not only PN *per se* but also the type of lipid constituent affects microbiome composition in newborns. As expected, the gut microbial composition of PN-dependent piglets differed from those fed with sow milk, but the microbiota further clustered according to ω-3 or ω-6 PUFA content in the nutrition mixture. Piglets fed with ω-3 PUFA-rich PN were more similar to the sow milk-fed group than those administered ω-6 PUFA. The group with prevailing ω-6 PUFA on PN showed a specific and significant increase in *Parabacteroides*, while the ω-3 group showed an increase in *Enterobacteriaceae* [16]. The limitation of this study is that the antibiotic treatment was administered only to piglets exhibiting signs of sepsis, but not globally to the whole cohort. Nevertheless, this innovative study points out an unexpected aspect of PN, namely the interplay of the gut microbiota and lipid components of the nutrition mixture.

2.4. Patients with Small Intestinal Resections: Fed vs. Enterally Deprived Portions of the Intestine

The common denominator for all of the above therapeutic or experimental settings is the absence of enteral nutrition, which leaves the intestinal microbiota in a state of acute nutrient withdrawal. No animal study comparing the effect of PN alone or PN in combination with enteral nutrition has been carried out. Ralls et al. published an interesting study comparing microbial diversity and differences in microbial characteristics in enterally fed and enterally deprived portions of the small bowel obtained after surgical resection [18]. The restraint of this study was the low number of samples used and the highly heterogeneous population of the patients. However, some valuable implications can be derived. Although only a partial stratification of microbial communities between fed and enterally deprived groups was found, some groups tended to expand in the fed group (*Staphylococcus, Pseudomonas, Campylobacter, Propionibacterium, Chryseomonas*) in comparison to others in the enterally deprived group (*Enterobacter, Shigella, Klebsiella* and *Fusobacterium*). A close correlation was identified in patients with low levels of enteric microbial diversity and those who developed post-operative enteric-derived infections.

2.5. Adult SBS Patients: The Specific Intestinal Environment

Patients diagnosed with short bowel syndrome (SBS) represent a specific group that are dependent on total parenteral nutrition. SBS occurs in patients with an extensive resection of the short bowel, leaving less than 150 cm. These patients suffer from severely decreased absorption capacity for water, electrolytes, and nutrients, while intravenous supplementation is required to maintain vital functions [24]. General adaptations following intestinal resection include compensatory hyperphagia, mucosal remodelling of the remaining part of the intestine and major modifications of the microbiota [25]. In contrast to previously described patient groups and animal models, these subjects do intake food per os, whereby the residual lumen of the gut is supplied with abundant but poorly digested substrates. In addition to the excessive nutrient delivery, the gut ecological system of SBS patients is altered in several other ways. Faecal pH has been shown to be lower in patients than in controls, with mean faecal pH at approx. 5.6 in type II SBS patients in comparison to the normal laboratory range of pH (pH = 6 to pH = 7) [19]. Acidic pH creates a specific environment that favours low pH-tolerant microorganisms [26]. In SBS patients, it is possible that because of the short length of the remnant small intestine and colon, the level of oxygen becomes too high, and thus anaerobic bacteria are discriminated in favour of more tolerant facultative anaerobes. The disruption of enterohepatic circulation may result in disturbed bile acid metabolism and a preference for microbiota that are tolerant to bile acids.

2.6. Adult SBS Patients: Microbiota Composition

Original studies that describe the microbiome in SBS patients are remarkably consistent in their findings. The common feature of the SBS microbiota is significantly reduced α-diversity when compared with healthy controls [21,27,28], which positively correlates with remaining small bowel length [21] and PN dependence duration [28]. SBS patients harbour a specific faecal microbiota that is enriched in the *Lactobacillus/Leuconostoc* group and depleted in anaerobic microorganisms, especially those of the *Clostridiaceae* family [19,20]. A characteristic feature of this microbiota is its high abundance of *Proteobacteria*, especially *Enterobacteriaceae* [21,28]. The expansion of *Proteobacteria* may be linked to altered nutrition supply, as *Proteobacteria* can metabolise broader classes of substrates (including amino acids) and are therefore more flexible than other phyla. The decrease of *Bacteroidetes* has been reported both for mucosa [19] and luminal content [28]. The important feature of the SBS microbiome is the alteration of the *Firmicutes* community. *Firmicutes* is a dominant phylum of the healthy gut microbiota. In SBS patients, this phylum is still highly abundant but some important families of butyrate-producers, such as *Lachnospiraceae, Ruminococcaceae* and others, are almost entirely absent [21].

The severe dysbiosis found in SBS patients has a significant impact on the faecal metabolome and seriously affects the host metabolism. The bioconversion of macromolecules into metabolites is carried out by the bacteria of various functional groups, resulting in metabolic trophic chains. In SBS, the trophic chains and fermentation end-products are produced by the lactobiota, and are thus different from those produced by the healthy microbiota. The dominance of the carbohydrate-fermenting *Lactobacillus/Leuconostoc* taxa and the depletion of lactate-consuming anaerobic bacteria result in the excessive formation of both D- and L-lactate. Mayeur et al. [27] demonstrated that the individual lactic acid bacteria composition predicts whether or not a particular SBS patient will accumulate D-lactate in stools. In healthy humans, the lactate produced by the gut microbiota is not accumulated in faeces but it is readily absorbed by intestinal cells or converted to other metabolites, particularly the short-chain fatty acids (SCFA) [29,30]. Furthermore, in healthy humans, D-lactate is efficiently metabolised in the liver, and is thus eliminated from circulation. SBS patients who often suffer from compromised liver function are at an increased risk of lactate acidosis and D-lactate encephalopathy. Another consequence of the profound shift in microbiota composition, particularly the elimination of butyrate-producing anaerobes, is the significant decrease in SCFA production. This SCFA shortage may have multiple impacts on the gut immune system, intestinal wall integrity, and endocrine signalling.

3. PN and the Immune System

The gut microbiota profoundly influences the host immune system [31]. Numerous microbial products—including proteins, polysaccharides, and molecules that activate pattern recognition receptors—activate Toll-like receptors (TLRs) and NOD-like receptors (NODs) and stimulate the mucosal immune system [32]. The gut microbiota has an irreplaceable role in mucosal and systemic immunity maturation [33–35]. It also promotes a tolerogenic state in the intestinal mucosa (stimulation of Treg lymphocytes, attenuation of NF-κB signalling, etc.) [36–40], and instigates mechanisms that prevent bacterial overgrowth (induction of IgA secretion) [41–44]. Some commensals even produce targeted antimicrobial peptides themselves [45]. The healthy gut microbiota provides its host with a physical barrier to incoming pathogens and stimulates it to produce various antimicrobial compounds [31].

3.1. The Microbiota and TLR Signalling

The loss of diversity associated with prolonged PN administration has several adverse impacts on immune functions. The extinction of normally robust commensals facilitates the expansion of pathogenic strains due to the alleviation of competitive exclusion. For instance, the *Proteobacteria* found in the intestines of PN patients includes the opportunistic pathogens *E. coli*, *Salmonella*, *Yersinia*, *Helicobacter*, and *Vibrio*, all of which are commonly associated with infection [46]. Concurrently, some beneficial commensals that normally stimulate immunotolerance are underrepresented in the PN-associated microbiota. The shift in the intestinal microbiota (particularly the enrichment in *Proteobacteria* expressing many TLR ligands) and the activation of MyD88-dependent TLR signalling are suspected as causes of pro-inflammatory status in the PN-associated intestinal mucosa. Nevertheless, results obtained from mice models deficient in TLR signalling in intestinal epithelial cells are contradictory. Several authors have shown the protective effects of MyD88-targeted deletion in intestinal epithelial cells. MyD88 deletion inhibited colitis development in a model of spontaneous colitis (SHP-2 IEC-KO mice), rescued the goblet/intermediate cell ratio and prevented NFκB hyperactivation and inflammation [47]. In a model of diet-induced obesity, MyD88 KO mice exhibited increased anti-inflammatory endocannabinoids, antimicrobial peptide production, and intestinal regulatory T cells, and were partially protected against diet-induced obesity, diabetes, and inflammation [48]. Accordingly, enhanced MyD88 signalling (C57Bl/6 mice expressing a constitutively active form of TLR4 in the intestinal epithelium) resulted in an elevated bacterial translocation, impaired epithelial barrier function, different expression of antimicrobial peptide genes, and altered epithelial cell differentiation [49]. In contrast, Frantz et al. reported that a loss of epithelial MyD88 signalling caused the following effects: increased numbers of mucus-associated bacteria; the translocation of bacteria to mesenteric lymph nodes; reduced transmucosal electrical resistance; impaired mucus-associated antimicrobial activity; and, downregulated expression of polymeric immunoglobulin receptor (the epithelial IgA transporter), mucin-2 and the antimicrobial peptides RegIII and Defa-rs1. These mice were also more susceptible to experimental colitis [50]. MyD88 signalling has also been shown to stimulate gastrointestinal motility [51] and promote the differentiation of intestinal epithelial cells [52]. These rather contradictory outcomes suggest that (i) both low and excessive TLR4 signalling can promote intestinal inflammation and (ii) the interaction between the intestinal microbiota and the immune system is complex. Further research is needed in order to better understand these causal relationships.

3.2. The Microbiota and Intestinal Macrophages

An important population of innate immune cells are intestinal resident macrophages, which play a central role in the maintenance of homeostasis in the gastrointestinal tract [53]. Intestinal macrophages constitutively produce IL-10, one of the major anti-inflammatory cytokines that promotes differentiation and maintenance of Treg cells. They are also hyporesponsive to TLR stimulation [54] and are less prone to the secretion of pro-inflammatory cytokines after LPS stimulation [55]. Resident intestinal macrophages contribute to the attenuation of the immune response to various bacterial and food antigens, while maintaining anti-inflammatory tone in the intestine [56,57]. Recent studies have shown that circulating and tissue-resident macrophages (lung, brain, skin, liver) consist of populations of different embryonic origin, and are also independently maintained in a steady state in adulthood [58,59]. Intestinal macrophages seem to be the only exception to this rule. During the neonatal period, intestinal macrophages are derived from embryonic precursors (the yolk sac and foetal liver), but are gradually replaced by the progeny of conventional haematopoiesis (i.e., Ly6C^{hi} blood monocytes) in adulthood [54]. This process occurs in both the small intestine and the colon, but is regulated by different mechanisms. In the colon, the establishment of the gut microbiota and commensal-derived signals [54,57] drives the replenishment of resident macrophages. Consequently, the microbiota can stimulate macrophages to produce tolerogenic IL-10 either via TLR-signalling [60,61] or via activation of intestinal macrophage receptor GPR109a by microbial metabolites (butyrate, niacin). This setting helps to establish an "immunotolerogenic" feedback loop, whereby the gut microbiota actively promotes the recruitment of circulating macrophages into the intestinal mucosa. These macrophages in turn create a tolerant environment that facilitates the growth of these bacteria. In contrast to the colon, replenishment and IL-10 production of small intestine macrophages are not regulated by the gut microbiota but directly by dietary amino acids [62]. PN administration leads to a profound decline in the number of IL-10-producing macrophages in the small intestine [62]. The compromised replenishment of IL-10-producing macrophages together with the shift in microbial composition towards a more immunogenic phenotype (TLR ligand-rich *Proteobacteria*) may act in synergy towards generating a pro-inflammatory state in the PN-dependent small intestine. To our knowledge, no data are available regarding the direct effect of PN on colon macrophages. However, the facts we do have at our disposal, namely the shift in microbiota composition and the increase in the pro-inflammatory cytokine production, at least suggest a similar scenario.

3.3. The Microbiota and Paneth Cells

Paneth cells are important components of mucosal immunity. They occur at the base of small intestinal crypts and are the primary source of small peptides that exhibit antimicrobial activity (AMPs), such as secretory phospholipase A2 (sPLA2), lysozyme, and α and β-defensins [63–65]. Paneth cells sense bacteria via MyD88-dependent toll-like receptor (TLR) activation, which triggers antimicrobial action [66]. In the PN mouse model, the attenuated expression of Paneth cell antimicrobial proteins was associated with a compositional shift in the microbiome (decreased *Firmicutes*; increased *Bacteroidetes* and *Proteobacteria*), weaker bactericidal activity of mucosal secretions and greater susceptibility to enteroinvasion by *E. coli* [14]. Omata et al. demonstrated that PN feeding resulted in the suppressed secretion of sPLA2 and increased bacterial survival. Taking these data together, PN significantly impairs the innate immune response by suppressing Paneth cell function [67].

3.4. The Microbiota and B-Lymphocytes

The current paradigm supposes that the antibody response is directly or indirectly mediated through TLR signalling, and that it depends on the interaction of bacterial DNA, proteins, and cell wall components with TLR receptors [68,69]. Quite recently, Kim et al. reported a new mechanism whereby the gut microbiota affects host antibody responses via their fermentation products (SCFA) [70]. A positive correlation between dietary fibre intake and intestinal IgAs levels was shown previously [71]. Kim et al. tested the hypothesis that SCFA, the main fermentation product of dietary fibre, affects antibody production. They showed that in isolated mice spleen B-cells in vitro, SCFA increased acetyl-CoA and regulated metabolic sensors to increase oxidative phosphorylation, glycolysis and fatty acid synthesis. This in turn produced energy and building blocks that supported antibody production. In parallel, SCFA controlled gene expression and expressed molecules necessary for plasma B cell differentiation. The effects of all major SCFA (C2, C3 and C4) were comparable. In vivo, mice fed a low dietary fibre (DF) diet were more susceptible to *Citrobacter rodentium* infection compared with mice fed a high DF diet. In susceptible animals, supplementation with DF or propionate (C3) increased host resistance and the IgA response to *C. rodentium* [70].

4. PNALD and Bile Acid Metabolism

4.1. Bile Acid Metabolism and Function

Bile acids (BAs) are synthesised from cholesterol in the liver as primary BAs, which are represented by chenodeoxycholic (CDCA) acid and cholic (CA) acid in humans. Primary BAs are conjugated to taurine or glycine in the liver and as bile salts secreted into bile through bile-salt export proteins (BSEP, ABCB11). Approximately 95% of BAs are reabsorbed in the small intestine via enterohepatic circulation, while a minor fraction escapes before being further metabolised by the gut microbiota in the colon to the secondary BAs, such as deoxycholic (DCA), urodeoxycholic (UDCA), and lithocholic (LCA) acids in humans [72]. In rodents, muricholic (MCA) acid is synthesised as well [73]. Primary and secondary BAs fulfil multiple functions. First, they serve as physiological emulsifiers that facilitate enteral absorption of dietary fat and fat-soluble vitamins [74]. Second, they have direct antibacterial effects. Third, BAs are potent signalling molecules that regulate the host glucose and lipid metabolism as well as energy homeostasis [75,76]. This regulatory function depends on the interaction of BAs with specific receptors, predominantly farnesoid-X receptor (FXR) and G-protein-coupled receptor (TGR5) [77]. However, FXR and TGR5 have different affinities to individual BAs, as FXR is activated by CDCA > DCA > LCA >> CA and TGR5 is activated by LCA > DCA > CDCA > CA [78].

4.2. Interplay Between Bile Acids and the Gut Microbiota

Because the transformation of BAs is solely dependent on the gut microbiota, the extent of BA receptor activation is largely dependent on microbiota composition [79]. FXR is a key regulator of BA metabolism. Activated FXR inhibits CYP7A1, a rate-limiting enzyme of BA synthesis in hepatocytes, by two mechanisms. In hepatocytes, FXR forms a heterodimer with SHP (small heterodimer partner) to suppress the transcription of CYP7A1 [80]. In enterocytes, activated FXR stimulates production of FGF15/19. This cytokine binds to FGFR4 receptor on the hepatocyte surface, thus suppressing CYP7A1 and BA synthesis [81]. Myiata et al. showed that antibiotic treatment elevates hepatic BA synthesis in mice via the suppression of FGF15 expression in the ileum [82], which confirms the potent effect of the gut microbiome on BA metabolism. FXR also regulates enterohepatic BA circulation by regulating the expression of BA transporters. Bacterial modifications of BAs start with primary BA deconjugation by bacteria that exhibit bile salt hydrolase (BSH) activity, followed by the formation of secondary BAs by microbes that exhibit 7α-dehydroxylase and 7α-dehydrogense activity [83]. A wide array of bacteria exhibit BSH activity, enabling them to deconjugate BAs. However, there are a few bacteria belonging to the *Clostridium* clusters XI and XVIa (exhibiting 7α-dehydroxylase activity), which may catalyse the dehydrogenation of deconjugated BAs [84]. As mentioned above, BAs are themselves toxic to bacteria. First, they have direct antibacterial effects. BAs may cause damage to the bacterial membrane because of their detergent properties [85], promote bacterial protein unfolding and aggregation [86], and trigger oxidative/nitrosative stress [87]. Second, they may influence bacterial growth indirectly via FXR activation. Among other genes, FXR controls expression of Ang1, iNos and IL18, which either counteract microbial overgrowth or protect the intestinal mucosa [88]. Activated FXR stimulates the expression of cathelicidin, an antimicrobial peptide that is active in bile ducts [89]. Nevertheless, the sensitivity of bacteria to BAs varies significantly. The growth of bacteria such as *Alistipes*, *Bilophila wadsworthia*, *Escherichia coli*, *Listeria monocytogenes* and *Bacteroides* is even facilitated by BAs, which handicap other symbiotic microbes [84]. Some bacteria are at least BA-tolerant, such as some *Lactobacillus*, *Bifidobacteria* and *Clostridium* species [87].

4.3. Bile Acids and PNALD

In the 1990s, Ohkohchi et al. reported that SBS children patients suffering from intractable diarrhoea exhibited a significantly increased faecal BA excretion and altered bile acid composition. They also observed that primary bile acids accounted for more than 95% of total BAs, while taurine- and glycine-conjugated BAs accounted for only 10%. In these children, the loss of bile acids was strongly associated with a decrease in the actual absorptive surface area of the residual small intestine, while growth of the normal bacterial flora was disturbed in the residual intestine [90]. The relationships between parenteral nutrition, PNALD and BA dysmetabolism were recently studied using animal models. In one SBS-PNALD model, newborn piglets were subjected to a 75% proximal small bowl resection and fed solely via the parenteral route [13]. Two and six weeks post-resection, a significant alteration in microbiota composition was observed, particularly the loss of *Clostridiales*. This was coupled with a decrease in the overall bacterial diversity in the colon as well as a shift to a primary BA-dominant profile in bile, portal serum, and colonic content. The animals also exhibited hepatic fibrosis, steatosis and inflammation. These changes were associated with a blunted FXR activation response in the intestine, altered FXR signalling in the liver and upregulated hepatic BA synthesis [83,91]. Taken together, these data suggest that the altered BA composition following microbial dysbiosis may contribute to PNALD due to the direct physiological effects of toxic BAs and altered FXR signalling.

5. PN and Intestinal Barrier Permeability

Epithelial barrier function is essential in order for the intestine to maintain an effective defence against intraluminal toxins, foreign antigens, and bacteria, and also for enabling the epithelium to effectively absorb nutrients. Such a defence mechanism requires an intact epithelial layer [92]. Increased incidence of sepsis is a common complication in patients dependent on long-term parenteral nutrition, and it is acknowledged that organisms arising from enteric flora constitute a large percentage of these infections [93]. In 1988, Alverdy showed that PN administration in rats significantly increased bacterial translocation to the mesenteric lymph nodes by increasing caecal bacterial counts and impairing the intestinal defence [94]. In subsequent years, the loss of epithelial barrier function was identified as one of the key factors in the development of septic complications associated with long-term PN dependence [95]. PN-associated loss of the epithelial barrier function is probably the result of several underlying mechanisms. First, the morphology of the intestinal wall is altered and the functionality of epithelial cells is compromised. Studies performed using PN mouse models have revealed structural changes, including the atrophy of small bowel villi, an increase in epithelial cell apoptosis and a decrease in epithelial cell proliferation [96–98]. Second, PN administration is associated with increased production of pro-inflammatory cytokines [99,100], while in vitro studies have demonstrated that cytokines produced by immune cells can result in increased permeability of the intestinal mucosa [101]. In particular, the upregulation of IFNγ and TNFα expression in intraepithelial lymphocytes together with decreased production of IL-10 have been identified as the main factors contributing to this pathology [92,102]. Finally, tight junction proteins have an essential role in the maintenance of epithelial barrier function. Among them, ZO (1 and 2), claudins and occludins are the most important and critical components in the structural and functional organisation of tight junctions [103–105]. These proteins regulate the transport of ions and small proteins across the intestinal wall, while their expression is downregulated with PN [92]. Increased TNFα signalling due to PN-associated pro-inflammatory status results in the dissociation of structural protein ZO-1 from tight junctions and worsens barrier function [106]. The exact mechanism underlying the aggravation of epithelial barrier function has not been fully elucidated yet, but there is strong evidence to suggest that an alteration in TLR signalling may represent a link between PN-induced changes in intestinal permeability and changes in microbiota composition.

It is important to stress that all of the above results have been obtained using PN models combined with complete enteral nutrient deprivation. The deprivation of enteral nutrients available to the intraluminal bacteria alters the selection pressure for determining the dominant species in the microbiota. In environments of relative starvation, *Proteobacteria* tend to dominate [107], while *Firmicutes* are usually the predominant group in enterally fed states [108]. Wildhaber et al. [97] showed that limited enteral feeding (covering only 25% of total caloric requirements), completely reversed the unfavourable phenotype associated with parenteral nutrition (increased bacterial translocation, elevated production of pro-inflammatory cytokines, T-subpopulation representation in the intestinal epithelium). Unfortunately, the authors did not determine microbiota composition, so it is not possible to discern whether the beneficial effect arose only from the provision of nutrients to intestinal epithelial cells or whether it was co-associated with a shift in microbiota composition.

6. PN and Pro/Prebiotic Treatment

We recently showed that the microbiota of adult SBS patients dependent on total parenteral nutrition is depleted of anaerobic butyrate producers and that the amount of SCFA (particularly propionate and butyrate) in luminal content is accordingly very low [32]. Intestinal dysbiosis is often treated with probiotics, which are defined as live microorganisms that confer a health benefit on the host when administered in adequate amounts [108]. Positive results have been reported for probiotic use in the management of postsurgical inflammatory bowel disease [109,110], antibiotic-associated diarrhoea [111], and necrotising enterocolitis [112]. The most popular components of probiotic preparations are the members of the *Lactobacillus* and *Bifidobacterium* genera, and their usage is usually safe. Nevertheless, in cases where probiotics have been administered to SBS children patients, positive as well as adverse effects have been reported. The only available double-blind, placebo-controlled randomised crossover clinical trial focusing on the effects of probiotics (*Lactobacillus rhamnosus* LCG) on intestinal permeability in SBS children was unable to prove any beneficial or negative effects [113]. A case-control study performed by Uchida et al. [114] evaluated the effects of treatment on *Bifidobacterium breve*, *Lactobacillus casei* and galacto-oligosaccharides. They proved elevation of stool SCFA in 3 out of 4 patients as well as a trend for increases in height and weight velocity. Five of the nine case studies delivered evidence on the positive effects of probiotic supplementation, while the remaining four reported adverse effects, such as *Lactobacillus* sepsis and D-lactic acidosis [115]. The variable outcomes of probiotic intervention are not surprising, bearing in mind the prevalence of *Lactobacilli* in the SBS microbiome. SBS patients suffer, not because of the lack of lactate-producers, but because of the virtual absence of butyrate-producers that use lactate in the healthy gut. In this setting, further supplementation with lactate-producing bacteria or their substrates (indigestible oligosaccharides) would not provide any benefit, and, with respect to microbiota composition in some cases, could even be detrimental. Supplementation of strictly anaerobic butyrate producers such as *Lachnospiraceae*, *Ruminococcaceae* and others could be theoretically more effective, but because of the significantly altered short-bowel environment (higher oxygen levels, more acidic pH, shorter transit time) the effectiveness of this treatment would be questionable. An interesting option for bypassing all of these obstacles is to supplement SCFA directly to the nutrition mixture. Using neonatal piglets that had undergone 80% proximal jejunoileal resection, Bartholome et al. demonstrated that the supplementation of a mixture with SCFA (acetate, propionate, and butyrate) or butyrate alone enhanced structural adaptations in the developing intestine [116]. In a mouse model, PN enriched with butyric acid partially reversed the parenteral nutrition-associated atrophy of gut-associated lymphoid tissue and improved IgA secretion in the intestinal and extraintestinal mucosae. In addition, it moderately recovered mucosal atrophy [117]. Other studies report that the intravenous butyrate improves the mechanical strength of colonic anastomosis [118], moderately increases mucosal protein synthesis [119] and ameliorates small-intestinal mucosal atrophy (PN rat model) [120]. Taken together, these data advocate intravenous SCFA (particularly butyrate) supplementation as a new option for the treatment of PN-associated intestinal complications.

7. Role of the Microbiota in PNALD Development

In the previous sections, we discussed the essential role of the gut microbiota in the maintenance of homeostasis in the intestinal environment and the adverse effects of dysbiosis (Figure 1). Recent results suggest that the overall decrease in microbial diversity and the overgrowth of the specific bacterial groups in the colonic microbiota are associated with PNALD. Wang et al. [121] showed that gut microbiota composition in SBS infant patients reflects the occurrence of complications like PNALD or central line-associated bloodstream infection (CLABSI). Although the overall diversity and number of bacterial species in samples from the asymptomatic group was similar to those from healthy control infants, there were striking differences in children suffering from PNALD and CLABSI. In addition to the decrease in diversity and the number of bacterial species, there was a shift from Gram-positive *Firmicutes* to Gram-negative *Proteobacteria* (mainly *Enterobacteriaceae*). Many *Proteobacteria* produce bacterial lipopolysaccharide (LPS), a potent hepatotoxic compound, and prolonged exposure to higher LPS concentrations may result in liver injury. Furthermore, the microbiome, when enriched in *Proteobacteria*, was demonstrated to accelerate liver fibrogenesis, which may contribute to PNALD development [122]. El Kasmi et al. demonstrated the interplay between intestinal injury and the intestinal microbiota in the development of PNALD. In mice, intestinal injury and increased permeability were induced by short-term (4 days) oral treatment with low doses of dextran sulphate sodium (DSS), followed by the continuous infusion of a soy lipid-based PN solution for 7 or 28 days. After 7 days on PN, the mice showed an increased intestinal permeability, elevated portal vein LPS levels, evidence of hepatocyte injury (elevated serum aspartate aminotransferase, alanine aminotransferase), cholestasis (elevated serum bile acids, total bilirubin), and an increased expression of interleukin-6, tumour necrosis factor alpha and transforming growth factor beta in Kupffer cells. Markers of liver injury remained elevated and were associated with lobular inflammation, hepatocyte apoptosis, peliosis and Kupffer cell hypertrophy and hyperplasia after 28 days on PN [123]. Interestingly, PN infusion without DSS pretreatment or DSS pretreatment alone did not result in liver injury or Kupffer cell activation. Suppression of the intestinal microbiota with broad-spectrum antibiotics and ablation of TLR4 signalling in *Tlr4* mutant mice prevented PNALD development, which strongly suggests the role of the microbiota in its etiopathogenesis. In a subsequent study, Harris et al. identified the specific microbial taxa associated with PNALD development in this model. Among those, members of the *Erysipelotrichaceae* family and representatives of the Gram-negative S24-7 lineage of *Bacteroidetes* were identified as candidates that might play a causal role in the pathogenesis of PNALD [124]. Interestingly, mice treated only with PN without intestinal injury did not develop PNALD, despite the similar composition of their intestinal microbiota. Taken together, these experiments suggest that at least two independent conditions must be met concurrently; (i) overgrowth of specific bacteria due to PN administration and (ii) increased intestinal permeability allowing MAMPs (microbe-associated molecular pattern) derived from these taxa to reach the liver and subsequently activate Kupffer cells [124,125].

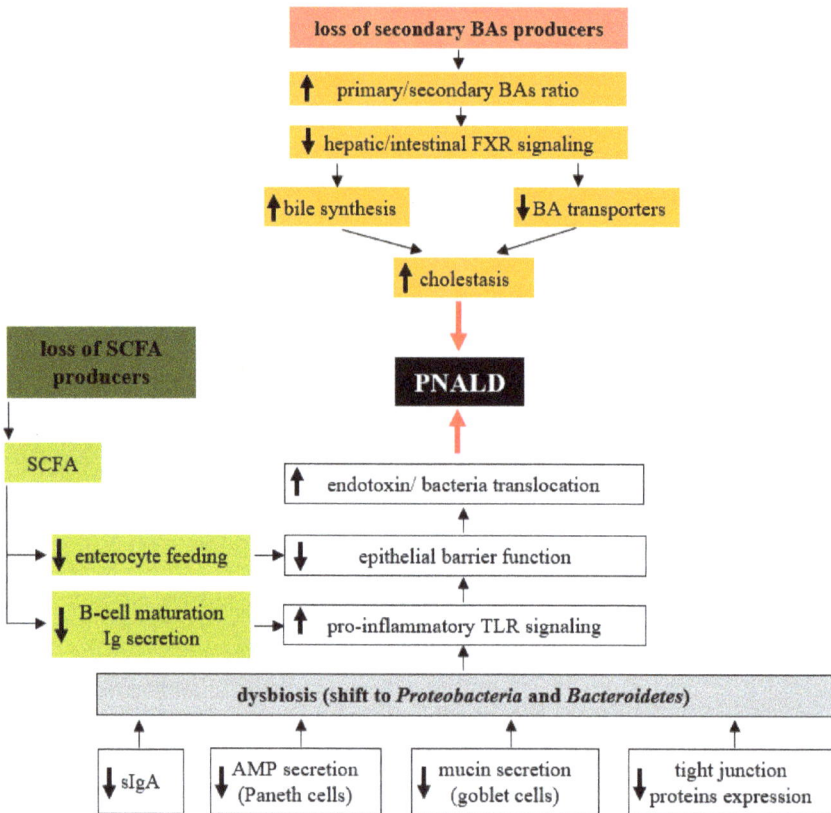

Figure 1. Gut microbiota-related factors contributing to PNALD development. Administration of parenteral nutrition (PN) is associated with decreased production of sIgA, reduced mucin synthesis in goblet cells and impaired antimicrobial function of Paneth cells. All these factors favour the growth of pathogenic bacteria (mostly from *Proteobacteria*) at the expense of beneficial commensals. In addition, the reduction in sIgA enables greater microbial access to the host epithelium and triggers an inflammatory response in the lamina propria. Enhanced toll-like receptors (TLR)-signalling due to the increased presence of potential pathogens stimulates the synthesis of pro-inflammatory cytokines in immune cells. Altogether, these factors contribute toward compromised epithelial barrier function (EBF) and increased translocation of endotoxins and even whole bacteria to the portal circulation and the liver, thereby inducing the inflammatory response. The lower abundance of SCFA producers results in decreased short-chain fatty acids (SCFA) availability, which attenuates B-cell maturation, specific antibody production and increased susceptibility to pathogens. The specific loss of secondary bile acids (BA) producers (*Clostridiales*) results in a significant shift towards primary BAs in faeces and impaired hepatic and intestinal farnesoid-X receptor (FXR) signalling. Consequently, bile acid synthesis in the liver becomes upregulated and expression of bile acid transporters becomes downregulated, resulting in the attenuation of BA transport to bile and the development of cholestasis.

8. Conclusions

A growing amount of evidence suggests that the deterioration of hepatic function in conjunction with long-term PN dependence is not the consequence of PN administration *per se* but because of intestinal failure and associated complications. The prominent factors seem to be increased permeability of the intestinal barrier, which facilitates massive translocation of bacterial toxins and even microorganisms into the portal circulation, mesenteric lymph nodes and liver, and overall pro-inflammatory status in the compromised intestine. The gut microbiota plays a profound role in the maintenance of intestinal barrier function and the establishment of either an immunotolerant or inflammatory setting of intestinal immunity. Therapeutic strategies focus on microbiota composition itself through the targeted delivery of beneficial microbiota products or by supplementation with immunomodulators. Nevertheless, understanding the complex interactions between the gut microbiota and the modified intestinal environment in PN patients is a crucial condition for efficient treatment.

Acknowledgments: This study was supported by the Ministry of Health of the Czech Republic, grant No. 15-28745A AZV CR. All rights reserved.

Author Contributions: Monika Cahova: manuscript design, manuscript writing, critical review of the manuscript; Miriam Bratova: material collection, critical review; Petr Wohl: critical review. All authors discussed and agreed upon the final manuscript.

Conflicts of Interest: The authors declare no conflict of interest.

References

1. Mizock, B.A. Immunonutrition and critical illness: An update. *Nutrition* **2010**, *26*, 701–707. [CrossRef] [PubMed]
2. Beath, S.V.; Kelly, D.A. Total Parenteral Nutrition-Induced Cholestasis: Prevention and Management. *Clin. Liver Dis.* **2016**, *20*, 159–176. [CrossRef] [PubMed]
3. Drongowski, R.A.; Coran, A.G. An analysis of factors contributing to the development of total parenteral nutrition-induced cholestasis. *J. Parenter. Enter. Nutr.* **1989**, *13*, 586–589. [CrossRef] [PubMed]
4. Luman, W.; Shaffer, J.L. Prevalence, outcome and associated factors of deranged liver function tests in patients on home parenteral nutrition. *Clin. Nutr.* **2002**, *21*, 337–343. [CrossRef] [PubMed]
5. Bharadwaj, S.; Gohel, T.; Deen, O.J.; DeChicco, R.; Shatnawei, A. Fish oil-based lipid emulsion: Current updates on a promising novel therapy for the management of parenteral nutrition-associated liver disease. *Gastroenterol. Rep.* **2015**, *3*, 110–114. [CrossRef] [PubMed]
6. Orso, G.; Mandato, C.; Veropalumbo, C.; Cecchi, N.; Garzi, A.; Vajro, P. Pediatric parenteral nutrition-associated liver disease and cholestasis: Novel advances in pathomechanisms-based prevention and treatment. *Dig. Liver Dis.* **2016**, *48*, 215–222. [CrossRef] [PubMed]
7. Mateu de Antonio, J.; Florit-Sureda, M. Effects unrelated to anti-inflammation of lipid emulsions containing fish oil in parenteral nutrition for adult patients. *Nutr. Hosp.* **2017**, *34*, 193–203. [CrossRef] [PubMed]
8. Burcelin, R.; Serino, M.; Chabo, C.; Garidou, L.; Pomie, C.; Courtney, M.; Amar, J.; Bouloumié, A. Metagenome and metabolism: The tissue microbiota hypothesis. *Diabetes Obes. Metab.* **2013**, *15*, 61–70. [CrossRef] [PubMed]
9. Kverka, M.; Tlaskalova-Hogenova, H. Intestinal Microbiota: Facts and Fiction. *Dig. Dis.* **2017**, *35*, 139–147. [CrossRef] [PubMed]
10. Hodin, C.M.; Visschers, R.G.; Rensen, S.S.; Boonen, B.; Olde Damink, S.W.; Lenaerts, K.; Buurman, W.A. Total parenteral nutrition induces a shift in the Firmicutes to Bacteroidetes ratio in association with Paneth cell activation in rats. *J. Nutr.* **2012**, *142*, 2141–2147. [CrossRef] [PubMed]
11. Miyasaka, E.A.; Feng, Y.; Poroyko, V.; Falkowski, N.R.; Erb-Downward, J.; Gillilland, M.G.; Mason, K.L.; Huffnagle, G.B.; Teitelbaum, D.H. Total parenteral nutrition-associated lamina propria inflammation in mice is mediated by a MyD88-dependent mechanism. *J. Immunol.* **2013**, *190*, 6607–6615. [CrossRef] [PubMed]
12. Heneghan, A.F.; Pierre, J.F.; Tandee, K.; Shanmuganayagam, D.; Wang, X.; Reed, J.D.; Steele, J.L.; Kudsk, K.A. Parenteral nutrition decreases paneth cell function and intestinal bactericidal activity while increasing susceptibility to bacterial enteroinvasion. *J. Parenter. Enter. Nutr.* **2014**, *38*, 817–824. [CrossRef] [PubMed]
13. Lapthorne, S.; Pereira-Fantini, P.M.; Fouhy, F.; Wilson, G.; Thomas, S.L.; Dellios, N.L.; Scurr, M.; O'Sullivan, O.; Ross, R.P.; Stanton, C.; et al. Gut microbial diversity is reduced and is associated with colonic inflammation in a piglet model of short bowel syndrome. *Gut Microbes* **2013**, *4*, 212–221. [CrossRef] [PubMed]
14. Harvey, R.B.; Andrews, K.; Droleskey, R.E.; Kansagra, K.V.; Stoll, B.; Burrin, D.G.; Sheffield, C.L.; Anderson, R.C.; Nisbet, D.J. Qualitative and quantitative comparison of gut bacterial colonization in enterally and parenterally fed neonatal pigs. *Curr. Issues Intest. Microbiol.* **2006**, *7*, 61–64. [PubMed]

15. Deplancke, B.; Vidal, O.; Ganessunker, D.; Donovan, S.M.; Mackie, R.I.; Gaskins, H.R. Selective growth of mucolytic bacteria including Clostridium perfringens in a neonatal piglet model of total parenteral nutrition. *Am. J. Clin. Nutr.* **2002**, *76*, 1117–1125. [PubMed]

16. Lavallee, C.M.; MacPherson, J.A.; Zhou, M.; Gao, Y.; Wizzard, P.R.; Wales, P.W.; Turner, J.M.; Willing, B.P. Lipid Emulsion Formulation of Parenteral Nutrition Affects Intestinal Microbiota and Host Responses in Neonatal Piglets. *J. Parent. Enteral. Nutr.* **2016**. [CrossRef] [PubMed]

17. Parm, U.; Metsvaht, T.; Ilmoja, M.L.; Lutsar, I. Gut colonization by aerobic microorganisms is associated with route and type of nutrition in premature neonates. *Nutr. Res.* **2015**, *35*, 496–503. [CrossRef] [PubMed]

18. Ralls, M.W.; Miyasaka, E.; Teitelbaum, D.H. Intestinal microbial diversity and perioperative complications. *J. Parenter. Enter. Nutr.* **2014**, *38*, 392–399. [CrossRef] [PubMed]

19. Joly, F.; Mayeur, C.; Bruneau, A.; Noordine, M.L.; Meylheuc, T.; Langella, P.; Messing, B.; Duée, P.H.; Cherbuy, C.; Thomas, M. Drastic changes in fecal and mucosa-associated microbiota in adult patients with short bowel syndrome. *Biochimie* **2010**, *92*, 753–761. [CrossRef] [PubMed]

20. Dibaise, J.K.; Young, R.J.; Vanderhoof, J.A. Enteric microbial flora, bacterial overgrowth, and short-bowel syndrome. *Clin. Gastroenterol. Hepatol.* **2006**, *4*, 11–20. [CrossRef] [PubMed]

21. Huang, Y.; Guo, F.; Li, Y.; Wang, J.; Li, J. Fecal microbiota signatures of adult patients with different types of short bowel syndrome. *J. Gastroenterol. Hepatol.* **2017**. [CrossRef] [PubMed]

22. Siggers, R.H.; Siggers, J.; Thymann, T.; Boye, M.; Sangild, P.T. Nutritional modulation of the gut microbiota and immune system in preterm neonates susceptible to necrotizing enterocolitis. *J. Nutr. Biochem.* **2011**, *22*, 511–521. [CrossRef] [PubMed]

23. Wang, S.; Ng, L.H.; Chow, W.L.; Lee, Y.K. Infant intestinal Enterococcus faecalis down-regulates inflammatory responses in human intestinal cell lines. *World J. Gastroenterol.* **2008**, *14*, 1067–1076. [CrossRef] [PubMed]

24. Messing, B.; Lémann, M.; Landais, P.; Gouttebel, M.C.; Gérard-Boncompain, M.; Saudin, F.; Vangossum, A.; Beau, P.; Guédon, C.; Barnoud, D.; et al. Prognosis of patients with nonmalignant chronic intestinal failure receiving long-term home parenteral nutrition. *Gastroenterology* **1995**, *108*, 1005–1010. [CrossRef]

25. Mayeur, C.; Gillard, L.; Le Beyec, J.; Bado, A.; Joly, F.; Thomas, M. Extensive Intestinal Resection Triggers Behavioral Adaptation, Intestinal Remodeling and Microbiota Transition in Short Bowel Syndrome. *Microorganisms* **2016**, *4*, 1. [CrossRef] [PubMed]

26. Duncan, S.H.; Louis, P.; Thomson, J.M.; Flint, H.J. The role of pH in determining the species composition of the human colonic microbiota. *Environ. Microbiol.* **2009**, *11*, 2112–2122. [CrossRef] [PubMed]

27. Mayeur, C.; Gratadoux, J.J.; Bridonneau, C.; Chegdani, F.; Larroque, B.; Kapel, N.; Corcos, O.; Thomas, M.; Joly, F. Faecal D/L lactate ratio is a metabolic signature of microbiota imbalance in patients with short bowel syndrome. *PLoS ONE* **2013**, *8*, e54335. [CrossRef] [PubMed]

28. Lilja, H.E.; Wefer, H.; Nystrom, N.; Finkel, Y.; Engstrand, L. Intestinal dysbiosis in children with short bowel syndrome is associated with impaired outcome. *Microbiome* **2015**, *3*, 18. [CrossRef] [PubMed]

29. Belenguer, A.; Holtrop, G.; Duncan, S.H.; Anderson, S.E.; Calder, A.G.; Flint, H.J.; Lobley, G.E. Rates of production and utilization of lactate by microbial communities from the human colon. *FEMS Microbiol. Ecol.* **2011**, *77*, 107–119. [CrossRef] [PubMed]

30. Bourriaud, C.; Robins, R.J.; Martin, L.; Kozlowski, F.; Tenailleau, E.; Cherbut, C.; Michel, C. Lactate is mainly fermented to butyrate by human intestinal microfloras but inter-individual variation is evident. *J. Appl. Microbiol.* **2005**, *99*, 201–212. [CrossRef] [PubMed]

31. Sekirov, I.; Russell, S.L.; Antunes, L.C.; Finlay, B.B. Gut microbiota in health and disease. *Physiol. Rev.* **2010**, *90*, 859–904. [CrossRef] [PubMed]

32. Abreu, M.T. Toll-like receptor signalling in the intestinal epithelium: How bacterial recognition shapes intestinal function. *Nat. Rev. Immunol.* **2010**, *10*, 131–144. [CrossRef] [PubMed]

33. Mazmanian, S.K.; Liu, C.H.; Tzianabos, A.O.; Kasper, D.L. An immunomodulatory molecule of symbiotic bacteria directs maturation of the host immune system. *Cell* **2005**, *122*, 107–118. [CrossRef] [PubMed]

34. Christensen, H.R.; Frokiaer, H.; Pestka, J.J. Lactobacilli differentially modulate expression of cytokines and maturation surface markers in murine dendritic cells. *J. Immunol.* **2002**, *168*, 171–178. [CrossRef] [PubMed]

35. Ivanov, I.I.; de Llanos Frutos, R.; Manel, N.; Yoshinaga, K.; Rifkin, D.B.; Sartor, R.B.; Finlay, B.B.; Littman, D.R. Specific microbiota direct the differentiation of IL-17-producing T-helper cells in the mucosa of the small intestine. *Cell Host Microbe* **2008**, *4*, 337–349. [CrossRef] [PubMed]

36. Beutler, B.; Rietschel, E.T. Innate immune sensing and its roots: The story of endotoxin. *Nat. Rev. Immunol.* **2003**, *3*, 169. [CrossRef] [PubMed]
37. Kelsall, B.L.; Leon, F. Involvement of intestinal dendritic cells in oral tolerance, immunity to pathogens, and inflammatory bowel disease. *Immunol. Rev.* **2005**, *206*, 132–148. [CrossRef] [PubMed]
38. Kelly, D.; Campbell, J.I.; King, T.P.; Grant, G.; Jansson, E.A.; Coutts, A.G.; Pettersson, S.; Conway, S. Commensal anaerobic gut bacteria attenuate inflammation by regulating nuclear-cytoplasmic shuttling of PPAR-gamma and RelA. *Nat. Immunol.* **2004**, *5*, 104. [CrossRef] [PubMed]
39. Lee, J.; Mo, J.H.; Katakura, K.; Alkalay, I.; Rucker, A.N.; Liu, Y.T.; Hyun-Ku, L.; Shen, C.; Cojocaru, G.; Shenouda, S.; et al. Maintenance of colonic homeostasis by distinctive apical TLR9 signalling in intestinal epithelial cells. *Nat. Cell Biol.* **2006**, *8*, 1327. [CrossRef] [PubMed]
40. Iwasaki, A.; Kelsall, B.L. Freshly isolated Peyer's patch, but not spleen, dendritic cells produce interleukin 10 and induce the differentiation of T helper type 2 cells. *J. Exp. Med.* **1999**, *190*, 229–239. [CrossRef] [PubMed]
41. Macpherson, A.J.; Uhr, T. Induction of protective IgA by intestinal dendritic cells carrying commensal bacteria. *Science* **2004**, *303*, 1662–1665. [CrossRef] [PubMed]
42. Peterson, D.A.; McNulty, N.P.; Guruge, J.L.; Gordon, J.I. IgA response to symbiotic bacteria as a mediator of gut homeostasis. *Cell Host Microbe* **2007**, *2*, 328–339. [CrossRef] [PubMed]
43. Suzuki, K.; Meek, B.; Doi, Y.; Muramatsu, M.; Chiba, T.; Honjo, T.; Fagarasan, S. Aberrant expansion of segmented filamentous bacteria in IgA-deficient gut. *Proc. Natl. Acad. Sci. USA* **2004**, *101*, 1981–1986. [CrossRef] [PubMed]
44. Yanagibashi, T.; Hosono, A.; Oyama, A.; Tsuda, M.; Hachimura, S.; Takahashi, Y.; Itoh, K.; Hirayama, K.; Takahashi, K.; Kaminogawa, S. Bacteroides induce higher IgA production than Lactobacillus by increasing activation-induced cytidine deaminase expression in B cells in murine Peyer's patches. *Biosci. Biotechnol. Biochem.* **2009**, *73*, 372–377. [CrossRef] [PubMed]
45. Zipperer, A.; Konnerth, M.C.; Laux, C.; Berscheid, A.; Janek, D.; Weidenmaier, C.; Burian, M.; Schilling, N.A.; Slavetinsky, C.; Marschal, M.; et al. Human commensals producing a novel antibiotic impair pathogen colonization. *Nature* **2016**, *535*, 511–516. [CrossRef] [PubMed]
46. Pierre, J.F. Gastrointestinal immune and microbiome changes during parenteral nutrition. *Am. J. Physiol. Gastrointest. Liver Physiol.* **2017**, *312*, G246–G256. [CrossRef] [PubMed]
47. Coulombe, G.; Langlois, A.; De Palma, G.; Langlois, M.J.; McCarville, J.L.; Gagné-Sanfaçon, J.; Perreault, N.; Feng, G.S.; Bercik, P.; Boudreau, F.; et al. SHP-2 Phosphatase Prevents Colonic Inflammation by Controlling Secretory Cell Differentiation and Maintaining Host-Microbiota Homeostasis. *J. Cell. Physiol.* **2016**, *231*, 2529–2540. [CrossRef] [PubMed]
48. Everard, A.; Geurts, L.; Caesar, R.; van Hul, M.; Matamoros, S.; Duparc, T.; Denis, R.G.; Cochez, P.; Pierard, F.; Castel, J.; et al. Intestinal epithelial MyD88 is a sensor switching host metabolism towards obesity according to nutritional status. *Nat. Commun.* **2014**, *5*, 5648. [CrossRef] [PubMed]
49. Dheer, R.; Santaolalla, R.; Davies, J.M.; Lang, J.K.; Phillips, M.C.; Pastorini, C.; Vazquez-Pertejo, M.T.; Abreu, M.T. Intestinal Epithelial Toll-Like Receptor 4 Signalling Affects Epithelial Function and Colonic Microbiota and Promotes a Risk for Transmissible Colitis. *Infect. Immun.* **2016**, *84*, 798–810. [CrossRef] [PubMed]
50. Frantz, A.L.; Rogier, E.W.; Weber, C.R.; Shen, L.; Cohen, D.A.; Fenton, L.A.; Bruno, M.E.C.; Kaetzel, C.S. Targeted deletion of MyD88 in intestinal epithelial cells results in compromised antibacterial immunity associated with downregulation of polymeric immunoglobulin receptor, mucin-2, and antibacterial peptides. *Mucosal Immunol.* **2012**, *5*, 501. [CrossRef] [PubMed]
51. Anitha, M.; Vijay-Kumar, M.; Sitaraman, S.V.; Gewirtz, A.T.; Srinivasan, S. Gut microbial products regulate murine gastrointestinal motility via Toll-like receptor 4 signalling. *Gastroenterology* **2012**, *143*, 1006–1016. [CrossRef] [PubMed]
52. Cheesman, S.E.; Neal, J.T.; Mittge, E.; Seredick, B.M.; Guillemin, K. Epithelial cell proliferation in the developing zebrafish intestine is regulated by the Wnt pathway and microbial signalling via Myd88. *Proc. Natl. Acad. Sci. USA* **2011**, *108*, 4570–4577. [CrossRef] [PubMed]
53. Cerovic, V.; Bain, C.C.; Mowat, A.M.; Milling, S.W. Intestinal macrophages and dendritic cells: What's the difference? *Trends Immunol.* **2014**, *35*, 270–277. [CrossRef] [PubMed]

54. Bain, C.C.; Bravo-Blas, A.; Scott, C.L.; Perdiguero, E.G.; Geissmann, F.; Henri, S.; Malissen, B.; Osborne, L.C.; Artis, D.; Mowat, A.M. Constant replenishment from circulating monocytes maintains the macrophage pool in the intestine of adult mice. *Nat. Immunol.* **2014**, *15*, 929–937. [CrossRef] [PubMed]

55. Smith, P.D.; Smythies, L.E.; Shen, R.; Greenwell-Wild, T.; Gliozzi, M.; Wahl, S.M. Intestinal macrophages and response to microbial encroachment. *Mucosal Immunol.* **2011**, *4*, 31–42. [CrossRef] [PubMed]

56. Denning, T.L.; Norris, B.A.; Medina-Contreras, O.; Manicassamy, S.; Geem, D.; Madan, R.; Karp, C.L.; Pulendran, B. Functional specializations of intestinal dendritic cell and macrophage subsets that control Th17 and regulatory T cell responses are dependent on the T cell/APC ratio, source of mouse strain, and regional localization. *J. Immunol.* **2011**, *187*, 733–747. [CrossRef] [PubMed]

57. Rivollier, A.; He, J.; Kole, A.; Valatas, V.; Kelsall, B.L. Inflammation switches the differentiation program of Ly6Chi monocytes from antiinflammatory macrophages to inflammatory dendritic cells in the colon. *J. Exp. Med.* **2012**, *209*, 139–155. [CrossRef] [PubMed]

58. Schulz, C.; Perdiguero, E.G.; Chorro, L.; Szabo-Rogers, H.; Cagnard, N.; Kierdorf, K.; Prinz, M.; Wu, B.; Jacobsen, S.E.W.; Pollard, J.W.; et al. A lineage of myeloid cells independent of Myb and hematopoietic stem cells. *Science* **2012**, *336*, 86–90. [CrossRef] [PubMed]

59. Hashimoto, D.; Chow, A.; Noizat, C.; Teo, P.; Beasley, M.B.; Leboeuf, M.; Becker, C.D.; See, P.; Price, J.; Lucas, D.; et al. Tissue-resident macrophages self-maintain locally throughout adult life with minimal contribution from circulating monocytes. *Immunity* **2013**, *38*, 792–804. [CrossRef] [PubMed]

60. Ueda, Y.; Kayama, H.; Jeon, S.G.; Kusu, T.; Isaka, Y.; Rakugi, H.; Yamamoto, M.; Takeda, K. Commensal microbiota induce LPS hyporesponsiveness in colonic macrophages via the production of IL-10. *Int. Immunol.* **2010**, *22*, 953–962. [CrossRef] [PubMed]

61. Hayashi, A.; Sato, T.; Kamada, N.; Mikami, Y.; Matsuoka, K.; Hisamatsu, T.; Hibi, T.; Roers, A.; Yagita, H.; Ohteki, T.; et al. A single strain of Clostridium butyricum induces intestinal IL-10-producing macrophages to suppress acute experimental colitis in mice. *Cell Host Microbe* **2013**, *13*, 711–722. [CrossRef] [PubMed]

62. Ochi, T.; Feng, Y.; Kitamoto, S.; Nagao-Kitamoto, H.; Kuffa, P.; Atarashi, K.; Honda, K.; Teitelbaum, D.H.; Kamada, N. Diet-dependent, microbiota-independent regulation of IL-10-producing lamina propria macrophages in the small intestine. *Sci. Rep.* **2016**, *6*, 27634. [CrossRef] [PubMed]

63. Bevins, C.L. Paneth cell defensins: key effector molecules of innate immunity. *Biochem. Soc. Trans.* **2006**, *34*, 263–266. [CrossRef] [PubMed]

64. Porter, E.M.; Bevins, C.L.; Ghosh, D.; Ganz, T. The multifaceted Paneth cell. *Cell Mol. Life Sci.* **2002**, *59*, 156–170. [CrossRef] [PubMed]

65. Ouellette, A.J. Defensin-mediated innate immunity in the small intestine. *Best Pract. Res. Clin. Gastroenterol.* **2004**, *18*, 405–419. [CrossRef] [PubMed]

66. Vaishnava, S.; Behrendt, C.L.; Ismail, A.S.; Eckmann, L.; Hooper, L.V. Paneth cells directly sense gut commensals and maintain homeostasis at the intestinal host-microbial interface. *Proc. Natl. Acad. Sci. USA* **2008**, *105*, 20858–20863. [CrossRef] [PubMed]

67. Omata, J.; Pierre, J.F.; Heneghan, A.F.; Tsao, F.H.; Sano, Y.; Jonker, M.A.; Kudsk, K.A. Parenteral nutrition suppresses the bactericidal response of the small intestine. *Surgery* **2013**, *153*, 17–24. [CrossRef] [PubMed]

68. Kirkland, D.; Benson, A.; Mirpuri, J.; Pifer, R.; Hou, B.; DeFranco, A.L.; Yarovinsky, F. B cell-intrinsic MyD88 signalling prevents the lethal dissemination of commensal bacteria during colonic damage. *Immunity* **2012**, *36*, 228–238. [CrossRef] [PubMed]

69. Teng, F.; Klinger, C.N.; Felix, K.M.; Bradley, C.P.; Wu, E.; Tran, N.L.; Umesaki, Y.; Wu, H.J.J. Gut Microbiota Drive Autoimmune Arthritis by Promoting Differentiation and Migration of Peyer's Patch T Follicular Helper Cells. *Immunity* **2016**, *44*, 875–888. [CrossRef] [PubMed]

70. Kim, M.; Qie, Y.; Park, J.; Kim, C.H. Gut Microbial Metabolites Fuel Host Antibody Responses. *Cell Host Microbe* **2016**, *20*, 202–214. [CrossRef] [PubMed]

71. Kudoh, K.; Shimizu, J.; Wada, M.; Takita, T.; Kanke, Y.; Innami, S. Effect of indigestible saccharides on B lymphocyte response of intestinal mucosa and cecal fermentation in rats. *J. Nutr. Sci. Vitaminol.* **1998**, *44*, 103–112. [CrossRef] [PubMed]

72. Bjorkhem, I. Mechanism of degradation of the steroid side chain in the formation of bile acids. *J. Lipid Res.* **1992**, *33*, 455–471. [PubMed]

73. Zhang, Y.; Limaye, P.B.; Renaud, H.J.; Klaassen, C.D. Effect of various antibiotics on modulation of intestinal microbiota and bile acid profile in mice. *Toxicol. Appl. Pharmacol.* **2014**, *277*, 138–145. [CrossRef] [PubMed]

74. Chiang, J.Y. Bile acid regulation of gene expression: Roles of nuclear hormone receptors. *Endocr. Rev.* **2002**, *23*, 443–463. [CrossRef] [PubMed]
75. Fan, M.; Wang, X.; Xu, G.; Yan, Q.; Huang, W. Bile acid signalling and liver regeneration. *Biochim. Biophys. Acta* **2015**, *1849*, 196–200. [CrossRef] [PubMed]
76. Duboc, H.; Tache, Y.; Hofmann, A.F. The bile acid TGR5 membrane receptor: From basic research to clinical application. *Dig. Liver Dis.* **2014**, *46*, 302–312. [CrossRef] [PubMed]
77. Li, T.; Chiang, J.Y. Bile acids as metabolic regulators. *Curr. Opin. Gastroenterol.* **2015**, *31*, 159–165. [CrossRef] [PubMed]
78. Jones, M.L.; Martoni, C.J.; Ganopolsky, J.G.; Labbe, A.; Prakash, S. The human microbiome and bile acid metabolism: Dysbiosis, dysmetabolism, disease and intervention. *Expert Opin. Biol. Ther.* **2014**, *14*, 467–482. [CrossRef] [PubMed]
79. Ridlon, J.M.; Kang, D.J.; Hylemon, P.B. Bile salt biotransformations by human intestinal bacteria. *J. Lipid Res.* **2006**, *47*, 241–259. [CrossRef] [PubMed]
80. Goodwin, B.; Jones, S.A.; Price, R.R.; Watson, M.A.; McKee, D.D.; Moore, L.B.; Galardi, C.; Wilson, J.G.; Lewis, M.C.; Roth, M.E.; et al. A regulatory cascade of the nuclear receptors FXR, SHP-1, and LRH-1 represses bile acid biosynthesis. *Mol. Cell* **2000**, *6*, 517–526. [CrossRef]
81. Holt, M.P.; Cheng, L.; Ju, C. Identification and characterization of infiltrating macrophages in acetaminophen-induced liver injury. *J. Leukoc. Biol.* **2008**, *84*, 1410–1421. [CrossRef] [PubMed]
82. Miyata, M.; Takamatsu, Y.; Kuribayashi, H.; Yamazoe, Y. Administration of ampicillin elevates hepatic primary bile acid synthesis through suppression of ileal fibroblast growth factor 15 expression. *J. Pharmacol. Exp. Ther.* **2009**, *331*, 1079–1085. [CrossRef] [PubMed]
83. Pereira-Fantini, P.M.; Lapthorne, S.; Joyce, S.A.; Dellios, N.L.; Wilson, G.; Fouhy, F.; Thomas, S.L.; Scurr, M.; Hill, C.; Gahan, C.G.; et al. Altered FXR signalling is associated with bile acid dysmetabolism in short bowel syndrome-associated liver disease. *J. Hepatol.* **2014**, *61*, 1115–1125. [CrossRef] [PubMed]
84. Nie, Y.F.; Hu, J.; Yan, X.H. Cross-talk between bile acids and intestinal microbiota in host metabolism and health. *J. Zhejiang Univ. Sci. B* **2015**, *16*, 436–446. (In Chinese) [CrossRef] [PubMed]
85. Islam, K.S.; Fukiya, S.; Hagio, M.; Fujii, N.; Ishizuka, S.; Ooka, T.; Ogura, Y.; Hayashi, T.; Yokota, A. Bile acid is a host factor that regulates the composition of the cecal microbiota in rats. *Gastroenterology* **2011**, *141*, 1773–1781. [CrossRef] [PubMed]
86. Cremers, C.M.; Knoefler, D.; Vitvitsky, V.; Banerjee, R.; Jakob, U. Bile salts act as effective protein-unfolding agents and instigators of disulfide stress in vivo. *Proc. Natl. Acad. Sci. USA* **2014**, *111*, E1610–E1619. [CrossRef] [PubMed]
87. Begley, M.; Gahan, C.G.; Hill, C. The interaction between bacteria and bile. *FEMS Microbiol. Rev.* **2005**, *29*, 625–651. [CrossRef] [PubMed]
88. Inagaki, T.; Moschetta, A.; Lee, Y.K.; Peng, L.; Zhao, G.; Downes, M.; Ruth, T.Y.; Shelton, J.M.; Richardson, J.A.; Repa, J.J.; et al. Regulation of antibacterial defense in the small intestine by the nuclear bile acid receptor. *Proc. Natl. Acad. Sci. USA* **2006**, *103*, 3920–3925. [CrossRef] [PubMed]
89. D'Aldebert, E.; Mve, M.J.B.B.; Mergey, M.; Wendum, D.; Firrincieli, D.; Coilly, A.; Fouassier, L.; Corpechot, C.; Poupon, R.; Housset, C.; et al. Bile salts control the antimicrobial peptide cathelicidin through nuclear receptors in the human biliary epithelium. *Gastroenterology* **2009**, *136*, 1435–1443. [CrossRef] [PubMed]
90. Ohkohchi, N.; Andoh, T.; Izumi, U.; Igarashi, Y.; Ohi, R. Disorder of bile acid metabolism in children with short bowel syndrome. *J. Gastroenterol.* **1997**, *32*, 472–479. [CrossRef] [PubMed]
91. Pereira-Fantini, P.M.; Bines, J.E.; Lapthorne, S.; Fouhy, F.; Scurr, M.; Cotter, P.D.; Gahan, C.G.; Joyce, S.A. Short bowel syndrome (SBS)-associated alterations within the gut-liver axis evolve early and persist long-term in the piglet model of short bowel syndrome. *J. Gastroenterol. Hepatol.* **2016**, *31*, 1946–1955. [CrossRef] [PubMed]
92. Sun, X.; Yang, H.; Nose, K.; Nose, S.; Haxhija, E.Q.; Koga, H.; Feng, Y.; Teitelbaum, D.H. Decline in intestinal mucosal IL-10 expression and decreased intestinal barrier function in a mouse model of total parenteral nutrition. *Am. J. Physiol. Gastrointest. Liver Physiol.* **2008**, *294*, G139–G147. [CrossRef] [PubMed]
93. Deitch, E.A. Gut-origin sepsis: Evolution of a concept. *Surgeon* **2012**, *10*, 350–356. [CrossRef] [PubMed]
94. Alverdy, J.C.; Aoys, E.; Moss, G.S. Total parenteral nutrition promotes bacterial translocation from the gut. *Surgery* **1988**, *104*, 185–190. [PubMed]

95. Demehri, F.R.; Barrett, M.; Ralls, M.W.; Miyasaka, E.A.; Feng, Y.; Teitelbaum, D.H. Intestinal epithelial cell apoptosis and loss of barrier function in the setting of altered microbiota with enteral nutrient deprivation. *Front. Cell. Infect. Microbiol.* **2013**, *3*, 105. [CrossRef] [PubMed]

96. Feng, Y.; Sun, X.; Yang, H.; Teitelbaum, D.H. Dissociation of E-cadherin and beta-catenin in a mouse model of total parenteral nutrition: A mechanism for the loss of epithelial cell proliferation and villus atrophy. *J. Physiol.* **2009**, *587*, 641–654. [CrossRef] [PubMed]

97. Wildhaber, B.E.; Yang, H.; Spencer, A.U.; Drongowski, R.A.; Teitelbaum, D.H. Lack of enteral nutrition—Effects on the intestinal immune system. *J. Surg. Res.* **2005**, *123*, 8–16. [CrossRef] [PubMed]

98. Demehri, F.R.; Barrett, M.; Teitelbaum, D.H. Changes to the Intestinal Microbiome With Parenteral Nutrition: Review of a Murine Model and Potential Clinical Implications. *Nutr. Clin. Pract.* **2015**, *30*, 798–806. [CrossRef] [PubMed]

99. Feng, Y.; Teitelbaum, D.H. Tumour necrosis factor—Induced loss of intestinal barrier function requires TNFR1 and TNFR2 signalling in a mouse model of total parenteral nutrition. *J. Physiol.* **2013**, *591*, 3709–3723. [CrossRef] [PubMed]

100. Yang, H.; Fan, Y.; Teitelbaum, D.H. Intraepithelial lymphocyte-derived interferon-gamma evokes enterocyte apoptosis with parenteral nutrition in mice. *Am. J. Physiol. Gastrointest. Liver Physiol.* **2003**, *284*, G629–G637. [CrossRef] [PubMed]

101. Clayburgh, D.R.; Shen, L.; Turner, J.R. A porous defense: The leaky epithelial barrier in intestinal disease. *Lab. Investig.* **2004**, *84*, 282–291. [CrossRef] [PubMed]

102. Yang, H.; Kiristioglu, I.; Fan, Y.; Forbush, B.; Bishop, D.K.; Antony, P.A.; Zhou, H.; Teitelbaum, D.H. Interferon-gamma expression by intraepithelial lymphocytes results in a loss of epithelial barrier function in a mouse model of total parenteral nutrition. *Ann. Surg.* **2002**, *236*, 226–234. [CrossRef] [PubMed]

103. Mitic, L.L.; Anderson, J.M. Molecular architecture of tight junctions. *Annu. Rev. Physiol.* **1998**, *60*, 121–142. [CrossRef] [PubMed]

104. Prasad, S.; Mingrino, R.; Kaukinen, K.; Hayes, K.L.; Powell, R.M.; MacDonald, T.T.; Collins, J.E. Inflammatory processes have differential effects on claudins 2, 3 and 4 in colonic epithelial cells. *Lab. Investig.* **2005**, *85*, 1139–1162. [CrossRef] [PubMed]

105. Fanning, A.S.; Jameson, B.J.; Jesaitis, L.A.; Anderson, J.M. The tight junction protein ZO-1 establishes a link between the transmembrane protein occludin and the actin cytoskeleton. *J. Biol. Chem.* **1998**, *273*, 29745–29753. [CrossRef] [PubMed]

106. Chen, C.; Wang, P.; Su, Q.; Wang, S.; Wang, F. Myosin light chain kinase mediates intestinal barrier disruption following burn injury. *PLoS ONE* **2012**, *7*, e34946. [CrossRef] [PubMed]

107. Sinclair, J.L.; Alexander, M. Role of resistance to starvation in bacterial survival in sewage and lake water. *Appl. Environ. Microbiol.* **1984**, *48*, 410–415. [PubMed]

108. Costello, E.K.; Gordon, J.I.; Secor, S.M.; Knight, R. Postprandial remodeling of the gut microbiota in Burmese pythons. *ISME J.* **2010**, *4*, 1375–1385. [CrossRef] [PubMed]

109. Gionchetti, P.; Rizzello, F.; Helwig, U.; Venturi, A.; Lammers, K.M.; Brigidi, P.; Vitali, B.; Poggioli, G.; Miglioli, M.; Campieri, M. Prophylaxis of pouchitis onset with probiotic therapy: A double-blind, placebo-controlled trial. *Gastroenterology* **2003**, *124*, 1202–1209. [CrossRef]

110. Mimura, T.; Rizzello, F.; Helwig, U.; Poggioli, G.; Schreiber, S.; Talbot, I.C.; Nicholls, R.J.; Gionchetti, P.; Campieri, M.; Kamm, M.A. Once daily high dose probiotic therapy (VSL#3) for maintaining remission in recurrent or refractory pouchitis. *Gut* **2004**, *53*, 108–114. [PubMed]

111. Szajewska, H.; Ruszczynski, M.; Radzikowski, A. Probiotics in the prevention of antibiotic-associated diarrhea in children: A meta-analysis of randomized controlled trials. *J. Pediatr.* **2006**, *149*, 367–372. [CrossRef] [PubMed]

112. Barclay, A.R.; Stenson, B.; Simpson, J.H.; Weaver, L.T.; Wilson, D.C. Probiotics for necrotizing enterocolitis: A systematic review. *J. Pediatr. Gastroenterol. Nutr.* **2007**, *45*, 569–576. [CrossRef] [PubMed]

113. Sentongo, T.A.; Cohran, V.; Korff, S.; Sullivan, C.; Iyer, K.; Zheng, X. Intestinal permeability and effects of Lactobacillus rhamnosus therapy in children with short bowel syndrome. *J. Pediatr. Gastroenterol. Nutr.* **2008**, *46*, 41–47. [CrossRef] [PubMed]

114. Uchida, K.; Takahashi, T.; Inoue, M.; Morotomi, M.; Otake, K.; Nakazawa, M.; Tsukamoto, Y.; Miki, C.; Kusunoki, M. Immunonutritional effects during synbiotics therapy in pediatric patients with short bowel syndrome. *Pediatr. Surg. Int.* **2007**, *23*, 243–248. [CrossRef] [PubMed]

115. Reddy, V.S.; Patole, S.K.; Rao, S. Role of probiotics in short bowel syndrome in infants and children—A systematic review. *Nutrients* **2013**, *5*, 679–699. [CrossRef] [PubMed]

116. Bartholome, A.L.; Albin, D.M.; Baker, D.H.; Holst, J.J.; Tappenden, K.A. Supplementation of total parenteral nutrition with butyrate acutely increases structural aspects of intestinal adaptation after an 80% jejunoileal resection in neonatal piglets. *J. Parenter. Enter. Nutr.* **2004**, *28*, 210–222. [CrossRef] [PubMed]

117. Murakoshi, S.; Fukatsu, K.; Omata, J.; Moriya, T.; Noguchi, M.; Saitoh, D.; Koyama, I. Effects of adding butyric acid to PN on gut-associated lymphoid tissue and mucosal immunoglobulin A levels. *J. Parenter. Enter. Nutr.* **2011**, *35*, 465–472. [CrossRef] [PubMed]

118. Rolandelli, R.H.; Buckmire, M.A.; Bernstein, K.A. Intravenous butyrate and healing of colonic anastomoses in the rat. *Dis. Colon Rectum* **1997**, *40*, 67–70. [CrossRef] [PubMed]

119. Stein, T.P.; Yoshida, S.; Schluter, M.D.; Drews, D.; Assimon, S.A.; Leskiw, M.J. Comparison of intravenous nutrients on gut mucosal proteins synthesis. *J. Parenter. Enter. Nutr.* **1994**, *18*, 447–452. [CrossRef] [PubMed]

120. Koruda, M.J.; Rolandelli, R.H.; Bliss, D.Z.; Hastings, J.; Rombeau, J.L.; Settle, R.G. Parenteral nutrition supplemented with short-chain fatty acids: Effect on the small-bowel mucosa in normal rats. *Am. J. Clin. Nutr.* **1990**, *51*, 685–689. [PubMed]

121. Wang, P.; Wang, Y.; Lu, L.; Yan, W.; Tao, Y.; Zhou, K.; Jie, J.; Wei, C. Alterations in intestinal microbiota relate to intestinal failure-associated liver disease and central line infections. *J. Pediatr. Surg.* **2017**, *52*, 1318–1326. [CrossRef] [PubMed]

122. De Minicis, S.; Rychlicki, C.; Agostinelli, L.; Saccomanno, S.; Candelaresi, C.; Trozzi, L.; Mingarelli, E.; Facinelli, B.; Magi, G.; Palmieri, C.; et al. Dysbiosis contributes to fibrogenesis in the course of chronic liver injury in mice. *Hepatology* **2014**, *59*, 1738–1749. [CrossRef] [PubMed]

123. El Kasmi, K.C.; Anderson, A.L.; Devereaux, M.W.; Fillon, S.A.; Harris, J.K.; Lovell, M.A.; Finegold, M.J.; Sokol, R.J. Toll-like receptor 4-dependent Kupffer cell activation and liver injury in a novel mouse model of parenteral nutrition and intestinal injury. *Hepatology* **2012**, *55*, 1518–1528. [CrossRef] [PubMed]

124. Harris, J.K.; El Kasmi, K.C.; Anderson, A.L.; Devereaux, M.W.; Fillon, S.A.; Robertson, C.E.; Wagner, B.D.; Stevens, M.J.; Pace, N.R.; Sokol, R.J. Specific microbiome changes in a mouse model of parenteral nutrition associated liver injury and intestinal inflammation. *PLoS ONE* **2014**, *9*, e110396. [CrossRef] [PubMed]

125. Lee, W.S.; Sokol, R.J. Intestinal Microbiota, Lipids, and the Pathogenesis of Intestinal Failure-Associated Liver Disease. *J. Pediatr.* **2015**, *167*, 519–526. [CrossRef] [PubMed]

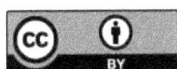

![nutrients logo] *nutrients*

MDPI

Review

Nutritional Therapies in Congenital Disorders of Glycosylation (CDG)

Peter Witters [1,2,*], David Cassiman [3] and Eva Morava [1,2,4]

1   Metabolic Center, University Hospitals Leuven, B-3000 Leuven, Belgium; emoravakozicz@tulane.edu
2   Department of Development and Regeneration, Faculty of Medicine, KU Leuven, B-3000 Leuven, Belgium
3   Department of Gastroenterology-Hepatology and Metabolic Center, University Hospitals Leuven,
     B-3000 Leuven, Belgium; david.cassiman@kuleuven.be
4   Hayward Genetics Center, Tulane University School of Medicine, New Orleans, LA 70112, USA
*   Correspondence: peter.witters@uzleuven.be; Tel.: +32-1634-3843

Received: 16 October 2017; Accepted: 1 November 2017; Published: 7 November 2017

Abstract: Congenital disorders of glycosylation (CDG) are a group of more than 130 inborn errors of metabolism affecting N-linked, O-linked protein and lipid-linked glycosylation. The phenotype in CDG patients includes frequent liver involvement, especially the disorders belonging to the N-linked protein glycosylation group. There are only a few treatable CDG. Mannose-Phosphate Isomerase (MPI)-CDG was the first treatable CDG by high dose mannose supplements. Recently, with the successful use of D-galactose in Phosphoglucomutase 1 (PGM1)-CDG, other CDG types have been trialed on galactose and with an increasing number of potential nutritional therapies. Current mini review focuses on therapies in glycosylation disorders affecting liver function and dietary intervention in general in N-linked glycosylation disorders. We also emphasize now the importance of early screening for CDG in patients with mild hepatopathy but also in cholestasis.

Keywords: galactose; mannose; congenital disorders of glycosylation (CDG); treatment; glycosylation; diet

1. Introduction

Congenital disorders of glycosylation (CDG) are a family of diseases with the common denominator that they all affect the most important posttranslational modification of proteins, i.e., glycosylation [1]. They were initially described by Jaak Jaeken and currently compromise a group of more than 130 separate entities [1]. The most abundant type of CDG affect N-linked glycosylation. Most of these CDG are multisystemic diseases with hepatic involvement [2].

N-glycosylation is initiated with the activation of sugars in the cytoplasm of the cell. These phosphorylated sugars are subsequently transferred to the lipid dolichol, in the membrane of the endoplasmic reticulum (ER). This stepwise enzymatic assembly process leads to the formation of a glycan molecule. The base of this glycan consists of N-acetyl glucosamines (GlcNac), followed by several mannose (Man) residues. It is first assembled at the cytoplasmic surface and later inside the ER. Finally, the addition of glucose molecules is a signal to release the glycan from dolichol, followed by the attachment of the glycan to a protein. In the case of N-glycosylation, the glycan is linked to an amino group of an asparagine (N). The final steps of the glycosylation process take place in the Golgi apparatus with tailoring of the glycan molecule to its mature form by trimming away some of the mannose units and adding galactose and sialic acid [3,4].

While the assembly process in the ER is almost fully understood because it is conserved down to yeast and the consecutive building steps mirror each other, the process in the Golgi is very complicated as the success of the end product depends on several other factors outside the classic glycosylation steps. This glycosylation relies on the proper function of several transporters making the activated sugars available for synthesis. Defects in Golgi proteins that affect the trafficking and the transport of glycoproteins throughout the Golgi (functioning for example in the transport of protons and trace elements) can also lead to hypoglycosylation [3]. This is a rapidly growing family of newly described CDG [1,5].

The diagnosis of *N*-linked glycosylation disorders is made by serum transferrin isoelectric focusing, or mass spectrometry of transferrin isoforms. Depending on whether the defect is localized in the cytoplasm or endoplasmic reticulum (E.R.) or in the Golgi compartment, a different pattern can be observed, (type I and type II, respectively) [6].

In *O*-linked glycosylation, the glycan is linked to the OH-group of serine or threonine. *O*-linked glycan defects are often tissue specific. The mucin type of *O*-glycosylation is Golgi related and frequently associated with *N*-linked glycosylation defects. It can be screened by isoelectric focusing of serum apolipoprotein C-III, that is only *O*-glycosylated [3]. A well-known group of tissue specific *O*-glycosylation defects are the dystroglycanopathies [1,7].

Glycosylphosphatidylinositol (GPI)-anchored glycosylation defects is a growing group of genetic disorders clinically characterized by intellectual disability and biochemically by hyperphosphatasia. GPI anchors attach a number of proteins, including alkaline phosphatase, to membranes. Hyperphopsphatasia reflects the inability of the ectoenzyme (alkaline phosphatase) to anchor to the membrane and hence this will continue to circulate causing the hyperphosphatasia [3]. Lipid linked glycosylation is also important for the correct anchoring of T-cell antigens. The best known GPI-anchor defect, paroxysmal nocturnal hemoglobinuria, is a somatic disorder [4,7].

In CDG there is an important role of the dolichol phosphate mutase (DPM) complex. This complex is involved in the activation of mannose. Activated mannose is needed in all three glycosylation pathways *N*-linked, *O*-linked, and GPI-anchored [3]. The DPM complex has three subunits (DPM1, DPM2 and DPM3). Genetic defects in the DPM complex result in severe multisystem phenotypes, with biochemical anomalies of all three pathways (combined glycosylation defects) [3]. The phenotype consists of typical *N*-glycosylation symptoms, such as seizures, microcephaly, strabismus and developmental disability, but also eye anomalies and brain migration defects, seen in the dystroglycanopathies [8].

Liver disease is a feature of nearly all *N*-linked CDG. It mostly involves increased levels of transaminases (for example in the most prevalent CDG, PMM2-CDG). But sometimes it can manifest as hepatomegaly, cholestasis or liver failure. Histologically, liver fibrosis, ductal plate malformation, cirrhosis and steatosis have been observed. Especially the recently described CDG subtypes involving the Golgi can have liver disease, as their predominant feature (ATP6AP1-CDG, TMEM199-CDG and CCDC1115-CDG) [2,9–11]. In several *N*-linked CDG, liver transplantation has been necessary, due to progressive cirrhosis, for instance in MPI-CDG, or CCDC1115-CDG. Not only is transferrin, central to the diagnosis of *N*-linked CDG, produced by the liver, but so are a myriad of secreted and glycosylated proteins. For example, coagulation factors, except for factor VIII, are solely produced by the liver. In many CDG, there are disturbances of the coagulation profile. Usually this is due to a synthesis defect with decreased levels of factor IX, XI, protein C, antithrombin III and protein S, and also decreased glycosylation of these factors [12].

Dietary therapy is an important intervention in CDG [13]. Only a few CGD subtypes are "treatable". This article focuses on the different treatment options in *N*-linked glycosylation disorders with liver involvement.

2. Materials and Methods

The present literature review started with the search of the Medline database, using PubMed as search engine (last accessed October 2017). AND and OR operators were used in the database search to combine the keywords "therapy", "treatment", "supplement" or "diet" in combination with CDG or the two common full names for CDG: (a) carbohydrate-deficient glycoprotein syndrome(s) and (b) congenital disorder(s) of glycosylation. For the search algorithm see Supplementary File S1.

Papers were included in present review if they contained information on potential nutritional treatments in CDG that are known to affect the liver. Additionally, clinical trials were searched on www.ClincalTrials.gov using the same keywords.

3. Results

Two hundreds and forty-three articles matching these search terms were identified. Selection of the articles on *N*-glycosylation and describing nutritional therapy in at least 1 patient or a relevant animal model. Forty-nine articles were selected for further study. This information was complemented with the information presented at the World CDG-conference 2017 and the registered trials on Clinicaltrials.gov.

3.1. Specific Dietary Therapies in Selected CDG Types

Several CDG were found to be (at least partially) treatable by nutritional interventions such as mannose, galactose, etc. (Table 1).

Table 1. Specific dietary treatments in *N*-linked disorders of glycosylation.

	PMM2-CDG	MPI-CDG	PGM1-CDG	SLC 35A2-CDG	SLC39A8-CDG	TMEM165-CDG
Mannose	-	X	-	-	-	-
Galactose	-	-	X	X	X	X
Frequent complex carbohydrate feeding	+/−	+/−	X	-	-	-
Manganese	-	-	-	-	X	? *

Abbreviations: CDG: congenital disorders of glycosylation, PMM2: phosphomannomutase 2; MPI: Mannosephosphate Isomerase. * Manganese only trialed in vitro, cautious use is potentially useful as oral therapy. X Clinically trialed dietary supplement with positive biochemical and clinical effects. +/− This therapy has shown beneficiary effect in some of the patients.

3.2. Mannose in PMM2-CDG (MIM # 212065)

PMM2-CDG is the first described CDG and is due to phosphomannomutase-2 (PMM2) deficiency. It has two clinical presentations. The neurological subtype presents with cerebellar atrophy with ataxia, intellectual disability, seizures, retinopathy, stroke like episodes and peripheral neuropathy [14]. The more severe and potentially lethal multisystem phenotype, also has organ involvement such as hepato-gastrointestinal (chronic diarrhea, protein-losing enteropathy, liver failure, cirrhosis), cardiac and kidney disease [15]. Liver involvement (mainly hepatomegaly and raised transaminases) is present in up to 50% of patients [2].

Nutritional therapy has been considered and trialed in the past in these patients. In vitro, there was a clear improvement observed in the glycosylation pattern by treating patient fibroblast lines with mannose [16,17]. However, clinically, based on multiple clinical reports (but no structural therapy trials), there has been no confirmed clinical improvement, nor biochemical improvement at the level of the defective glycosylation, in patients [17,18].

As of now we have to conclude that mannose therapy is not effective in PMM2-CDG. Evaluating the reported laboratory data in PMM2 deficient patients is also difficult, since in older patients, transferrin isoforms may normalize spontaneously, and in many patients with PMM2-CDG there is a gradual improvement of transaminases over time [15], parallel with clinical stabilization. There is an absolute need for future nutritional therapeutic trials; ideally double blind randomized controlled trials, in PMM2-CDG.

3.3. Mannose in MPI-CDG (MIM # 602579)

MPI-CDG is longest known treatable CDG-type. It is characterized by bleeding diathesis, increased risk for thrombotic events, abnormal liver function, hyperinsulinism and chronic diarrhea.

Patients have a normal intellect. Transferrin analysis shows a type I pattern. On liver histology congenital hepatic fibrosis, microvesicular steatosis and fibrosis or cirrhosis has been documented.

Initial investigations showed successful restoration of glycosylation by mannose in vitro which was followed by compassionate use of mannose in MPI-CDG patients [19]. This is not surprising because mannose can be phosphorylated by the hexokinase so that the defective phophomannose isomerase (MPI) that converts fructose-6-phosphate to mannose-6-phosphate can be bypassed. The dose of 200 mg/kg 4–6 times/day was suggested to keep serum mannose levels high enough to alleviate endocrine abnormalities, coagulation defects and the chronic protein-losing enteropathy [19–21]. In some of the patients, a higher dosage was needed for full recovery. In a low percentage of patients high doses of mannose led to hemolysis and jaundice. It can also lead to seizures [22]. Coagulation abnormalities and hyperinsulinism usually improve within a few weeks of mannose supplements, both on intravenous and on oral therapy. Chronic diarrhea may recur in exceptional cases. Mannose therapy does not prevent further hepatic injury and about 1/3 of the patients develop liver cirrhosis, sometimes requiring liver transplantation [21,23]. Formal placebo-controlled clinical studies of oral or IV mannose in MPI-CDG patients have not been performed so far, so the data is anecdotal.

3.4. Galactose in PGM1-CDG (MIM # 614921)

PGM1-CDG is a combined disorder of glycogenolysis, glycolysis and glycosylation. Most patients are born with a midline defect of the palate, cardiomyopathy and multiple laboratory abnormalities including abnormal coagulation, endocrine parameters and liver function tests. Hypoglycemia is partially due to hyperinsulinism and the abnormal glycogenolysis in patients. Short stature is associated with feeding difficulties. Patients have normal intellect [24].

Phosphoglucomutase 1 (PGM1) deficiency is a unique glycosylation disorder showing a mixed type of glycosylation defect (type I/II). The most characteristic finding is decreased galactosylation additional to a global decrease in glycan synthesis. Based on the decreased number of galactose molecules in truncated glycans and the success of galactose supplements in vitro in patient fibroblasts, recently clinical trials were initiated to evaluate the success of galactose treatment in PGM1 patients [24]. Pilot studies showed an improvement in liver transaminases, coagulation factors (antithrombin III and factor XI) and in a variable degree of endocrine parameters. The frequency of rhabdomyolysis decreased, however, the treatment did not affect muscle weakness and creatine kinase (CK) levels [25,26]. A frequent complex carbohydrate rich diet remains necessary to keep blood glucose levels in the normal range in all patients. In three patients, transient tube feeding had been needed due to severe recurrent hypoglycemic episodes. The frequency of hypoglycemic episodes however did improve on D-galactose therapy.

3.5. Galactose in SLC35A2-CDG (UDP-Galactose Transporter) (MIM # 300896)

This CDG is due to a deficiency of the UDP-galactose transporter (solute carrier (SLC) 35A2) in the Golgi leading to a type II pattern on transferrin analysis. Clinically it manifests as an early infantile epilepsy with developmental delay, hypotonia, variable ocular anomalies, and brain malformations (cerebellar atrophy, delayed myelination and a thin corpus callosum) [27]. Many of the patients have a mosaic form of the mutation, not showing transferrin abnormalities. Non-mosaic patients have significant elevation of the transaminases.

In one patient, glycosylation could be nearly completely restored by galactose supplementation [28]. Although seizures tend to improve on galactose therapy, transaminases remain elevated (personal communication, European Metabolic Group conference 2016).

3.6. Galactose in SLC39A8-CDG (Manganese transporter) (MIM # 616721)

This type II CDG is a recently described multi-systemic neurodevelopmental disorder with phenotypes ranging from cranial synostosis, hypsarrhythmia and disproportionate dwarfism to strabismus, cerebellar atrophy, hypotonia, intellectual disability and recurrent infections [1]. Liver transaminases can be chronically mildly elevated. SLC39A8 is required for the manganese homeostasis in the Golgi, where manganese is a cofactor of the β-1,4-Galactosyltransferase. Unsurprisingly, manganese supplementation [29] and galactose supplementation [30,31] have been attempted. Galactose generally improves glycosylation and high dose manganese treats the epilepsy.

3.7. Galactose in TMEM165-CDG (MIM # 614727)

TMEM165-CDG, a type II CDG, combines impaired *N* and *O*-glycosylation and manifests with striking osseous changes as epiphyseal, metaphyseal, and diaphyseal dysplasia. Other features that accompany this peculiar skeletal phenotype are muscular hypotrophy, fat excess, partial growth hormone deficiency, and, in some patients, episodes of unexplained fever. Biochemically there is a mild to moderate increases of serum transaminases (particularly of aspartate transaminase (AST)), CK, and lactate dehydrogenase (LDH), as well as decreased coagulation factors VIII, IX, XI, and protein C [32,33].

Galactose therapy has very recently shown to be beneficial in patient fibroblasts improved glycosylation as well as biochemical parameters (blood coagulation) [5]. This could be due to an upregulation of manganese dependent transferases in the Golgi, such as B4GALT1 (β-1,4-Galactosyltransferase 1).

3.8. General Symptom Directed Dietary Therapy in CDG

Next to the specific treatment of several *N*-linked CDG, there are also nutritional treatments of certain syndromes that are often present in CDG.

For instance, hyperinsulism is a well-known feature of MPI-CDG, PGM1-CDG and PMM2-CDG. This can be treated by dietary interventions, such as using foods with a low glycemic index, nocturnal tube feeding and the use of uncooked corn-starch in children above 1 year of age [25]. Most patients need additional diazoxide therapy [25].

There is often a component of failure to thrive in CDG patients. In these patients complimentary feeding and tube feeding can be necessary. Moreover, an elementary diet can prove to be useful.

Protein losing enteropathy is a main feature of MPI-CDG but can also be present in the most prevalent CDG (PMM2-CDG). In some patients lymphangiectasia have been documented and a MCT diet has shown to be useful [12,34]. Somatostatin treatment is an additional non-nutritional intervention.

MAN1B1-CDG is the only known CDG (type II) that is known to be associated with obesity in addition to slight facial dysmorphism and psychomotor retardation [35]. In this CDG, caloric restriction can be necessary.

Similar to MELAS (mitochondrial encephalomyopathy, lactic acidosis, and stroke-like episodes) syndrome, L-arginine has been used to treat stroke-like episodes in CDG. L-arginine could improve NO production and hence vasodilation in these patients (personal communications, Prof P de Lonlay). However, no formal trials have been performed.

In CDG presenting with cholestasis (such as ALG8-CDG, COG6-CDG, COG7-CDG, CCDC115-CDG and ATP6AP1-CDG), nutritional interventions such as in other causes of cholestasis can be necessary [2]. These entail the supplementation of fat-soluble vitamins and MCT (medium-chain triglycerides) that are more easily absorbed in the absence of bile [36].

In pediatric neurology, the ketogenic diet has proven to be useful in controlling refractory seizures [37]. In CDG refractory seizure are rare, but the ketogenic diet could also be used. One issue complicating this is the occurrence of hyperinsulinism in some CDG often leading to hypoglycemia [15] while on the ketogenic diet as this contains a low amount of carbohydrates [37].

Dietary treatment of CDG has been mostly successful with the traditional method (fructose and lactose restrictions), however no clinical trial is available about the efficacy of this diet. Alcohol use worsens the liver phenotype in CDG significantly, and oppresses lipid linked oligosaccharide synthesis. The alcohol-related glycosylation abnormality is reversible.

4. Discussion

Congenital Disorders of Glycosylation are usually multisystem disorders, mostly affecting the central nervous system, in addition to diverse laboratory anomalies. *N*-linked glycosylation defects are always affecting liver function, leading to abnormal synthesis of secretory proteins, including albumin, hormone transporters, and coagulation and anticoagulation factors, partially due to abnormal synthetic function of the liver, but also due to a disturbed glycosylation and insufficient posttranslational regulation of important functional proteins [12]. Alpha 1 antitrypsin, ceruloplasmine and other liver proteins are frequently abnormal. Liver transaminase levels are almost always elevated, although spontaneous recovery is common. Hepatomegaly is uncommon and only a few *N*-linked disorders lead to cholestasis, fibrosis or cirrhosis [2,9].

Jaundice is rarely present. In fact, only two recently described disorders (CCDC115-CDG and ATP6VAP1-CDG) are cholestatic conditions. In addition, some patients had to undergo liver transplantation [9,10].

This is also the case for MPI-CDG, where a cryptogenic liver disease can progress to liver cirrhosis without overt symptoms, even on successful dietary therapy.

The biochemical background of dietary monosaccharide therapy in CDG is not completely understood. Mannose therapy has been for long the only treatment in Mannose-Phosphate Isomerase (MPI) deficiency. The background of the therapy is that the enzyme block in MPI-CDG does not allow producing sufficient amount of mannose-6-phosphate for the endoplasmic reticulum (ER) related glycosylation. Using a very high concentration of mannose, administered every 4 hours, could salvage this [20]. By this concentration mannose can be directly activated (phosphorylated) by hexokinase. This phosphorylation step requires a higher than physiologic concentration of mannose since the enzyme's natural substrate is glucose, and hexokinase is only moonlighting in this reaction under these conditions. Mannose supplements unfortunately do not solve the clinical problem in PMM2 deficiency where a lack of mannose-1-phosphate makes further mannose activation impossible [38]. Experimental treatments in fibroblasts using chemically disguised mannose-1-phosphate are ongoing [13].

The theory behind oral galactose treatment is different. In SLC35A2-CDG the galactose transporter appears to be upregulated by excess of galactose, which leads to an increase in galactose transport to the Golgi in vitro [28]. This mechanism is similar to that seen by defects of the fucose transporter SLC35A1 (SLC35A1-CDG), which also shows an improved function on oral fucose therapy, with improving glycosylation. In both cases, transferrin glycosylation increases significantly but also some of the clinical features improve [13].

Galactose mode of action is different in PGM1-CDG. The hypothesis is that increasing galactose concentrations in blood increase galactose-1-phosphate and UDP-galactose levels, which restore the altered balance within abnormal nucleotide sugar pools. This would improve hypogalactosylation in the Golgi. Interestingly, in some unknown way, galactose supports the ER related glycosylation as well in PGM1 deficiency, where it has been shown that lipid linked oligosaccharide synthesis is arrested, but recovers on in vitro galactose treatment [24–26]. Galactose might offer extra energy substrate for patients, since some of the adults with PGM1 deficiency also show an improvement of their muscle disease [39].

In TMEM165, galactose's positive effect is suspected secondary through B4GALT1, a Golgi enzyme, which is both manganese and galactose concentration sensitive. TMEM165 defect leads to abnormal manganese transport to the Golgi, affecting Golgi oligotransferases, which apparently improve their function with extra galactose, and increase galactosylation [5]. This is similar to galactose effect in SCLA39A8-CDG, providing manganese for the Golgi, and also for B4GALT1, where both manganese and galactose therapy restores glycosylation, however a cautiously administered high dose of oral manganese therapy is clinically more efficient [29].

Dietary intervention is an evolving and increasingly used therapy in CDG. More and more subtypes are trialed on monosaccharide supplementation, due to the relatively high safety, especially compared to experimental drug trials, and the ease of supplementation. Monosaccharides can be mixed with any type of food and usually have a pleasant, if any taste. Previous experience with monosaccharide therapy in individual cases showed that increasing the concentration of specific monosaccharides can lead to an increase in Golgi availability. This has been demonstrated by improvement in galactosylation on galactose therapy in SLC35A2-CDG [27,28]. Similar results were observed on fucose therapy in fucose transporter deficiency [40]. Based on these observations one should hypothesize a potential beneficial effect of sialic acid in SLC35A1-CDG, or of *N*-acetyl Glucosamine (GlcNAc) in SLC35A3-CDG as GlcNAc has been already used in the past safely in patients with different medical conditions, for example as supportive therapy in chronic osteoarthritis, as a health supplement. Oral sialic acid supplementation, however has not yet been proven to be efficient and its long acting form was recently withdrawn from clinical trials, due to not reaching any of the study end-points in GNE-CDG [13]. The problem with the dietary use of sialic acid is that this molecule is not efficiently taken up by the cell and in the Golgi compartment as an oral therapy.

Additional dietary therapies could aim at increasing UDP concentrations in the cell, to have sufficient UDP available for the synthesis of UDP-sugars [24]. This novel approach has been successfully used in CAD-CDG [41]. This has not been systematically trialed in other CDGs. Other possible therapies include manganese supplementation in CDGs related to defective manganese transport, already shown to be effective in two cases of SLC39A8-CDG [29], and manganese can be probably a potential adjuvant therapy for TMEM165-CDG [5].

The question is, whether these dietary interventions are sufficient, and potentially the most efficient interventions in CDG? We learnt from the lesson on MPI-CDG, that mannose therapy is not only risky, when applied in higher doses, but also cannot prevent the progressive fibrotic liver disease in about one third of the patients [23]. Galactose therapy has beneficial effects in several CDGs but does not fully alleviate all clinical symptoms. The long term future of CDG therapy is most likely the use of activated monosaccharides instead of using single dietary sugars. In order to increase substrate concentrations, or supplement missing substrates, we should administer a more specific therapy by ingesting only a small amount of the active compound, compared to the currently used large amounts of simple sugars (in some cases 50 g/monosaccharide added to the diet daily). The efficacy of these novel potential drugs should be however carefully evaluated, for toxicity. The use of animal models is imperative instead of using cell culture models, since a successful cellular delivery of monosaccharides in fibroblasts does not mean that the oral supplementation would be effective [18,38].

5. Conclusions

In summary, in our current mini review we evaluated the different nutritional therapy options, associated with a positive effect on liver function in CDG. We believe this new type of nutritional therapy holds great promise for the future and over the last decade numerous CDG have been transformed to at least partially treatable disorders.

Supplementary Materials: The following are available online at www.mdpi.com/2072-6643/9/11/1222/s1, File S1: Search algorithm used in Pubmed (https://www.ncbi.nlm.nih.gov/pubmed/), accessed on 1 October 2017.

Acknowledgments: P.W. is supported by the clinical research fund, University Hospitals Leuven, Leuven, Belgium. E.M. and D.C. are recipients of the clinical investigatorship, FWO Flanders, Belgium.

Author Contributions: P.W., E.M. and D.C. conceived and designed the research; P.W., E.M. and D.C. analyzed the data; P.W., E.M. and D.C. wrote the paper.

Conflicts of Interest: The authors declare no conflict of interest.

Abbreviations

CDG   Congenital disorders of glycosylation
ER   Endoplasmic reticulum
GlcNac   *N*-acetyl glucosamines
Man   Mannose
GPI   Glycosylphosphatidylinositol
DPM   Dolichol phosphate mutase
PMM2   Phosphomannomutase-2
MPI   Phophomannose isomerase
PGM1   Phosphoglucomutase 1
CK   Creatine kinase
SLC   Solute carrier
AST   Aspartate transaminase
LDH   Lactate dehydrogenase
MELAS   Mitochondrial encephalomyopathy, lactic acidosis, and stroke-like episodes

References

1. Jaeken, J.; Peanne, R. What is new in CDG? *J. Inherit. Metab. Dis.* **2017**, *40*, 569–586. [CrossRef] [PubMed]
2. Marques-da-Silva, D.; Dos Reis Ferreira, V.; Monticelli, M.; Janeiro, P.; Videira, P.A.; Witters, P.; Jaeken, J.; Cassiman, D. Liver involvement in congenital disorders of glycosylation (CDG). A systematic review of the literature. *J. Inherit. Metab. Dis.* **2017**, *40*, 195–207. [CrossRef] [PubMed]
3. Witters, P.; Morava, E. Congenital disorders of glycosylation (CDG): Review. *eLS* **2016**, 1–6. [CrossRef]
4. Jaeken, J.; Hennet, T.; Matthijs, G.; Freeze, H.H. CDG nomenclature: Time for a change! *Biochim. Biophys. Acta* **2009**, *1792*, 825–826. [CrossRef] [PubMed]
5. Morelle, W.; Potelle, S.; Witters, P.; Wong, S.; Climer, L.; Lupashin, V.; Matthijs, G.; Gadomski, T.; Jaeken, J.; Cassiman, D.; et al. Galactose supplementation in patients with tmem165-CDG rescues the glycosylation defects. *J. Clin. Endocrinol. Metab.* **2017**, *102*, 1375–1386. [CrossRef] [PubMed]
6. Lefeber, D.J.; Morava, E.; Jaeken, J. How to find and diagnose a CDG due to defective *N*-glycosylation. *J. Inherit. Metab. Dis.* **2011**, *34*, 849–852. [CrossRef] [PubMed]
7. Freeze, H.H. Congenital disorders of glycosylation: CDG-I, CDG-II, and beyond. *Curr. Mol. Med.* **2007**, *7*, 389–396. [CrossRef] [PubMed]
8. Barone, R.; Aiello, C.; Race, V.; Morava, E.; Foulquier, F.; Riemersma, M.; Passarelli, C.; Concolino, D.; Carella, M.; Santorelli, F.; et al. DPM2-CDG: A muscular dystrophy-dystroglycanopathy syndrome with severe epilepsy. *Ann. Neurol.* **2012**, *72*, 550–558. [CrossRef] [PubMed]
9. Jansen, E.J.; Timal, S.; Ryan, M.; Ashikov, A.; van Scherpenzeel, M.; Graham, L.A.; Mandel, H.; Hoischen, A.; Iancu, T.C.; Raymond, K.; et al. ATP6AP1 deficiency causes an immunodeficiency with hepatopathy, cognitive impairment and abnormal protein glycosylation. *Nat. Commun.* **2016**, *7*, 11600. [CrossRef] [PubMed]
10. Jansen, J.C.; Cirak, S.; van Scherpenzeel, M.; Timal, S.; Reunert, J.; Rust, S.; Perez, B.; Vicogne, D.; Krawitz, P.; Wada, Y.; et al. CCDC115 deficiency causes a disorder of Golgi homeostasis with abnormal protein glycosylation. *Am. J. Hum. Genet.* **2016**, *98*, 310–321. [CrossRef] [PubMed]
11. Jansen, J.C.; Timal, S.; van Scherpenzeel, M.; Michelakakis, H.; Vicogne, D.; Ashikov, A.; Moraitou, M.; Hoischen, A.; Huijben, K.; Steenbergen, G.; et al. TMEM199 deficiency is a disorder of Golgi homeostasis characterized by elevated aminotransferases, alkaline phosphatase, and cholesterol and abnormal glycosylation. *Am. J. Hum. Genet.* **2016**, *98*, 322–330. [CrossRef] [PubMed]
12. Scott, K.; Gadomski, T.; Kozicz, T.; Morava, E. Congenital disorders of glycosylation: New defects and still counting. *J. Inherit. Metab. Dis.* **2014**, *37*, 609–617. [CrossRef] [PubMed]
13. Peanne, R.; de Lonlay, P.; Foulquier, F.; Kornak, U.; Lefeber, D.J.; Morava, E.; Perez, B.; Seta, N.; Thiel, C.; Van Schaftingen, E.; et al. Congenital disorders of glycosylation (CDG): Quo vadis? *Eur. J. Med. Genet.* **2017**. [CrossRef] [PubMed]

14. De Diego, V.; Martinez-Monseny, A.F.; Muchart, J.; Cuadras, D.; Montero, R.; Artuch, R.; Perez-Cerda, C.; Perez, B.; Perez-Duenas, B.; Poretti, A.; et al. Longitudinal volumetric and 2D assessment of cerebellar atrophy in a large cohort of children with phosphomannomutase deficiency (PMM2-CDG). *J. Inherit. Metab. Dis.* **2017**. [CrossRef]

15. Schiff, M.; Roda, C.; Monin, M.L.; Arion, A.; Barth, M.; Bednarek, N.; Bidet, M.; Bloch, C.; Boddaert, N.; Borgel, D.; et al. Clinical, laboratory and molecular findings and long-term follow-up data in 96 french patients with PMM2-CDG (phosphomannomutase 2-congenital disorder of glycosylation) and review of the literature. *J. Med. Genet.* **2017**. [CrossRef] [PubMed]

16. Panneerselvam, K.; Freeze, H.H. Mannose corrects altered *N*-glycosylation in carbohydrate-deficient glycoprotein syndrome fibroblasts. *J. Clin. Investig.* **1996**, *97*, 1478–1487. [CrossRef] [PubMed]

17. Kjaergaard, S.; Kristiansson, B.; Stibler, H.; Freeze, H.H.; Schwartz, M.; Martinsson, T.; Skovby, F. Failure of short-term mannose therapy of patients with carbohydrate-deficient glycoprotein syndrome type 1A. *Acta Paediatr.* **1998**, *87*, 884–888. [CrossRef] [PubMed]

18. Mayatepek, E.; Kohlmuller, D. Mannose supplementation in carbohydrate-deficient glycoprotein syndrome type I and phosphomannomutase deficiency. *Eur. J. Pediatr.* **1998**, *157*, 605–606. [CrossRef] [PubMed]

19. Harms, H.K.; Zimmer, K.P.; Kurnik, K.; Bertele-Harms, R.M.; Weidinger, S.; Reiter, K. Oral mannose therapy persistently corrects the severe clinical symptoms and biochemical abnormalities of phosphomannose isomerase deficiency. *Acta Paediatr.* **2002**, *91*, 1065–1072. [CrossRef] [PubMed]

20. De Lonlay, P.; Seta, N. The clinical spectrum of phosphomannose isomerase deficiency, with an evaluation of mannose treatment for CDG-Ib. *Biochim. Biophys. Acta* **2009**, *1792*, 841–843. [CrossRef] [PubMed]

21. Mention, K.; Lacaille, F.; Valayannopoulos, V.; Romano, S.; Kuster, A.; Cretz, M.; Zaidan, H.; Galmiche, L.; Jaubert, F.; de Keyzer, Y.; et al. Development of liver disease despite mannose treatment in two patients with CDG-Ib. *Mol. Genet. Metab.* **2008**, *93*, 40–43. [CrossRef] [PubMed]

22. Schroeder, A.S.; Kappler, M.; Bonfert, M.; Borggraefe, I.; Schoen, C.; Reiter, K. Seizures and stupor during intravenous mannose therapy in a patient with CDG syndrome type 1b (MPI-CDG). *J. Inherit. Metab. Dis.* **2010**, *33* (Suppl. S3), S497–S502. [CrossRef] [PubMed]

23. Janssen, M.C.; de Kleine, R.H.; van den Berg, A.P.; Heijdra, Y.; van Scherpenzeel, M.; Lefeber, D.J.; Morava, E. Successful liver transplantation and long-term follow-up in a patient with MPI-CDG. *Pediatrics* **2014**, *134*, e279–e283. [CrossRef] [PubMed]

24. Tegtmeyer, L.C.; Rust, S.; van Scherpenzeel, M.; Ng, B.G.; Losfeld, M.E.; Timal, S.; Raymond, K.; He, P.; Ichikawa, M.; Veltman, J.; et al. Multiple phenotypes in phosphoglucomutase 1 deficiency. *N. Engl. J. Med.* **2014**, *370*, 533–542. [CrossRef] [PubMed]

25. Morava, E. Galactose supplementation in phosphoglucomutase-1 deficiency; review and outlook for a novel treatable CDG. *Mol. Genet. Metab.* **2014**, *112*, 275–279. [CrossRef] [PubMed]

26. Wong, S.Y.; Gadomski, T.; van Scherpenzeel, M.; Honzik, T.; Hansikova, H.; Holmefjord, K.S.B.; Mork, M.; Bowling, F.; Sykut-Cegielska, J.; Koch, D.; et al. Oral D-galactose supplementation in PGM1-CDG. *Genet. Med.* **2017**. [CrossRef] [PubMed]

27. Kodera, H.; Nakamura, K.; Osaka, H.; Maegaki, Y.; Haginoya, K.; Mizumoto, S.; Kato, M.; Okamoto, N.; Iai, M.; Kondo, Y.; et al. De novo mutations in SLC35A2 encoding a UDP-galactose transporter cause early-onset epileptic encephalopathy. *Hum. Mutat.* **2013**, *34*, 1708–1714. [CrossRef] [PubMed]

28. Dorre, K.; Olczak, M.; Wada, Y.; Sosicka, P.; Gruneberg, M.; Reunert, J.; Kurlemann, G.; Fiedler, B.; Biskup, S.; Hortnagel, K.; et al. A new case of UDP-galactose transporter deficiency (SLC35A2-CDG): Molecular basis, clinical phenotype, and therapeutic approach. *J. Inherit. Metab. Dis.* **2015**, *38*, 931–940. [CrossRef] [PubMed]

29. Park, J.H.; Hogrebe, M.; Fobker, M.; Brackmann, R.; Fiedler, B.; Reunert, J.; Rust, S.; Tsiakas, K.; Santer, R.; Gruneberg, M.; et al. SLC39A8 deficiency: Biochemical correction and major clinical improvement by manganese therapy. *Genet. Med.* **2017**. [CrossRef] [PubMed]

30. Park, J.H.; Hogrebe, M.; Gruneberg, M.; DuChesne, I.; von der Heiden, A.L.; Reunert, J.; Schlingmann, K.P.; Boycott, K.M.; Beaulieu, C.L.; Mhanni, A.A.; et al. SLC39A8 deficiency: A disorder of manganese transport and glycosylation. *Am. J. Hum. Genet.* **2015**, *97*, 894–903. [CrossRef] [PubMed]

31. Riley, L.G.; Cowley, M.J.; Gayevskiy, V.; Roscioli, T.; Thorburn, D.R.; Prelog, K.; Bahlo, M.; Sue, C.M.; Balasubramaniam, S.; Christodoulou, J. A SLC39A8 variant causes manganese deficiency, and glycosylation and mitochondrial disorders. *J. Inherit. Metab. Dis.* **2017**, *40*, 261–269. [CrossRef] [PubMed]

32. Foulquier, F.; Amyere, M.; Jaeken, J.; Zeevaert, R.; Schollen, E.; Race, V.; Bammens, R.; Morelle, W.; Rosnoblet, C.; Legrand, D.; et al. TMEM165 deficiency causes a congenital disorder of glycosylation. *Am. J. Hum. Genet.* **2012**, *91*, 15–26. [CrossRef] [PubMed]

33. Zeevaert, R.; de Zegher, F.; Sturiale, L.; Garozzo, D.; Smet, M.; Moens, M.; Matthijs, G.; Jaeken, J. Bone dysplasia as a key feature in three patients with a novel congenital disorder of glycosylation (CDG) type II due to a deep intronic splice mutation in tmem165. *JIMD Rep.* **2013**, *8*, 145–152. [PubMed]

34. Theodore, M.; Morava, E. Congenital disorders of glycosylation: Sweet news. *Curr. Opin. Pediatr.* **2011**, *23*, 581–587. [CrossRef] [PubMed]

35. Rymen, D.; Peanne, R.; Millon, M.B.; Race, V.; Sturiale, L.; Garozzo, D.; Mills, P.; Clayton, P.; Asteggiano, C.G.; Quelhas, D.; et al. MAN1B1 deficiency: An unexpected CDG-II. *PLoS Genet.* **2013**, *9*, e1003989. [CrossRef] [PubMed]

36. Los, E.L.; Lukovac, S.; Werner, A.; Dijkstra, T.; Verkade, H.J.; Rings, E.H. Nutrition for children with cholestatic liver disease. *Nestle Nutr. Workshop Ser. Pediatr. Program.* **2007**, *59*, 147–157. [PubMed]

37. Neal, E.G.; Chaffe, H.; Schwartz, R.H.; Lawson, M.S.; Edwards, N.; Fitzsimmons, G.; Whitney, A.; Cross, J.H. The ketogenic diet for the treatment of childhood epilepsy: A randomised controlled trial. *Lancet Neurol.* **2008**, *7*, 500–506. [CrossRef]

38. Freeze, H.H. Towards a therapy for phosphomannomutase 2 deficiency, the defect in CDG-IA patients. *Biochim. Biophys. Acta* **2009**, *1792*, 835–840. [CrossRef] [PubMed]

39. Schrapers, E.; Tegtmeyer, L.C.; Simic-Schleicher, G.; Debus, V.; Reunert, J.; Balbach, S.; Klingel, K.; Du Chesne, I.; Seelhofer, A.; Fobker, M.; et al. News on clinical details and treatment in PGM1-CDG. *JIMD Rep.* **2016**, *26*, 77–84. [PubMed]

40. Marquardt, T.; Luhn, K.; Srikrishna, G.; Freeze, H.H.; Harms, E.; Vestweber, D. Correction of leukocyte adhesion deficiency type II with oral fucose. *Blood* **1999**, *94*, 3976–3985. [PubMed]

41. Koch, J.; Mayr, J.A.; Alhaddad, B.; Rauscher, C.; Bierau, J.; Kovacs-Nagy, R.; Coene, K.L.; Bader, I.; Holzhacker, M.; Prokisch, H.; et al. CAD mutations and uridine-responsive epileptic encephalopathy. *Brain* **2017**, *140*, 279–286. [CrossRef] [PubMed]

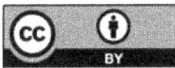

MDPI

St. Alban-Anlage 66

4052 Basel

Switzerland

Tel. +41 61 683 77 34

Fax +41 61 302 89 18

www.mdpi.com

Nutrients Editorial Office

E-mail: nutrients@mdpi.com

www.mdpi.com/journal/nutrients

www.ingramcontent.com/pod-product-compliance
Lightning Source LLC
Chambersburg PA
CBHW041218220326
41597CB00033BA/6030